"Surviving and Thriving in the Real World represents one of the few evidence-based approaches to support the transition to adulthood for autistic teens. Using a combination of parent coaching and teen goal setting, STRW incorporates current best practices to support autistic teens in learning everyday life skills that are crucial to helping them attain their future goals. This is a wonderful resource for families, educators, and clinicians."

Laura Grofer Klinger, *Ph.D., Director of the University of North Carolina at Chapel Hill TEACCH Autism Program and Professor of Psychiatry*

"Research clearly shows that, for many youth with autism, everyday living skills lag significantly behind other areas. This contributes to low levels of functional independence and reduced quality of life in adulthood, even among people with high cognitive and language abilities. The STRW intervention directly addresses the critical deficit in daily living skills that is so common among teens with autism, using evidence-based strategies to promote age-appropriate skills that are essential for successful independent living. Interventions like STRW, which are built on a strong research base and prioritize skills that are actually important to youth with autism and their families, are exactly what we need to promote well-being in this growing population."

Somer L. Bishop, *Ph.D., Professor in Residence, Department of Psychiatry and Behavioral Sciences, University of California San Francisco*

"Surviving and Thriving in the Real World (STRW) provides a much-needed and comprehensive intervention to explicitly and systematically address daily living skills – skills that are often overlooked yet are critical for adult life. The STRW manual presents thoughtfully designed and detailed lessons based on current evidence-based practices. I highly recommend STRW for therapists and educators who support neurodivergent individuals in different contexts."

Nancy Bagatell, *Ph.D., Professor of Occupational Science and Occupational Therapy, University of North Carolina at Chapel Hill*

Surviving and Thriving in the Real World

This interactive manual provides clinicians (e.g., psychologists, occupational therapists, social workers, educators) with a structured curriculum to target the acquisition and mastery of age-appropriate daily living skills using evidence-based strategies for neurodivergent adolescents (e.g., autism, ADHD).

The Surviving and Thriving in the Real World (STRW) curriculum has been iteratively developed over the last 12 years and is the first evidence-based daily living skills intervention for autistic adolescents with average or above cognitive abilities. The 15-week STRW intervention builds essential daily living skills including personal hygiene, cleaning, laundry, cooking, grocery shopping, and spending, saving, and budgeting money using strategies such as a direct instruction and feedback, naturalistic teaching, a specific contract with goals and rewards, task analysis, visual supports, video modelling, and technology. The manual consists of a general overview and specific chapters on each of the 15 intervention sessions that target specific daily living skills during separate caregiver group sessions and individual caregiver/teen dyad sessions. The manual also includes the handouts for each session and provides clinicians with access to the PowerPoint slides that are utilized in all of the telehealth sessions.

This manual will equip practitioners with the skills to help their neurodivergent adolescent clients learn and practice daily living skills to prepare them for successful adult outcomes in work, college, independent living, and social connectedness.

Amie Duncan is a Clinical Psychologist at Cincinnati Children's Hospital Medical Center and a Professor of Pediatrics at the University of Cincinnati College of Medicine.

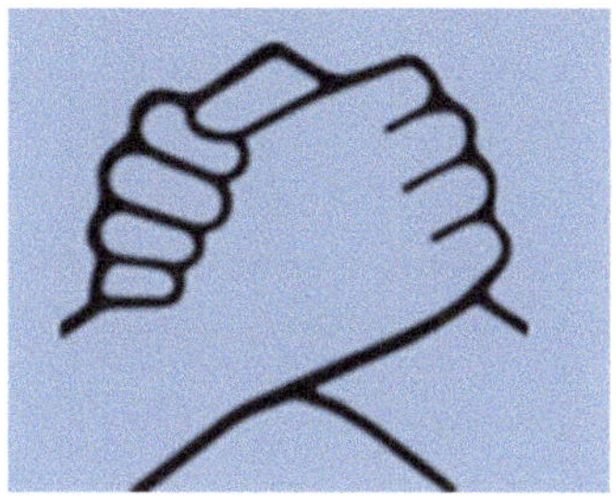

Surviving and Thriving in the Real World (STRW)

A Daily Living Skills Intervention for Neurodivergent Teens

Amie Duncan, Ph.D.

Routledge
Taylor & Francis Group
NEW YORK AND LONDON

Disclaimer

The information expressed in this publication are solely those of the author and do not represent the views of Cincinnati Children's Hospital.

This work was partially supported by a grant from the Eunice Kennedy Shriver National Institute of Child Health and Human Development (NICHD K23HD094855–01) and the Department of Defense Autism Research Program (W81XWH-17-ARP). The content is solely the responsibility of the authors and does not necessarily represent the official views of the U.S. National Institutes of Health (NIH).

Designed cover image: Getty Images

First published 2026
by Routledge
605 Third Avenue, New York, NY 10158

and by Routledge
4 Park Square, Milton Park, Abingdon, Oxon, OX14 4RN

Routledge is an imprint of the Taylor & Francis Group, an informa business

ISBN: 978-1-032-59966-3 (pbk)
ISBN: 978-1-003-45883-8 (ebk)

DOI: 10.4324/9781003458838

Typeset in Palatino
by Apex CoVantage, LLC

This manual is dedicated to all of the autistic teens and their families who have graciously allowed us to work alongside them as they have worked on building the daily living skills that will further propel them to achieve their goals as they transition from high school to adulthood.

Contents

About the Author

Amie Duncan, Ph.D., is a licensed clinical psychologist with training and expertise in working with autistic teens as they strive to make a successful transition from high school to the adult world of work, college, independent living, social connectedness, and community participation. She is Professor of Pediatrics in the College of Medicine at the University of Cincinnati and is a clinical psychologist in the Division of Behavioral Medicine and Clinical Psychology at Cincinnati Children's Hospital Medical Center (CCHMC). She received her doctoral degree from the University of Alabama and completed her post-doctoral fellowship at CCHMC. She has been a principal or co-principal investigator on several federally funded research studies (National Institute for Child Health and Human Development, Department of Defense Autism Research Program, and Department of Education) that seek to develop and evaluate interventions for autistic teens in the areas of daily living skills and executive functioning. She lives in Cincinnati, Ohio, with her husband and three children. More information about Dr. Duncan and the STRW intervention can be found at www.STRW.org.

Preface

The idea for developing the Surviving and Thriving in the Real World (STRW) intervention was inspired by the work I did in graduate school with autistic undergraduate students at the University of Alabama. I was struck by how daily living skills such as waking up on time, keeping one's dorm room clean and organized, doing laundry, personal hygiene, and managing money were so very critical to successfully transitioning to college and achieving a high quality of life for the autistic young adults.

The STRW intervention has been iteratively developed over the last 12 years through a series of research studies focused on its development, evaluation, and refinement. After taking a faculty position at Cincinnati Children's Hospital Medical Center (CCHMC), I received funding from the Jack Rubinstein Foundation within the Division of Developmental and Behavioral Pediatrics at CCHMC to develop and pilot an intervention for autistic adolescents in the outpatient clinic setting and school setting. I then obtained funding from the Center for Clinical and Translational Science and Training K Scholars program (supported by CCHMC and Grant #UL1TR001425) to pilot the refined STRW daily living skills intervention with autistic adolescents and their caregivers in the outpatient setting. Our team then received funding from both the Eunice Kennedy Shriver National Institute of Child Health and Human Development (Grant #K23HD094855) and the Department of Defense Autism Research Program (Grant #W81XWH-17) to further our understanding of the efficacy of the STRW intervention for a large sample of autistic teens as compared to an active control group. The current STRW manual has been refined after each of these studies with significant input and feedback from autistic adolescents and their caregivers and the therapists who facilitated the intervention.

Acknowledgments

As a strong believer in the importance of daily living skills for building independence, autonomy, and self-efficacy in all children and adolescents, I am particularly grateful to my three children, who have allowed me to trial out many, many strategies and ideas for building daily living skills at home, school, and in the community. All three of them have provided me with countless inspiration for how to teach a new skill, build motivation or buy-in when working on "boring" skills, and create and adapt a system to make it feasible for busy families and teens to still work on critical life skills on a regular basis. I am also beyond grateful to my husband, who is supportive of me incorporating so many of my ideas for building daily living skills into our family's routines and rhythms. He has also been my champion as I have worked to write this manual with the hopes that it will inspire others to teach daily living skills to facilitate a successful transition to the adult world.

Over the course of my career, I have been lucky enough to receive invaluable mentorship from other women researchers and clinicians. First and foremost, Dr. Lori Stark saw my passion and potential as a new faculty member and helped me carve my ideas into a clear line of research. Dr. Stark was such a champion, and the time, energy, and direct feedback she gave when meeting with me weekly and reviewing grant applications and manuscripts has truly catapulted me to where I am today. I can only say that I promise to pay it forward and mentor others in the same way that she mentored me. I also want to acknowledge my mentors and collaborators who have worked with me on the iterative development of the STRW intervention, including Dr. Jareen Meinzen-Derr, Dr. Lisa Ruble, Dr. Judy Reaven, Dr. Avani Modi, Dr. Laura Klinger, Dr. Nancy Bagatell, and Dr. Susan Wiley. I want to thank Carrie Fassler, who is the most amazing clinical research coordinator and has been my partner on every single one of the research studies on the STRW intervention. Last, I want to express gratitude to the graduate students, post-doctoral fellows, psychologists, and clinical research coordinators at Cincinnati Children's Hospital Medical Center who have worked with me over the last 12 years on delivering the STRW intervention through our research studies.

Finally, I want to offer my gratitude to the autistic teens and their families who have participated in our research studies and provided invaluable feedback as we refined the content of the STRW intervention. Our hope is that this manual can help neurodivergent teens with building age-appropriate daily living skills to increase the likelihood of a successful transition to the adult world of work, college, independent living, and community participation.

Using the STRW Intervention Manual

- The *Surviving and Thriving in the Real World* (STRW) intervention manual has the following components:
  - **Overview of the STRW Intervention** – This section discusses specific components of the STRW intervention, including purpose and content, evidence-based strategies, key treatment ingredients, parent/caregiver and adolescent involvement, and the role of the STRW therapist. This section also includes information for STRW therapists to effectively facilitate sessions, including session logistics, the structure of dyad and caregiver sessions, how to prepare for sessions, and how to track progress. The "Therapist Resources" section references handouts and resources for the facilitation of each STRW session that are available via the STRW website (www.STRW.org) including the PowerPoint presentation slides for each session, the regularly updated STRW Resources handout, and the Real World Practice Tracking Sheet. The final section includes information on the research evidence of the STRW intervention.
  - **STRW Session Overviews** – This section discusses the objectives and content of each STRW session in detail. This information is meant to supplement the PowerPoint presentations that are utilized to facilitate the caregiver group sessions and caregiver/teen dyad sessions. The handouts for each caregiver group session and each dyad session are included within each session overview. Both caregivers and teens should be provided with their own STRW workbook (see "Therapist Resources"), which consists of all of the handouts that are referred to in each session.
    - *Preparing for STRW* – this chapter will describe how to prepare an adolescent and their caregiver for beginning treatment. During the Pre-STRW session, the therapist will meet with the caregiver/teen dyad to discuss the teen's profile of daily living skill (DLS) strengths and challenges and begin to prepare for upcoming STRW sessions by setting goals and discussing expectations (e.g., commitment, motivation, time, and effort) of the STRW intervention.
    - *STRW Sessions 1–14* – the next 14 chapters will describe each of STRW's 14 sessions in detail for both the caregiver group sessions and the caregiver/teen dyad sessions. Specifically, the chapter will begin by describing the session's primary aims and will then describe the structure, supplies, and preparation for both the caregiver group session and the caregiver/teen dyad session. Notes for successfully facilitating each session will also be included (e.g., how to increase motivation/buy-in of teen, how to easily

incorporate new DLS goals into the family's weekly schedule, etc.). The content (e.g., activities, discussion, instruction) is described in detail in each STRW session overview. Each caregiver group session and caregiver/teen dyad session has a corresponding set of PowerPoint slides and handouts that the therapist utilizes when facilitating the intervention via telehealth. Caregivers and teens will each receive a STRW workbook that contains all of the handouts corresponding to all STRW sessions that are included in each chapter.

- **References**
- **Appendix**
- **Index**

Overview of the Surviving and Thriving Intervention

This overview includes the following sections that are meant to provide a comprehensive understanding of the Surviving and Thriving in the Real World (STRW) intervention and how to facilitate the caregiver group sessions and caregiver/teen dyad sessions.

- Importance of Targeting Daily Living Skills
- Evidence-Based Strategies Used in STRW
- STRW Treatment Ingredients
- Parent/Caregiver and Adolescent Involvement and Commitment
- STRW Therapist Roles and Responsibilities
- Session Logistics
- Structure of the STRW Session Overviews
- Therapist Resources
- Tracking Progress
- Flexible Delivery of the STRW Intervention
- Research Evidence on the STRW Intervention

Importance of Targeting Daily Living Skills

- **What are daily living skills (DLS)?**
  - Daily living skills (DLS) are the everyday tasks that people do to take care of themselves at home, school, and work and in the community (Saulnier & Klaiman, 2022). These skills are often categorized into three main categories:
    - Personal – includes self-care and hygiene (e.g., showering, brushing teeth, changing clothes, putting on deodorant) and healthcare (e.g., taking medications, caring for cuts and injuries, making doctor appointments)
    - Domestic – includes cleaning (e.g., vacuuming, dusting, taking out the trash), laundry, cooking (e.g., using appliances, making meals, planning meals), and household maintenance (e.g., changing lightbulbs, making home repairs)

DOI: 10.4324/9781003458838-1

- Community – includes navigating the community (e.g., going grocery shopping), transportation (e.g., using a map to get from one place to another, taking the bus, driving a car), and money management (e.g., saving, spending, and budgeting money, paying bills).

♦ **Why are DLS important for adolescents?**

- Developing age-appropriate DLS increases the likelihood of having positive adult outcomes in employment, college, independent living, social connectedness, and quality of life (Lythcott-Haims, 2015; McCauley et al., 2020; Taylor et al., 2015; Taylor & Seltzer, 2011; Vaillant, 2012). For example, in order to be successful in the workplace, individuals need to wake up, shower regularly, wear clean clothing, prepare and eat breakfast, and navigate to their job on time. Thus, targeting critical DLS in adolescence may make the transition to the adult world easier because teens are given the opportunity to learn, practice, and master these skills with support from a caregiver in their home environment.

♦ **What is the purpose of the STRW intervention?**

- Surviving and Thriving in the Real World is an intervention (Duncan et al., 2021) that was developed for autistic teens that targets the acquisition of age-appropriate DLS, including hygiene and self-care, cleaning, laundry, cooking, grocery shopping, and money management (see Figure 0.1). A range of evidence-based strategies (e.g., visual strategies, task analysis, video modeling, technology) are introduced and then individualized based on the teen's strengths, challenges, and DLS goals. Key treatment ingredients such as the DLS contract and Real World Practice homework assignments are implemented to increase the likelihood of achieving specific DLS goals. STRW strives to help adolescents and their caregivers build critical DLS that will allow them to make a successful transition from high school to the adult world of college, employment, independent living, and community participation.

♦ **What DLS are targeted in the STRW intervention?**

- The DLS targeted in STRW were chosen based on input and feedback from autistic adolescents and their caregivers because they are not only critical in adolescence but also essential for making a smooth transition from high school to the adult world. See Table 0.1 for a list of the DLS that are targeted in each session. The DLS that are taught fall into the categories of domestic (e.g., doing laundry from start to finish, cleaning one's bedroom, packing a lunch for school, cooking dinner), personal (e.g., brushing teeth, showering, taking vitamins and medications), and community (e.g., grocery shopping, using a checking account to purchase items).
- While specific DLS are taught in STRW sessions, they are individualized to the specific teen to increase the likelihood of acquiring skills. For example, teens are able to choose the recipes that they want to learn to cook in the microwave, stove, and oven. Teens and their caregivers also work with the therapist to identify the steps specific to their needs and to their home environment that need to be completed for complex tasks such as cleaning the bedroom (e.g., make bed, take out trash, vacuum rug, pick up all belongings off of the floor, etc.).

Figure 0.1 Elements of the STRW Intervention

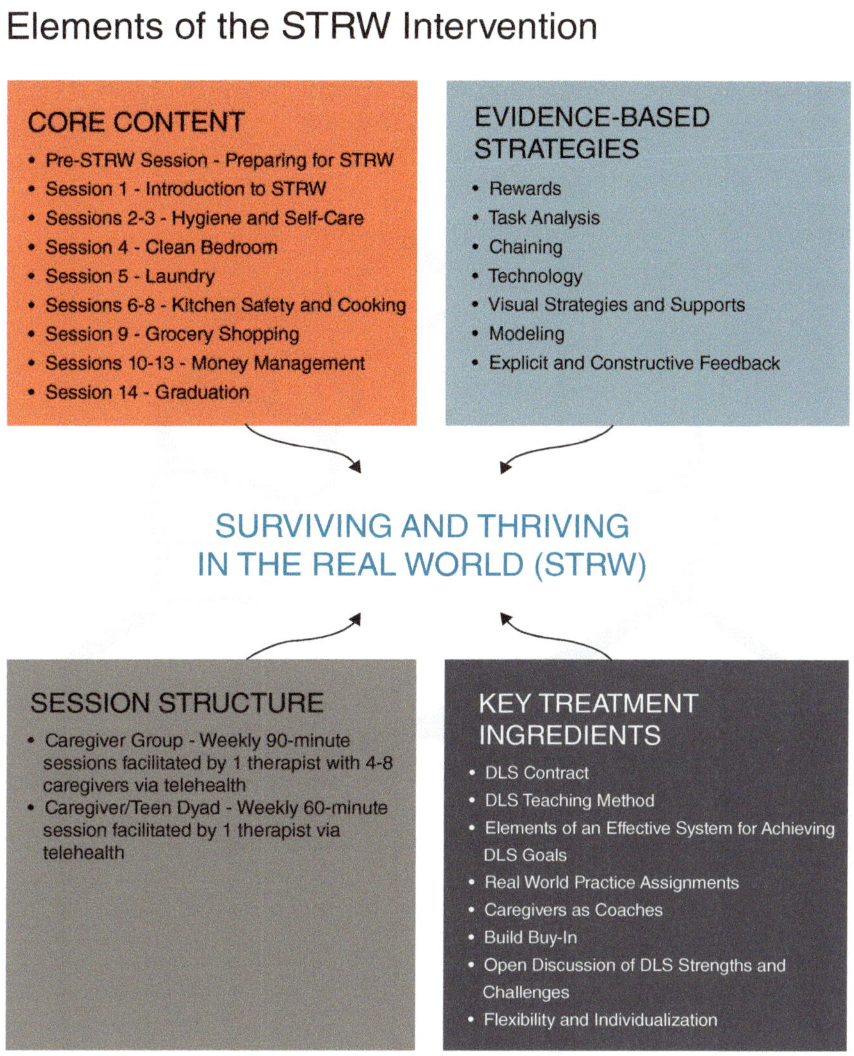

- **Does the STRW intervention lead to gains in DLS?**
  - Our team has completed a series of research studies on the STRW intervention in autistic teens (see "Research Evidence on the STRW Intervention"). We have consistently shown that teens who participate in the STRW gain 2–4 years of DLS from pre-treatment to post-treatment that are maintained at 6-month follow-up (Duncan et al., 2017, 2022, 2023, 2025, 2026). Overall, teens make clinically significant and meaningful gains in developing and mastering age-appropriate DLS after receiving the STRW intervention.

- **Who would benefit from the STRW intervention?**
  - Neurodivergent adolescents (e.g., teens with diagnoses such as autism and ADHD) (Armstrong, 2010) who have challenges in acquiring age-appropriate DLS would likely benefit from the STRW intervention. Several research studies (Duncan et al., 2021) have demonstrated that the STRW intervention has been shown to lead to significant gains in DLS for autistic adolescents (see "Research Evidence on the STRW Intervention"). However, STRW may also be effective for both neurodivergent and neurotypical adolescents who are struggling to

Table 0.1 Content of the STRW Intervention Sessions

SESSION	CONTENT
Preparing for STRW	• Setting DLS goals to work on in STRW • Reviewing results of DLS assessment
Session 1	• Overview of STRW
Session 2	• Personal hygiene and self-care skills
Session 3	• Morning routine
Session 4	• Cleaning one's bedroom
Session 5	• Doing laundry
Session 6	• Cooking in the microwave • Kitchen safety
Session 7	• Cooking in the oven • Mixing and measuring ingredients
Session 8	• Cooking on the stove top • Cleaning the kitchen
Session 9	• Grocery shopping
Session 10	• Understanding the cost of items • Purchasing items
Session 11	• Using a checking and savings account
Session 12	• Budgeting for purchases
Session 13	• Budgeting for an event
Session 14	• Graduation • Evaluating whether DLS goals were met • Looking ahead and setting future DLS Goals

acquire age-appropriate DLS because the intervention targets critical DLS using individualized evidence-based strategies and incorporates treatment ingredients to support the development of DLS (e.g., caregivers as coaches).

Evidence-Based Strategies Used in STRW

The DLS targeted in STRW often appear easy or simple (e.g., putting dirty clothes in a hamper, bringing the hamper to the washing machine, loading the dirty clothes into the washing machine), but it is often challenging for teens to put together all of the "simple" DLS to form a more complex DLS (e.g., doing laundry from start to finish). Whether the DLS are simple or complex, STRW uses a set of evidence-based strategies that have been shown to be effective at acquiring DLS in autistic adolescents (Odom et al., 2021; Steinbrenner et al., 2020). Once a particular evidence-based strategy works for a teen, it can be applied to the development and mastery of other DLS. See the following for evidence-based strategies that are used throughout the STRW intervention.

- *Rewards* – External rewards are an essential evidence-based strategy that are used to reinforce teens as they make progress towards building DLS (Steinbrenner et al., 2020). While some teens may be intrinsically motivated to learn DLS so that they become more independent as they enter young adulthood, many teens need an additional incentive to work towards learning and mastering DLS. Teens and their caregivers work together to determine the reward for a specific goal on the DLS contract (see "Key Treatment Ingredients").
  - Rewards on the DLS contract should be:
    - *Specific* – Caregivers and teens should specifically define the reward that will be earned, and it should be appropriate for the DLS goal that they are working towards. For example, if a teen completes their DLS goal of doing a load of laundry, an appropriate reward may be 30 minutes of extra screen time (not 4 hours of extra screen time!).
    - *Consistent* – Rewards should be given each time that a DLS goal is met. If a teen trusts that they will be rewarded for meeting the DLS goal, they are more likely to do it, which leads to them mastering a DLS.
    - *Meaningful* – If a reward is valuable and meaningful, it will likely be strong enough to motivate the teen to work towards their DLS goal.
    - *Individualized* – It is important to consider what the teen's interests and preferences are when choosing a reward. It will be helpful to have a range of rewards, including:
      - Monetary – earn allowance or money for completing DLS that can be used to purchase items of their choice (e.g., clothing, Legos, books, music)
      - Electronic or screen based – may include extra screen time for video games, for television or movies, or for renting or streaming a movie
      - Social – going to the mall or a movie with a friend, having a friend come over or sleep over, or extra time to play a video game with a friend
      - Privilege based – may include getting to choose what movie to pick for family movie night, choosing what dinner is made on Friday, or sleeping in on the weekend
      - Relationship based – playing a board game with a parent/caregiver, playing basketball with a sibling, or going out to lunch with a family member
  - Important guidelines for implementing rewards on the DLS contract include:
    - If a teen's current rewards do not appear to be motivating them to work on their DLS goals, the caregiver and therapist should discuss and identify other rewards the teen may be more motivated to earn.
    - If a reward is earned for a DLS goal, it cannot be taken away for any other reason (e.g., fighting with a sibling, getting a bad grade, etc.).
    - As a teen begins to master a DLS (i.e., performing a skill independently the majority of the time), it will be important to increase the expectations on

the DLS contract for earning a reward. For example, if a teen is consistently meeting their morning routine goal, the caregiver and teen should increase the expectation for earning a reward on the DLS contract (e.g., must do all steps of morning routine 4 out of 5 days without any prompts to earn a reward).

- Consistent and meaningful rewards are particularly important when learning a new DLS but will eventually be faded as this skill becomes expected. Many caregivers will continue to provide teens with an "allowance" if they complete specific DLS because this also allows them to continue to get experience with spending, saving, and budgeting money. The process for fading rewards is discussed in the caregiver group session in Session 14.
- While rewards are important, it is also critical that the caregiver provide verbal praise and discusses the importance and value of building DLS. This is likely to increase the likelihood of building intrinsic motivation for building the DLS targeted in STRW and also continuing to work on DLS that are needed in adolescence and into adulthood.

♦ *Task Analysis* – Task analysis is a strategy in which a complex task is broken down into clear, simple, and specific steps (Steinbrenner et al., 2020). Throughout STRW sessions, adolescents and their caregivers will use a task analysis to break down complex tasks such as cleaning their bedroom and doing laundry from start to finish. Creating a task analysis also allows for the caregiver and teen to discuss what steps the teens are doing independently and then develop a plan for teaching and practicing any of the steps that are not acquired. Task analyses can be written down (e.g., on a piece of paper, whiteboard) and then posted in a convenient place (e.g., the laundry task analysis can be hung in the laundry room). Task analyses can also be electronic (e.g., to-do list app, list each step in an Excel worksheet) so that they can then be easily accessed on the teen's phone, computer, or tablet. Once a task analysis is created for a task, it can then be used as a checklist to ensure all steps are completed thoroughly, correctly, and in sequential order. While task analyses should be individualized (e.g., some teens may do all of their laundry using the cold water setting on the washer), there will also be steps that are common because they are critical to the task (e.g., loading the washer, using detergent, switching laundry from the washer to the dryer).

♦ *Chaining* – Chaining is often used to teach the steps that have been specified in a task analysis (Steinbrenner et al., 2020). It is a behavioral learning strategy that teaches one step of a skill at a time, and usually the first step or the last step is taught first. After a step is mastered, the adolescent continues learning each step in sequence until all steps of the task are learned and can be performed together. For example, for learning the complex skill of doing laundry, the adolescent may learn the first step of sorting the dirty clothing into lights and darks, and then the caregiver may demonstrate the remaining steps of laundry in order (e.g., loading the clothes into the washing machine, choosing the correct cycle, etc.).

♦ *Technology* – Technology strategies may include mobile phone apps, smart speakers (e.g., Amazon Echo), tablets or laptops, and smart watches. Technology is often intrinsically motivating for adolescents and may thus increase the likelihood that they will want to utilize it to practice specific DLS (Steinbrenner et al., 2020). Technology may also increase the teen's independence as they remember to complete DLS goals without prompting or reminding from their caregiver. Various technology strategies can be used to remind a teen to get started, persevere, or complete a DLS using alarms, calendar reminders, and/or checklists. For example, various phone apps can be used to wake a teen up in the morning, provide a checklist of steps that need to be done for the teen's morning hygiene routine, and remind the teen to do their laundry at a specific day and time.

- *Visual strategies and supports* – Each caregiver/teen dyad session begins with the therapist reviewing the visual schedule that provides an overview of all session activities. Visual supports are also used throughout STRW to increase the likelihood of DLS acquisition by clearly indicating the steps in a complex task or by reminding the teen to start, persevere, and/or complete a task (Hume et al., 2009, 2014; Steinbrenner et al., 2020). Examples of visual strategies and supports for teaching DLS include: (1) creating a checklist of a task analysis on a white board or laminated piece of paper; (2) putting a Post-It note on the bathroom mirror to serve as a reminder to complete a specific DLS (e.g., taking medication, using face wash); (3) hanging up the DLS contract to serve as a reminder of the goals being worked on, progress thus far, and the rewards that can be earned; and (4) utilizing resources that include both visual and verbal instructions for completing tasks (e.g., visual cookbooks).
- *Modeling* – Modeling is used throughout STRW as a way to build upon the direct instruction that teens receive for acquiring DLS and allows them to actually "see" how the specific steps of a DLS are completed. Peers (e.g., friend, sibling) or adults (e.g., caregiver, family member, neighbor, teacher) can serve as models to demonstrate and teach specific DLS (Hume et al., 2009; Steinbrenner et al., 2020). For example, an older sibling could demonstrate how they budget for household expenses each month or how they grocery shop using a list.
- *Video Modeling* – Teens may also benefit from video modeling such that they watch a video that details how to perform a specific skill (e.g., cooking scrambled eggs, shaving, folding laundry, cleaning one's bedroom). While there are many videos available on the Internet, some teens may also prefer to record their own video that has a caregiver, sibling, friend, or themselves performing the specific task. A task analysis could also be paired with the video so that the teen could use it as they learn a new DLS.
- *Explicit and Constructive Feedback* – As teens are learning and practicing new skills, their caregiver and the therapist provide explicit and constructive feedback about their performance (e.g., how to measure flour when baking cookies, how to make sure they are not overloading a washing machine). Specifically, caregivers provide this feedback during the review of the DLS contract in dyad sessions, when learning and practicing skills in the dyad session, and throughout the week as the teen works toward achieving their DLS goals. The therapist often models how to give direct feedback in a supportive manner with an emphasis on teaching skills and building independence when caregivers provide feedback on completion of a goal (e.g., quality), level of independence, and use of strategies. The therapist will discuss how to give feedback during the caregiver groups sessions and may also role play with caregivers on how they could give more effective feedback to their teen.

STRW Treatment Ingredients

In addition to incorporating evidence-based strategies in treatment sessions, the STRW intervention also has several key treatment ingredients that are meant to increase the likelihood of building age-appropriate and are used throughout the STRW intervention.

- *DLS Contract*
  - An essential strategy in the STRW intervention is a written DLS contract (see Figure 0.2) between the caregiver and adolescent that: (1) clearly defines the DLS goal, (2) defines the expectations and requirements for meeting the goal (e.g., how often, how much prompting, how much independence, etc.), and (3) specifies the reward to be earned for meeting the goal. The DLS contract leads to a clear understanding of what needs to be done by the teen (i.e., work on the DLS goal) and the caregiver (i.e., provide support as specified in the expectations and provide a reward). The DLS contract is introduced in Session 3 and is used in every subsequent session to define and refine goals and rewards as adolescents learn and practice specific DLS. The DLS contract is also used

Figure 0.2 Example of a Completed DLS Contract

Daily Living Skills Contract

Date September 6

Goal	Expectations	Reward	MONDAY	TUESDAY	WEDNESDAY	THURSDAY	FRIDAY	SATURDAY	SUNDAY
Morning Routine	Complete 10 of 11 steps without a reminder on 4/5 weekdays. Post checklist in room and bathroom. Check in with mom when done.	Choice of dinner on the weekend	✓	✓	✓		✓		
Cleaning Bedroom	Clean bedroom on Sunday using checklist. Check with mom when done.	1 hour of extra screen time							✓
Laundry	Do 1 load from start to finish. Set alarm for starting and switching loads.	30 minutes of extra screen time					✓		
Cooking	Help mom/dad cook dinner from start to finish on Wednesday nights.	Choice of dinner to cook and then eat			✓				
Grocery Shopping & Money	Assist with finding items on the family's grocery list. Pay for items with mom's debit card.	Choice of item at the grocery store						✓	

Teen ______________________ Parent / Caregiver ______________________ to track progress on goals so that any successes can be celebrated and any challenges can be addressed as goals and rewards are modified as needed. It is recommended that the contract be posted in the teen's home so that it can serve as a visual reminder of the DLS goals that they are working on and the progress they are making.

- *STRW DLS Teaching Method*
  - The STRW DLS Teaching Method is used throughout the STRW intervention to increase the likelihood of acquiring and mastering age-appropriate DLS that will foster the teen's independence with their caregiver's support. It incorporates evidence-based strategies such as direct instruction, reinforcement, task analysis, modeling, and explicit and constructive feedback to systematically teach DLS and increase the teen's level of independence (Steinbrenner et al., 2020). See Figure 0.3 for an example of how to use the DLS Teaching Method for the DLS of cleaning one's bedroom. The four main steps of the STRW DLS Teaching Method are:

Figure 0.3 DLS Teaching Method for Cleaning Your Bedroom

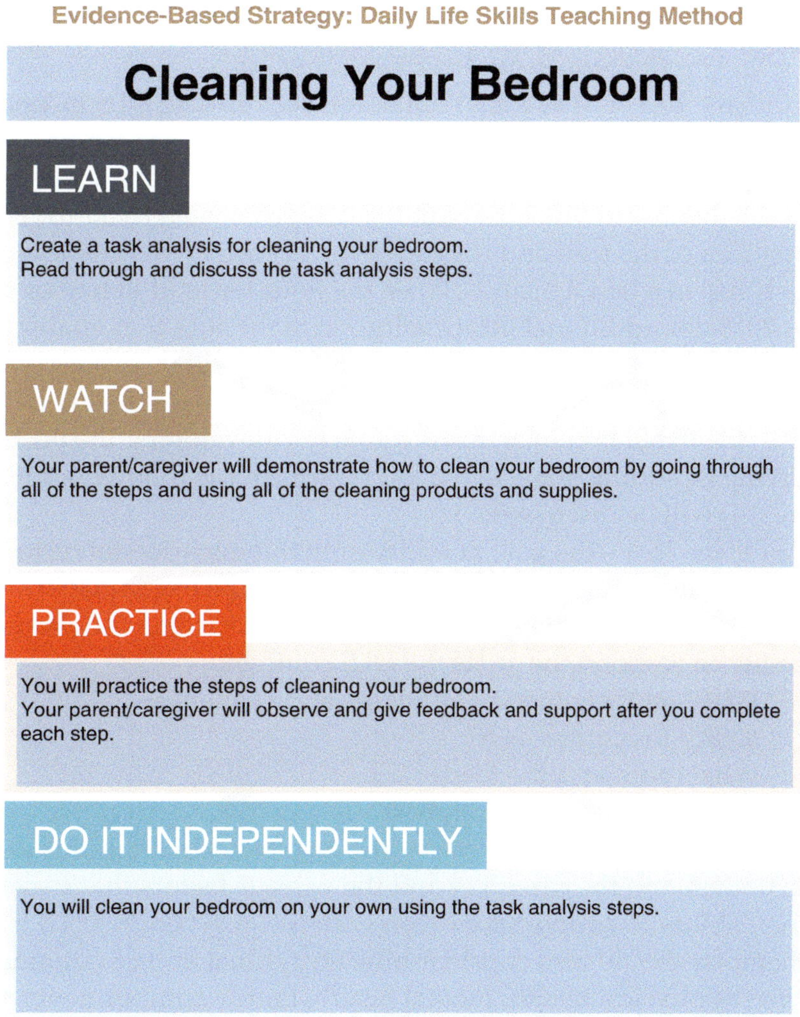

- *Learn* – teens will learn the specific steps of each DLS and how to complete each step. This may involve direct instruction on a topic, completing a task analysis to break down the steps of a skill, or reviewing safety rules. In STRW sessions, the therapist and the caregiver will primarily be involved in instructing and supporting the teen as they learn a new DLS.
- *Watch* – teens will watch (as needed) their caregiver complete a specific DLS. The caregiver will often use a completed task analysis to model and/or talk through each step of a DLS in detail, and the therapist will provide feedback as needed. The steps for Watch and Practice are often combined depending on the teen's experience (e.g., caregiver may demonstrate how to turn the burner on and then have the teen immediately practice it before cooking a grilled cheese on the stovetop).
- *Practice* – teens will practice completing some or all of the steps for a specific DLS. The caregiver will provide feedback and guidance as needed as they support the teen in learning the new skill. Practice occurs during the STRW dyad session and also between sessions (e.g., at home, at the grocery store, etc.).
- *Do It Independently* – teens will complete the DLS independently after they have had opportunities to practice and receive feedback from their caregiver. This will most often occur outside of the STRW dyad sessions as the teen makes progress on their DLS contract goals.

♦ *Elements of an Effective System for Achieving DLS Goals*
- The primary aim of STRW is to build age-appropriate DLS in teens by developing an effective and individualized system that can be used during the intervention and also in the future. In order to help teens achieve their DLS goals, the therapist will work with the caregiver/teen dyad to (1) consider the qualities of the teen and the caregiver; (2) use evidence-based strategies to teach and master DLS; and (3) use the Four Laws of Behavior Change (see Clear, 2018, for additional information) to make sure that goals are obvious, appealing, easy, and satisfying. These elements will be discussed in each session when reviewing the DLS contract and when creating the new DLS contract to increase the likelihood of achieving goals by developing the best system! When modifying or adding goals to the DLS contract, the following four elements (see Figure 0.4) will be discussed:
  - *Role of the Teen* – the goal of addressing this each session is to understand how the teen and what is going on in their life (e.g., final exams, extracurricular activities, vacations or breaks from school) may impact their ability to work on the goals the DLS contract.
    - What are their specific strengths and challenges that may affect their ability to acquire DLS?
    - What motivates the teen?
    - How does the teen learn best?
  - *Role and Impact of the Caregiver* – the goal of addressing this each session is to understand the caregiver and the various factors that may be impacting their ability to support their teen with the goals on their DLS contract. The therapist should also consider how individual and environmental factors such as physical health, mental health, family commitments, workload,

holidays, breaks from school or work, and local and national events may impact the caregiver.
    - How much time is available to dedicate to helping the teen achieve their DLS goals?
    - How much energy does the caregiver have to devote to targeting DLS?
    - Is the caregiver motivated to help the teen?
    - What is the level of commitment to working on DLS goals?
    - How will stress or conflict affect the caregiver's ability to help the teen learn and practice DLS?
  - *Evidence-Based Strategies* will be introduced to teens as they learn, practice, and master various DLS. It will be important to identify which strategies work best for the teen because they can be used again and again.
  - The *Four Laws of Behavior Change* (Clear, 2018) make it more likely that teens, in collaboration with their caregiver, will achieve their DLS goals.
    - *Obvious* – the cues to get started on a DLS goal should be as obvious as possible. This can typically be done by modifying the environment to make it more likely that goals will be met. For example, a teen could put all of their items needed for their morning hygiene routine in the same place on the bathroom counter to make it more likely that they will do all of the hygiene tasks while in the bathroom.
    - *Attractive* – the goal should be attractive or appealing to increase the teen's motivation and follow-through. For example, teens can do one of their favorite things right before (e.g., 15 minutes of screen time, watch favorite show) or at the same time (e.g., listen to music, bake brownies while waiting for laundry to finish) as their DLS goal. This can sometimes be difficult to do for every DLS goal, but it should always be considered.
    - *Easy* – achieving the goal should be as simple as possible. This is a critical law because it is important for teens to be successful when working towards DLS goals. For example, breaking down a complex DLS into simple, achievable steps makes it more likely that they will be able to meet their DLS goal.
    - *Satisfying* – it is critical to make achieving DLS goals satisfying and rewarding for teens because it increases the likelihood that they will continue to work on meeting their goals. For example, after preparing a meal, teens are intrinsically rewarded by being able to eat the meal. The rewards on the DLS contract will also make achieving a goal satisfying. Caregivers can also discuss how building these DLS now will pay off in the future because they will have increased independence.

- *Real World Practice Assignments*
  - Each week, teens and their caregivers are given a Real World Practice assignment to practice DLS at home, school, or in the community. Once the DLS contract is introduced in Session 3, adding and modifying DLS goals on the contract will always be included as one of the Real World Practice assignments. Each Real World Practice will also include an assignment that is meant to build the teen's understanding of purchasing items and basic money management

Figure 0.4 Elements of an Effective System for Achieving DLS Goals

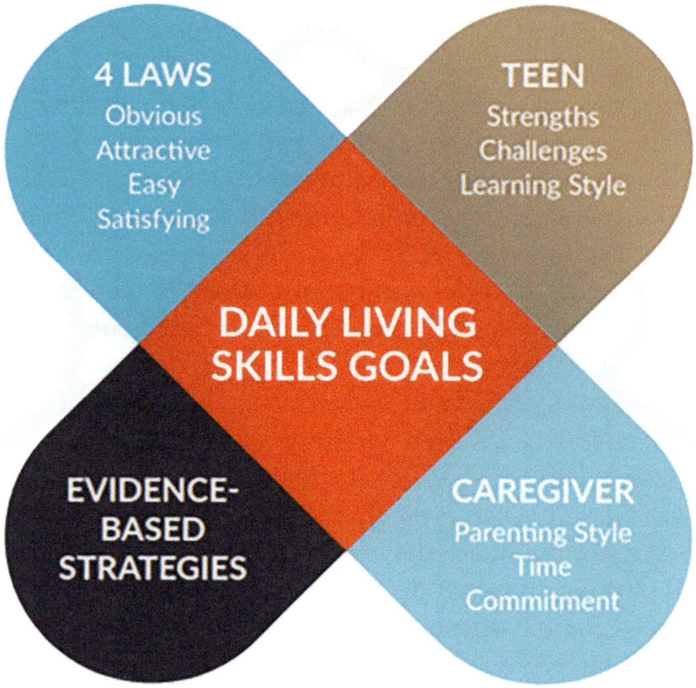

skills (e.g., understanding what things cost, comparing prices between two items, using cash to purchase an item, and making sure the correct change was received). These money assignments are meant to expose teens to purchasing items so that they are more equipped to then build their skills in areas such as saving and budgeting in STRW Sessions 10–13.

- *Caregivers as Coaches*
  - A primary role of caregivers in the STRW intervention is to be a DLS "coach" to their teen as they model, support, and generalize the DLS that are taught in each caregiver/teen dyad session. In caregiver group sessions, all caregivers are given ideas and feedback on how to be an effective DLS coach when the progress of each teen is discussed in detail while reviewing the Real World Practice assignments. For example, if a caregiver reports that their teen is not motivated to do their laundry, the therapist and the other caregivers may brainstorm possible ideas for increasing motivation (e.g., modify the reward, choose a different day/time to do the laundry when the caregiver has more time to support the teen, allow the teen to do something enjoyable while waiting to switch clothes from the washing machine to the dryer). The group sessions allow for in-depth discussions on how caregivers can support their teen and individualize the system for working towards a DLS goal to increase the likelihood of success. Notably, as the caregivers get to know one another, they often provide extremely valuable feedback and guidance to one another about how to target specific DLS goals. The therapist should strive to encourage a collaborative and supportive environment so that all caregivers feel comfortable sharing both successes and challenges and also contributing suggestions and ideas.

- *Build Buy-In*
  - DLS are often not inherently motivating skills to learn, practice, and then incorporate into one's daily life, especially if the adolescent has not had this as an expectation in the past. In addition, caregivers need to be aware of the time and energy needed to support their adolescent in building DLS so that they can commit to being a coach that provides instruction, modeling, feedback, and ongoing support. Thus, it is critical to build buy-in from both the adolescent and the caregiver so that they are more likely to reach their DLS goals. The Preparing for STRW session and the first three sessions of the STRW intervention are focused on building teen and caregiver buy-in.
    - In the Preparing for STRW session (also called the Pre-STRW session), which is held prior to the start of the intervention, adolescent and caregiver dyads go over the results of any DLS assessments that they completed. The dyad then collaborates to identify DLS goals in the areas of hygiene, cleaning, laundry, cooking, and money management. The therapist will work to ensure that the perspectives and opinions of both caregivers and teens are considered while also assisting with choosing goals that are realistic to achieve. Once the STRW intervention begins, both the caregiver and dyad sessions continue to address motivation and buy-in.
    - In Session 1, the therapist emphasizes the importance of working on building age-appropriate DLS in order to meet current goals (e.g., working a part-time job, increasing independence from caregivers) and long-term future goals (e.g., attending college, living in an apartment or dorm, saving up for large purchases).
    - During the Session 2 caregiver group, the therapist discusses the link between DLS and adult outcomes such as college, employment, independent living, and overall quality of life and then describes how to build an effective system to target DLS goals that incorporates the teen (e.g., strengths, challenges), caregiver (e.g., time, effort, competing demands, parenting style), evidence-based strategies, and the Four Laws of Behavior Change.
    - Building upon this foundation, the Session 3 caregiver group session and caregiver/teen dyad session both discuss how to use a DLS contract to target specific DLS goals, which will then lead to increased independence and facilitate a more successful transition to adulthood. If teens are not intrinsically motivated to work on DLS, the external rewards that are built into the DLS contract typically lead to buy-in and motivation to build and practice their DLS.

- *Open Discussion of DLS Strengths and Challenges*
  - Throughout all caregiver group and caregiver/teen dyad sessions, both adolescents and caregivers are encouraged to openly discuss challenges and successes that they have experienced with building their DLS, including the strategies that have worked and the strategies that have not worked. This is extremely valuable information that helps with developing an individualized plan for targeting specific DLS and also identifying evidence-based strategies that may lead to successful acquisition of DLS. The therapist should ensure that they are creating an environment in sessions in which both caregivers and

teens can be honest and openly share about whether they are meeting their DLS goals and what obstacles they may be facing. For example, in caregiver group sessions, it is common for caregivers to report that they are over-involved in their teen's DLS and need to take an intentional step back and evaluate how to better foster independence in their teen. This honest admission often leads to other caregivers normalizing that they have experienced similar struggles, which then presents an opportunity for the therapist and other caregivers to discuss strategies that may build autonomy and independence in the adolescents.

- While teens are not directly exposed to other teens who may struggle with acquiring age-appropriate DLS during the STRW intervention, it will be important for the therapist to engage in open, non-judgmental conversations about the teen's strengths (e.g., likes to cook), challenges (e.g., needs multiple reminders to complete personal hygiene tasks in the morning before school), preferences (e.g., interested in learning how to earn and save up money, likes keeping their room orderly), and possible motor, sensory, or other challenges that may impact DLS. The teen is more likely to be bought into working on DLS goals if they feel like they are being heard and that they are an integral part of developing the goals, expectations, and rewards that make up the DLS contract.

- *Flexibility and Individualization*
  - There is significant flexibility and individualization built into the caregiver/teen dyad sessions to increase the likelihood of the teen successfully acquiring the age-appropriate DLS that they are targeting on the DLS contract. Individualization and flexibility occur in the following ways:
    - Adapting evidence-based strategies to make it more likely the teen will utilize them (e.g., determining whether they prefer going through their morning routine checklist on a whiteboard or their phone's calendar app).
    - Providing choices to the teen when targeting DLS (e.g., choosing a recipe that they want to cook in the oven, identifying which upcoming event or activity they want to create a budget for)
    - Incorporating DLS into daily life (e.g., having the teen cut up vegetables for dinner alongside the caregiver, encouraging the teen to navigate the grocery store for the items that they need)
    - Providing choices regarding DLS contract goals (e.g., practice cooking by either packing their own lunch or by cooking dinner for the family)

Parent/Caregiver and Adolescent Involvement and Commitments

- Parents/caregivers participate in both weekly caregiver group sessions and dyad sessions with their adolescent. They also support their adolescent as they practice specific DLS throughout the week. During the STRW intervention, parents/caregivers will:

- Commit to putting in the time and effort to work on DLS with their teen during weekly caregiver/teen dyad sessions and throughout the week at home and in the community
- Share their experiences and engage in discussions with other parents/caregivers during the weekly group session
- Engage in problem solving to identify possible solutions for obstacles that are often faced when working on the development of DLS at home, at school, and in the community
- Collaborate with their adolescent to set specific DLS goals using individualized evidence-based strategies
- Support their adolescent during dyad sessions to acquire new DLS using evidence-based strategies
- Identify goals and assist with defining expectations and rewards on a weekly DLS contract
- Track and discuss progress on DLS goals during group and dyad sessions
- Provide guidance and feedback to their adolescent as new DLS are practiced during their everyday life

♦ Adolescents participate in the weekly dyad sessions with their parent/caregiver and also work on practicing specific DLS throughout the week in their everyday environment. During the STRW intervention, adolescents will:

- Identify their profile of DLS strengths and challenges
- Collaborate with their parent/caregiver during dyad sessions with a therapist to learn, practice, and master DLS
- Set specific DLS goals to work towards
- Use a weekly DLS contract to track progress on reaching DLS goals
- Practice DLS at home and in the community with support from their caregiver
- Understand what motivates them to work towards DLS goals
- Identify the evidence-based strategies and supports that facilitate the continued development of DLS

STRW Therapist Roles and Responsibilities

♦ **What personnel are needed to facilitate STRW?**

- It is recommended that one lead therapist facilitate both the weekly caregiver group session and the weekly caregiver/teen dyad sessions. For example, if a STRW group consisted of six adolescents and their caregivers, the lead therapist would conduct the weekly caregiver session with the six caregivers and would also conduct a total of six weekly caregiver/teen dyad sessions. One lead therapist facilitating all STRW sessions is beneficial because the therapist (1) gains critical and candid input from the caregiver about their teen's progress

on DLS goals during the week at the caregiver group session and (2) observes, interacts, and provides in the moment feedback to the caregiver and teen during the dyad session. Thus, the therapist can incorporate all of the observations and information from the caregiver, the teen, and the caregiver/teen interaction that is obtained from both the caregiver group and the dyad session to get a comprehensive conceptualization of how to assist with targeting specific DLS.
- Alternatively, two therapists could co-facilitate the weekly caregiver group sessions and then divide the facilitation of the dyad sessions. For example, if a STRW group consisted of six adolescents and their caregivers, the therapists would co-lead the weekly caregiver session and then each therapist would conduct three weekly caregiver/teen dyad sessions. This allows for flexibility if a therapist is sick or takes vacation during a STRW group and the other therapist can facilitate the caregiver group session and provide updates about any information discussed that may impact upcoming dyad sessions.

- **What are the qualifications of a STRW therapist?**
  - Ideal STRW therapists are psychologists, social workers, occupational therapists, and/or special education teachers who have experience working with adolescents and their caregivers to target the acquisition of specific skills using evidence-based strategies.
  - Therapists should also feel comfortable doing the following:
    - Building and maintaining rapport with adolescents and their caregivers
    - Knowing when and how to challenge caregivers and teens about issues such as setting realistic goals and prioritizing the practicing of DLS during the week
    - Providing supportive feedback and coaching to caregivers and teens as they practice DLS during dyad sessions
    - Strategically managing time during both the caregiver group sessions and the caregiver/teen dyad sessions to ensure that material is covered in appropriate detail while also allowing for caregivers and teens to share their experiences
    - Remaining positive and encouraging, even when teens are struggling to learn a new DLS.
  - Many STRW therapists frequently utilize components of motivational interviewing (Miller & Rollnick, 2012) as they build a relationship with the caregiver/teen dyad and collaborate with them to identify DLS goals and build effective systems of evidence-based strategies to target these DLS goals. For example, it is important for STRW therapists to partner with the caregiver/teen dyad by providing their expertise in teaching DLS but also to be aware that the caregiver and teen have expertise in themselves, including their strengths, challenges, and motivation for building age-appropriate DLS. The motivational interviewing processes of engaging, focusing, evoking, and planning may also be useful to STRW therapists.

- **What training do therapists need before facilitating the STRW intervention?**
  - It is highly recommended that all STRW therapists read the STRW manual and attend the STRW Therapist Training (see STRW website for training

opportunities). A list of certified STRW therapists can be found at the STRW website (www.STRW.org).

- **Should there be a trained back-up therapist?**
  - It can be extremely beneficial to have a back-up therapist who is able to facilitate both the STRW caregiver group sessions and/or the caregiver/teen dyad sessions.
  - Back-up therapists should have the same training as the lead therapist, including reading the STRW manual and participating in a STRW Therapist Training. Prior to facilitating a session, they should consult with the lead therapist about the session they will be leading and then adequately prepare by reading the manual and reviewing the PowerPoint presentation slides and session handouts.
  - It is particularly difficult to reschedule the caregiver group sessions, so it is beneficial to try to stick to the schedule of sessions that was provided to families at the start of treatment. If the lead therapist knows of a planned absence, they can provide the back-up therapist with information about the caregivers in preparation for the facilitation of the session. If feasible, it may be beneficial for back-up therapists to attend an entire caregiver group session or parts of a session so that caregivers can be introduced to the back-up therapist.
  - Back-up therapists can also fill in for the lead therapist for a caregiver/teen dyad session, but this is often not ideal because of the close therapeutic relationship that is established and built between the therapist and the caregiver/teen dyad. It may be more beneficial to reschedule the caregiver/teen dyad session rather than have a back-up therapist facilitate it.

- **Does one therapist need to facilitate both the STRW caregiver group sessions and the caregiver/teen dyad sessions?**
  - Ideally, the STRW intervention should be led by one lead therapist who facilitates both the caregiver group sessions and all of the caregiver/teen dyad sessions. This allows for the therapist to build a strong relationship with each caregiver/teen dyad while also getting a deep understanding of their strengths and challenges that may impact the acquisition of targeted DLS.
  - However, it is also feasible for one therapist to run the weekly caregiver group session and an additional one to two therapists to facilitate the caregiver/teen dyad sessions. For example, Therapist 1 may run the caregiver group, and then Therapists 1, 2, and 3 each see two to three caregiver/teen dyads. As another example, Therapist 1 may run the caregiver group, and then Therapists 1 and 2 each sees three caregiver/teen dyads. Of note, it is important for all STRW therapists to be in contact with one another about the details of each session (e.g., during a supervision session, writing treatment summary notes of the dyad sessions to discuss with the caregiver group therapist, etc.) because this will have implications for how the subsequent sessions are facilitated.

Session Logistics

- **What are the characteristics of adolescents and caregivers who may benefit from participating in the STRW intervention?**
  - Adolescents in STRW should be between the ages of 14 and 18. Adolescents are more likely to benefit if they have DLS that are in the low to below average range, which suggests they do not have DLS commensurate with same-aged peers. Assessments such as the Adaptive Behavior Assessment System, 3rd Edition (Harrison & Oakland, 2015), or the Vineland Adaptive Behavior Scales, 3rd Edition (Sparrow et al., 2016), may be helpful in identifying whether teens have DLS below the average range. Ideally, adolescents should also be motivated to work on DLS for both the short-term rewards (e.g., increased independence and autonomy) and long-term benefits (e.g., increased likelihood of going to college, working at a part-time or full-time job, and living independently). Adolescents should also be ready to commit to attending all dyad sessions and working on DLS goals throughout the 15-week STRW intervention.
  - The parents/caregivers of adolescents should be able to commit to (1) attending all caregiver group sessions and caregiver/teen dyad sessions for 15 weeks, (2) helping their adolescent practice their DLS goals throughout the week, and (3) tracking their adolescent's progress on DLS goals so that this can be discussed in STRW sessions. Ideally, the same caregiver should attend each caregiver group and dyad session, but if a caregiver cannot make it one week, another caregiver can attend with some preparation beforehand (e.g., if the mother consistently attends but is going out of town, she should update the father on the DLS contract and things that may be helpful to bring up in the caregiver group session). Two caregivers are also welcome to consistently attend (e.g., a mother and a father, a mother and a grandmother), especially if they are both working on DLS goals with the teen.

- **How many caregiver and adolescent dyads should be in a STRW group?**
  - The ideal number of participants is four to eight caregiver/teen dyads. However, it is important to note that the therapist running the caregiver group sessions with seven to eight caregivers may find it difficult to allow all caregivers to discuss their teen's progress and also cover all of the STRW intervention content. It can be helpful for the STRW therapist to first start running groups with four to six caregiver/teen dyads and then run the STRW intervention with seven to eight caregiver/teen dyads once they are familiar with the content, structure, and flow of the STRW intervention.

- **What is the frequency and timing of STRW sessions?**
  - Prior to beginning the intervention, the therapist will meet with each caregiver/teen dyad in the Preparing for STRW Session. This session will discuss the unique DLS strengths and challenges of the teen, and the caregiver and teen will collaborate to set goals that will be targeted during the STRW intervention.

- After the preparing for STRW Session, the STRW intervention consists of weekly caregiver group sessions and weekly caregiver/teen dyad sessions for 14 weeks.
- Ideally, the caregiver group should always happen before the dyad session so that caregivers are aware of the content that will be discussed in the session with their teen. This also allows caregivers the opportunity to openly discuss any challenges or barriers that may be affecting the teen as they work toward their DLS goals.
- The caregiver group session should be attended by caregivers of the adolescents only. This session is held on the same day and time each week for 90 minutes and is delivered online (e.g., via the HIPAA-compliant version of Zoom). The primary goals of these sessions are to (1) review the progress that adolescents have made with their DLS goals and (2) discuss the upcoming caregiver/teen dyad session content. Caregivers are also given an opportunity to openly share any challenges or barriers that they are facing when working on targeting specific DLS with their teen at home and in the community.
- The caregiver/teen dyad session is attended by one adolescent and their caregiver. This dyad session is typically held at the same day and time but can be rescheduled based on schedule changes for the adolescent, caregiver, or therapist. This session is also delivered online via a videoconferencing platform (e.g., Zoom). The primary goals of these dyad sessions are to (1) review and track the progress that adolescents have made with their goals on their DLS contract; (2) provide instruction, modeling, and practice of specific DLS; and (3) modify the DLS goals that are being targeted on the DLS contract based on the teen's performance and any new DLS that they learned in the session.

- **How are DLS taught in the adolescent's home during the weekly caregiver/teen dyad sessions?**
  - DLS will be taught in the caregiver and teen's home environment during dyad sessions via telehealth (e.g., a videoconferencing platform such as Zoom). This means that caregivers and teens should be prepared to learn and practice specific DLS in the teen's bedroom (e.g., morning routine, cleaning one's bedroom, putting laundry away), laundry area (e.g., practicing using the washing machine and dryer), and kitchen (e.g., cooking in the microwave, oven, and stovetop).
  - It is also helpful to have an area in the home (e.g., kitchen table, office, teen's bedroom) that can be used to discuss the teen's progress on their DLS contract at the beginning of the dyad session, revise the DLS contract, and discuss any preparation or planning for the next dyad session.
  - It may also be necessary to hold STRW sessions in other environments or settings based on where the teen performs specific DLS. For example, if the teen and caregiver do their laundry at a laundromat, it may be beneficial to practice using the washing machine and dryer at the laundromat that they typically go to. If it is not feasible to have the session in the laundromat, the therapist and caregiver/teen dyad can walk through the steps of doing laundry at home and have the caregiver and teen practice these skills the next time that they are doing laundry. As another example, if a teen does not have a stove or oven to practice cooking, they could practice these skills at the home of a neighbor or family member.

- Between STRW sessions, caregivers and teens will often need to practice their DLS outside of the home (e.g., practicing using a list to find and purchase items at the grocery store, opening up a checking account, using a debit card to purchase hygiene items at the store).

♦ **What materials are needed for facilitating STRW sessions?**

- The therapist needs the following materials to facilitate STRW caregiver groups sessions and dyad sessions:
  - Computer with HIPAA-compliant videoconferencing program (e.g., Zoom)
  - STRW manual with Session Overviews and session-specific handouts
  - PowerPoint presentation slides for caregiver group sessions and caregiver/teen dyad sessions (see "Therapist Resources" for additional information). The PowerPoint slides directly correspond to the content in the STRW manual's Session Overviews for each caregiver group and dyad session
  - Videos (links for videos are accessible via the STRW Resources handout that is available on the STRW website)
  - Several other resources needed for facilitating STRW sessions (e.g., Real World Practice Tracking Sheet) are available on the STRW website (see "Therapist Resources")

♦ **What materials do the teen and caregiver need when attending STRW sessions?**

- Computer or phone with capability to attend sessions via videoconferencing program.
- STRW workbooks:
  - Separate STRW workbooks for caregivers and teens that contain hard copies of session handouts should be mailed to them. Caregivers will receive one workbook that includes material from the caregiver group sessions and the dyad session. Teens will receive one workbook for the dyad session. These STRW workbooks are available on the STRW website (see also "Therapist Resources").
  - The workbooks have cover pages for each session and also have footers that clearly indicate the session and handout numbers.
  - Each session also has a blank page that can be used by teens or caregivers to take any additional notes.
  - The workbooks can also be provided electronically to caregivers.
- Session-specific materials – will depend on the session and may include ingredients to cook a recipe or laundry supplies (e.g., detergent). The therapist will review what materials are needed so that caregivers and teens are prepared for each dyad session.

♦ **How do caregivers and teens access STRW materials?**

- The therapist should provide caregivers and teens with a hard copy of the STRW workbook that contains the handouts that are needed for the STRW sessions. All handouts for caregivers and teens are also at the end of each Session Overview in the manual.
- An electronic copy of the workbooks can also be provided to caregivers and teens.
- Caregivers and teens can also access certain STRW materials (e.g., the DLS Contract, Task Analysis Steps) on the STRW website (www.STRW.org) under Parent Resources.

- **How should the therapist prepare for each session?**
  - The therapist should prepare for the session by reading the Session Overview in the STRW manual. It may be helpful to make notes, highlight, or underline concepts in the manual that may apply to specific caregivers or teens. Therapists may also find it helpful to jot down notes or helpful hints after they have facilitated a session so that they remember it for future sessions (e.g., a good microwave recipe, a to-do list phone app).
  - The therapist should also review the PowerPoint presentation prior to each caregiver group session and caregiver/teen dyad session. The notes in each PowerPoint presentation contain time estimates, content that is optional to cover, material that may be needed, and any preparation for the session, which is identical to what is in each Session Overview. Therapists are also able to edit the notes of the slides and can add, remove, or modify the notes to customize the information in the PowerPoint slides.
  - It may take several sessions for a therapist to get an understanding of how to facilitate the session using their manual and the PowerPoint slides. Some options include:
    - Utilizing just the PowerPoint slides and notes to facilitate sessions and using the manual to prepare for sessions.
    - Utilizing the PowerPoint slides to display content to the caregiver and teen and using the manual to facilitate the sessions.
  - The therapist may want to practice sharing their screen prior to the first session so that they feel comfortable with using the PowerPoint slides, displaying any handouts, and taking any notes.
  - Many therapists prefer to have two monitors such that they display the PowerPoint with the session notes on one monitor and then use the other monitor to take notes and record progress using the Real World Practice Tracker.

- **How are the STRW PowerPoint presentations for the caregiver group and dyad sessions organized?**
  - All STRW PowerPoint presentations can be accessed at the STRW website (see "Therapist Resources" for additional information).
  - The notes in each PowerPoint slide for the STRW caregiver and dyad sessions directly correspond to the information found in each Session Overview. Thus, the therapist can choose to use the manual when facilitating or just rely on the notes in the PowerPoint slides.
    - The PowerPoint presentation notes contain all the information that the therapist should say verbatim (e.g., instructions, discussion questions for caregivers and/or teens) and include information related to logistics of each session (e.g., time estimates, reminders, session materials, session prep, etc.).
    - Similar to the manual, any text that the therapist should say verbatim is bolded and italicized. All handouts are underlined.
    - The therapist can download the PowerPoint presentations and edit them as needed. In particular, it can be helpful for the therapist to edit the notes section of the slides so that the information and/or content is individualized for each teen. For example, the therapist can edit content such as the Guess the Price items to be individualized to the teen (e.g., items in the recipe that they are cooking for the stovetop session).

- **How should the therapist use the manual and PowerPoints to facilitate sessions?**
  - As noted, the PowerPoint presentations should be used to present the session material at each caregiver group session and caregiver/teen dyad session. The therapist can use the notes in each PowerPoint presentation slide, which are identical to what is in each Session Overview of the manual, to assist with facilitating the material.
  - The therapist should ensure that only they are able to view the notes on each PowerPoint slide and that caregivers and teens can only see the content on each slide.
  - The Session Overviews have more detail on how to facilitate the session (e.g., individualizing the material, modifying instruction of specific concepts, helpful tips) that will be beneficial for the therapist to read through prior to facilitating.

- **What additional tasks does the therapist need to do during sessions?**
  - While not required, it is helpful for the therapist to take notes during the dyad session on how the teen did with their Real World Practice assignment, description of the session (e.g., challenges, current skill level, etc.), and the goals on their DLS contract. It is also helpful to take notes during the caregiver session on issues or challenges that the teen or caregiver may be experiencing, current skill level of the teen for the upcoming dyad session, and possible modifications to the DLS contract for the upcoming dyad session.
  - Beginning in Session 4, the therapist will also need to complete the Real World Practice Tracker. This can be completed during the session or immediately after using any notes that the therapist took.
  - Many therapists find it helpful to modify/complete the DLS contract with the caregiver and teen at the end of each dyad session using an editable PDF of the DLS contract handout. The therapist can then email a copy of the DLS contract to the caregiver and teen. This may save time and also provide information about the goals, expectations, and rewards that the teen is working on. Further, the therapist can quickly incorporate any changes to the DLS contract in future sessions.

- **How does the therapist know how much time to spend on each section in the caregiver and caregiver/teen dyad sessions?**
  - Each section in the manual has time estimates for the therapist that indicate how much time should be spent on a particular section. If the therapist adheres to these estimates, they will be able to facilitate all sections within the allotted time for caregiver group sessions (90 minutes) and caregiver/teen dyad sessions (60 minutes). Thorough preparation by the therapist (e.g., reading the manual, reminding the caregiver and teen to complete any specific tasks to prepare) increases the likelihood of the therapist being able to adequately cover all sections of the session within the specified time period.

- **How should therapists handle rescheduling of sessions?**
  - If the therapist needs to cancel due to vacation or illness, they should inform the caregivers in the caregiver group session or the caregiver/teen dyad as soon as possible. See the following for possible rescheduling options:

  - Caregiver/teen dyad sessions
    - Can be rescheduled for a different day/time during the same week.
    - Two dyad sessions can be scheduled during the same week but several days apart so that the teen has time to work on their DLS contract goals.
    - Two dyad sessions can be combined for an extra-long session (90–120 minutes), and the teen will then likely have two new goals on their DLS contract that they need to work on before the next session.
    - Have the back-up therapist facilitate the dyad session as long as they have familiarity with the dyad (e.g., have attended or facilitated the caregiver group session, have attended or facilitated the dyad session).
  - Caregiver group session
    - Can be rescheduled for a different day/time during the same week that the majority of caregivers can attend.
    - Two caregiver group sessions can be combined for an extra-long session (120–150 minutes) to allow for coverage of all content and for caregivers to describe their teen's progress on the DLS contract.
    - Have the back-up therapist facilitate the caregiver group session as long as they have familiarity with the caregiver group (e.g., have attended or facilitated the caregiver group session previously).
- If the caregiver and/or teen need to reschedule a session, the therapist should identify whether any of the previous options would be feasible.
  - If the caregiver is not able to make the caregiver group session, the therapist can offer to meet with them prior to the next dyad session for 15–20 minutes to review the material that they missed.
  - If the caregiver and teen need to reschedule a dyad session, the options are to (1) reschedule it for a different day/time during the same week, (2) schedule two dyad sessions during the same week that are several days apart, or (3) schedule an extra-long dyad session (90–120 minutes) to cover the material in two sessions.

♦ **How should therapists handle the implementation of the DLS contract when caregivers and teens go on vacation or have a school break or holiday?**

- While it is understandable that the DLS contract may need to be adjusted during vacations or holidays (e.g., teen can wake up later when on vacation), consistency is important when building DLS. It is particularly critical for teens to continue personal hygiene tasks (e.g., brush teeth, change clothing, put on deodorant) so that they understand the importance of these skills at all times. This will also increase the likelihood of these DLS becoming acquired and integrated into the teen's routine.
- The therapist and caregiver/teen dyads should have a discussion when there will be a planned vacation or school holiday or break. It will be important to discuss what this change in the teen's schedule will entail and how it will affect the DLS that are being targeted on the DLS contract. Caregivers and teens should be encouraged to think through what DLS goals are realistic to continue to work on and how working on goals can be incorporated into the contract. For some families, a break or holiday may provide additional time to practice specific DLS (e.g., budgeting for a vacation, grocery shopping, preparing meals, doing

laundry). The teen's DLS contract may need to be altered for several weeks while they are on vacation or a school holiday such that the expectations of each goal are modified. Overall, the therapist should encourage the caregiver and teen to view holidays and vacations as opportunities for the teen to adjust to changing expectations and increase their flexibility while still targeting DLS contract goals.

- **Do therapists need to be in contact with the caregiver or teen outside of sessions?**
  - The therapist is encouraged to send a brief email or text message to caregivers and teens to remind them about the date and time of the upcoming sessions.
  - It is often beneficial for therapists to email any handouts that were completed during the session (e.g., the DLS contract, Individualized DLS goals).
  - While not mandatory, the therapist can also email the caregivers and teens a link to an anonymous satisfaction form to complete after each session or at the end of the intervention to provide feedback.
    - The questions to include in the satisfaction forms can be found on the STRW website (see also "Therapist Resources"). These questions can be used to create survey forms that can be emailed to caregivers and teens.

Structure of the STRW Session Overviews

The STRW manual has Session Overviews for each session that are structured in a consistent manner to allow for the therapist to quickly develop a flow for how to proceed through each session section (e.g., how much time to spend on reviewing the Real World Practice assignment, how much time to spend prepping for the next session, etc.). See the following for the sections in each Session Overview, which include how to facilitate the caregiver group and caregiver/teen dyad sessions.

- *Aims* – outlines the specific goals for both sessions or the individual caregiver group session and the caregiver/teen dyad session. By facilitating the session content as outlined in the manual, the aims will be achieved by the therapist.
- *Structure* – indicates how the caregiver group and caregiver/teen dyad sessions will be delivered.
- *Session Supplies* – identifies the handouts, resources, and links that are needed to facilitate the session.
- *Caregiver/Teen Preparation for Session* – indicates any preparation that needs to be completed by the caregiver and/or teen prior to the session. It can often be beneficial for the therapist to send a reminder to the caregiver and teen about any preparation (e.g., reminder to look up a recipe and gather ingredients for the stovetop cooking session).
- *Therapist Preparation for Session* – indicates any preparation that the therapist needs to do for the session. This typically involves using the Real World Practice Tracking Sheet (available on the STRW website) to track the teen's progress on the goals on their DLS contract. It also involves the therapist thinking through how a session

may need to be modified based on information obtained from the caregiver and/or teen (e.g., the teen does not have a microwave, so they will practice cooking skills with an air fryer instead).

- *Notes* – this section is particularly critical for the therapist to read over because it contains helpful information on effectively and efficiently facilitating the session content. It contains a section on overall session notes and notes specific to the caregiver group session and the caregiver/teen dyad session.
- *Caregiver Group Session Content* – includes all of the information needed to facilitate the caregiver group session, including instructions and verbatim text. Each bullet point corresponds to a PowerPoint slide, and there is also a "slide" icon to represent this. All text that the therapist should say verbatim is bolded and italicized. Any time a handout is referred to, it is underlined.
  - *Wrap-Up* – includes directions for the therapist to complete after the caregiver group session is over.
  - *Caregiver Group Session Handouts* – includes all handouts that are referred to in the session and also included in the STRW workbook for caregivers.

- *Caregiver/Teen Dyad Session Content* – includes all of the information needed to facilitate the caregiver/teen dyad session, including instructions and verbatim text. Each bullet point corresponds to a PowerPoint slide, and there is also a "slide" icon to represent this. All text that the therapist should say verbatim is bolded and italicized. Any time a handout is referred to, it is underlined.
  - *Wrap-Up* – this section includes directions for the therapist to complete after the caregiver/teen dyad session is over.
  - *Caregiver/Teen Dyad Session Handouts* – includes all handouts that are referred to in the session and also included in the STRW workbook for both caregivers and teens.

Caregiver Group Session Content – within each Session Overview, there are sections with detailed information on how to facilitate the caregiver group session.

- *Group Rules* – the group rules for each caregiver group session include: (1) be respectful, (2) pay attention to the material, (3) stay on topic, (4) raise your hand if you have a question, and (5) do not use your phone or other device during the sessions. These are meant to create an atmosphere in which other caregivers are involved, engaged, and participating in the session as the therapist facilitates and provides instruction and feedback. The therapist can add other rules that may be beneficial (e.g., reserving the last 5–10 minutes of each session to discuss "off topic" questions that are brought up throughout the group). It may be particularly important to go over these rules for the first three to four sessions and then review as necessary.
- *Videoconferencing Etiquette and Tips* – these are included for the therapist to review in the first few sessions in particular. Many of the tips are practical, especially for caregivers who are not familiar with videoconferencing platforms (e.g., Zoom). However, the etiquette guidelines are included to create an atmosphere that is collaborative and respectful and can be referred back to as needed.
- *Review – Real World Practice* – the majority of each caregiver group session will be spent discussing the experience each caregiver had with completing the Real World Practice assignments. Once the DLS contract is implemented in Session 3,

the therapist will be able to provide constructive feedback and individualized support on how to modify or refine the DLS goals, expectations, and rewards to the caregivers. This review allows for problem solving around challenges experienced by caregiver group members and also normalizes the issues that are commonly faced by caregivers of teens (e.g., decreased motivation to work on DLS, difficulties waking up in the morning, etc.). It is also an opportunity for caregivers to discuss their teen's progress without their teen present, which will allow for the therapist to understand how they may address goals on the DLS contract and other issues (e.g., motivation, commitment, etc.) in future dyad sessions. While the feedback is given to individual caregivers, much of it will be applicable to the other caregivers, either now or in the future. The therapist will need to manage time appropriately so that each caregiver is given the opportunity to discuss progress over the last week (e.g., goals on DLS contract, Real World Practice assignments), which also increases accountability to work on the DLS goals. It should take approximately 45–60 minutes to complete this section depending on the number of caregivers in the group.

- *Session Goals* – this section provides a brief overview of the goals for the specific session and what specific DLS will be targeted. It should take 1–2 minutes to complete this section and answer any questions.
- *Review of Dyad Session Content* – the therapist will review the content that will be discussed and taught in the upcoming dyad session. The goal of this section is to provide caregivers with an understanding of what they will need to do to prepare for the session as they instruct, model, and help their teen practice a new DLS in the home environment. The therapist should answer any questions and discuss if any modifications need to be made for specific dyads based on strengths, challenges, preferences, availability of materials (e.g., do not have a microwave and will instead practice cooking with an air fryer), fine or gross motor issues (e.g., will use a folding board to assist with folding and putting away laundry), sensory issues (e.g., will wear gloves when doing laundry), or skill level with a specific DLS (e.g., has experience using a checking account and will instead spend more time practicing how to use the banking app). It should take approximately 20–30 minutes to complete this section.
- *Real World Practice and Prep for the Next Session* – the therapist will review any Real World Practice assignments that need to be completed before the next caregiver group session. The therapist will also discuss any preparation that may need to be done before the next caregiver session (e.g., brainstorm possible recipes the teen may enjoy cooking on the stovetop). It should take 2–3 minutes to complete this section and answer any questions about the next caregiver session.

Caregiver/Teen Dyad Session Content – within each Session Overview, there are sections with detailed information on how to facilitate the caregiver/teen dyad session.

- *Session Schedule* – this section is meant to orient the caregiver and teen to all of the material that will be covered during the dyad session. The therapist should briefly go over each item on the Session Schedule. It should take about 1–2 minutes to complete this section.

- *Session Rules* – the rules for each dyad session include: (1) be respectful, (2) pay attention to the material, (3) listen to others, (4) work together, (5) stay on topic, and (6) do not use your phone or other device during the sessions. These are meant to create an atmosphere in which the caregiver and teen are involved, engaged, working together, and participating in the session as the therapist facilitates and provides instruction and feedback. The therapist can add other rules that may be beneficial (e.g., do not interrupt others when they are speaking). It may be particularly important to go over these rules for the first several sessions and then review as necessary.
- *Videoconferencing Etiquette and Tips* – these are included for the therapist to review in the first two sessions in particular. Many of the tips are practical, especially for caregivers and teens who are not familiar with videoconferencing (e.g., Zoom). However, the etiquette guidelines are included to create an atmosphere that is collaborative and respectful and can be referred back to as needed.
- *Real World Practice Check-In* – this is a critical part of the dyad session and is meant to provide an opportunity for the therapist to discuss how the teen is progressing with the goals on their DLS contract. After the DLS contract is introduced in Session 3, the focus of this check-in is to review each goal that is being targeted on the DLS contract and discuss what is working and what is not and do some brainstorming with the caregiver/teen dyad to address any challenges. The therapist should ask each question on the PowerPoint slide(s) to obtain an understanding of whether the DLS contract was used and whether goals were worked on and met over the course of the week. It will be important for the therapist to encourage caregivers and teens to be open and honest so that successes can be celebrated and any challenges can be addressed through discussion or modification of the DLS contract. It will be beneficial to discuss possible changes to goals, expectations, and rewards from the previous DLS contract that will then be incorporated into the next week's DLS contract that the teen will work on for the following week. The therapist should also be keeping track of the teen's progress on their DLS contract by recording the responses of caregivers and teens on the Real World Practice Tracking Sheet (see "Therapist Resources"), which allows for the monitoring of progress across sessions and as new goals are added to the DLS contract. Once the DLS contract has been introduced, the therapist will also conclude the Real World Practice Check-In by discussing whether the dyad is considering all of the critical elements of an effective system for achieving DLS goals (i.e., teen qualities; caregiver qualities; evidence-based strategies; Four Laws of Behavior Change to ensure that goals are obvious, appealing, easy, and satisfying). It should take about 10–15 minutes to complete this section.
- *Instruction, Modeling, and Practicing of Specific DLS* – this section varies depending on session content, but it may consist of DLS instruction (e.g., technique for cutting up vegetables safely), modeling (e.g., caregiver modeling how to cut up vegetables using a knife and cutting board), and practicing (e.g., teen using a knife and cutting board to cut up vegetables). While instruction occurs in each session using the DLS Teaching Method, modeling and practicing may be combined depending on the nature of the DLS and time constraints in the session. While the therapist will lead this portion of the session, caregivers will be actively engaged as they instruct, model, and individualize the content for their teen (e.g., the specific functions of

their microwave buttons). Teens will be actively engaged as they learn new skills and also watch and practice these skills with feedback and support from their caregiver and the therapist. Various evidence-based strategies will be introduced during this portion of the dyad session. It should take about 20–30 minutes to complete this section.

- *Elements of an Effective System for Achieving DLS Goals* – after a new DLS has been taught, modeled, and/or practiced, the therapist will encourage the caregiver/teen dyad to think through the elements of an effective system for achieving DLS goals to increase the likelihood of success as the new skill is added to the DLS contract. While it may take some time to go through these four elements, caregivers and teens will become increasingly adept at identifying whether there are any missing elements or things that should be taken into consideration. For example, teens will be asked if they have considered their strengths, challenges, learning style, and level of commitment, while caregivers will be asked if they have considered their parenting style (see Reaven et al., 2012 for more information), time and effort, and level of commitment. Going through these four elements will then make it easier to add or modify/refine the goals, expectations, and rewards on the DLS contract and increase the teen's likelihood of successfully meeting goals.
- *Developing Your DLS Contract* – beginning in Session 3, the therapist will guide the caregiver and teen dyad in adding new DLS goals or modifying/refining existing goals on the DLS contract. As the STRW intervention progresses, the therapist should fade back their level of support in developing the DLS contract so that caregivers and teens develop confidence in doing this independently. The goal is to have a completed DLS contract before the end of the session. Any modifications that were made to the DLS contract during the Real World Practice Check-In will be included in the new contract. It should take about 10-12 minutes to complete this section.
- *Real World Practice Assignment* – the therapist will review any Real World Practice assignments that need to be completed before the next caregiver/teen dyad session. After Session 3, the primary Real World Practice assignment will be to work on goals on the DLS contract. Each session will also have an assignment that is meant to work on specific money management skills (e.g., purchasing items, comparing prices, awareness of what things cost) prior to the sessions on money management. It should take about 3 minutes to complete this section.
- *Guess the Price* – at the end of each session, there is an opportunity for teens to get practice with identifying the prices of common hygiene items, household product items, and food items. This is meant to be a fun way to build awareness of what things cost. Caregivers and teens could compete against each other to guess the price of products that they may need to buy at the store. The items for Guess the Price can be individualized based on what products the teen and caregiver use. There are Guess the Price items in each session PowerPoint that can be used, and the therapist should look up the price prior to the session to make sure that it is accurate. This part of the session is optional and can be eliminated due to time constraints or lack of interest/need from the teen. It should take 2–3 minutes to complete this section.

- *Planning for the Next Session* – this section will remind caregivers and teens of the date/time of the next dyad session. If there is any preparation that needs to be done before the next dyad session (e.g., purchasing ingredients to cook a recipe, gathering a basket of clean clothes to practice laundry), it will be discussed here. It should take 2–3 minutes to complete this section.

Therapist Resources

- The following STRW Resources are available at the STRW Website (www.STRW.org) by clicking on the "For Therapists" tab and then navigating to the "Session Materials" page, which is a password-protected page that can be accessed using the case-sensitive password "thrive":
  - STRW session PowerPoint Presentations (caregiver group and dyad sessions)
  - Caregiver Group and Dyad Session STRW Workbooks (contains all session handouts)
  - Real World Practice Tracking Sheet (used beginning in Session 4)
  - STRW Resources handout (updated regularly)
  - STRW Budgeting Workbook (used in Sessions 10, 12, and 13)
  - STRW Graduation Certificate handout (used in Session 14)
  - Satisfaction Forms for Caregiver Group Sessions and Dyad Sessions (optional)
  - Fidelity Sheets for Caregiver Group Sessions and Dyad Sessions (optional)

- The appendix also has several resources that may be useful for STRW therapists, including:
  - Example DLS Contracts – includes examples of DLS contracts from previous STRW teen participants. These may be helpful to get an understanding of how to individualize goals, expectations, use of evidence-based strategies and supports, and rewards.
  - Example Task Analyses – includes examples of how STRW teen participants broke down the steps for the tasks of morning routine, nighttime routine, cleaning the bedroom, and laundry. These may be helpful to get an understanding of how detailed to get when creating task analyses with caregiver and teen participants.
  - Strategies Commonly Used to Target Goals on the DLS Contract – includes the evidence-based strategies, supports, and tools that teens utilize as they work on their DLS goals of morning routine, cleaning the bedroom, laundry, cooking, grocery shopping, and money management. It may be beneficial for therapists to review these prior to facilitating these sessions and developing the DLS contract with the caregiver/teen dyads.
  - Motivating Rewards Identified by Teens in the STRW Intervention – includes a list of rewards that were identified by previous STRW teen participants in categories including food, money, spending time with family, spending time with friends, screen time, shopping, outings, and privileges.

- Recipe Ideas for the STRW Cooking Sessions – includes ideas of recipes to cook if the caregiver/teen dyad is having trouble identifying what to cook in Sessions 6–8.
- Tips for STRW Therapists: How to Facilitate Achievement of DLS Goals – includes tips and guidelines that may be beneficial for STRW therapists as they begin facilitating the caregiver group sessions and the caregiver/teen dyad sessions. These tips were developed based on feedback from previous STRW therapists about how to effectively provide instruction and support to caregivers and teens while also actively partnering and collaborating with them so that they were motivated to build their DLS during STRW sessions and also after the intervention ends.
- Possible Solutions to Common Challenges that Arise for STRW Therapists – includes ideas for how STRW therapists can address common challenges that arise when facilitating the caregiver group and dyad sessions, including commitment; engagement; inattention; too much prompting; and family factors such as time, use of rewards, and caregiver/teen relationship.

Tracking Progress

- **Should DLS assessments be administered to the caregiver and teen before and after the intervention?**
  - It is recommended that specific assessments of DLS be utilized at the beginning of treatment to get an understanding of the teen's DLS strengths and challenges. Any assessments can be utilized by the therapist during the Pre-STRW session to get an understanding of the teen's DLS profile. This same assessment could then be administered at post-treatment to see if there was improvement in specific DLS areas and/or special skills.
  - Possible assessments that may be beneficial to administer include:
    - Adaptive Behavior Assessment System (Harrison & Oakland, 2015)
    - Vineland Adaptive Behavior Scales (Sparrow et al., 2016)
    - Teenager Survival Checklist, Updated (Erickson et al., 2013)
  - Notably, not all DLS assessments will capture some of the individualized progress that teens made during the STRW intervention. For example, if a teen still requires some prompts or reminders to complete specific DLS (e.g., laundry, cooking), this still may be significant progress for them, but the DLS assessment results may not demonstrate this improvement (e.g., does not include the particular skill they made progress on, does not give full credit for skill acquisition if prompting is still needed).

- **How is progress in DLS tracked during STRW sessions?**
  - There are several ways that DLS goals are tracked:
    - The Real World Practice Tracking Sheet (see "Therapist Resources") will be utilized beginning in Session 4 to track all goals on the DLS contract.

- The DLS contract is another way in which goals are tracked by the caregiver and teen. They are encouraged to use the DLS contract to indicate the days that they achieved goals throughout the week.
- In the Preparing for STRW session, the caregiver and teen also work together to set six DLS goals based on the results of the DLS assessments and their individual strengths and challenges. These goals are written down on the Individualized DLS Goals handout by the caregiver and teen and will be incorporated into the DLS contract in future sessions. In Session 14, the caregiver and teen will also revisit the goals they created together.

♦ **How do therapists use the Real World Practice Tracking Sheet in dyad sessions?**
  - Beginning in the Session 4 dyad session, the therapist should track the teen's progress on meeting the goals on their DLS contract. The Real World Practice Tracking Sheet (see "Therapist Resources") should be completed as the therapist asks the questions and corresponding follow-up questions for each DLS goal discussed in the Real World Practice Check-In section of each dyad session. The dyad PowerPoint slide has specific questions (e.g., "Did you work on your morning routine goal this week?") and follow-up questions (e.g., "How many days did your work on your morning routine?"), and the teen's responses should be transcribed directly onto the sheet. Caregivers and teens are encouraged to be honest about their reporting so that the information can be used to address challenges and brainstorm possible solutions.

Flexible Delivery of the STRW Intervention

Our team has only conducted research on the efficacy of the STRW intervention with autistic adolescents in the outpatient clinic setting and via telehealth. However, clinicians may find the content and structure of the STRW intervention useful for other age groups (e.g., elementary or middle school autistic students, autistic adults) or other populations (e.g., teens with ADHD, adolescents with an intellectual disability, neurotypical teens). Some possible options and ideas on administration include the following:

♦ **Elementary and Middle School Students** – Students in grades 1–8 who have DLS challenges will likely benefit from the content focused on the morning routine, cleaning the bedroom, cooking, and grocery shopping. Depending on the individual child, the money management sessions may be too complex or sophisticated based on their personal experience, so the therapist may want to eliminate them or simplify them (e.g., discuss the use of a money diary to build an understanding of how much money they spend when with their caregivers, create a savings contract to deposit a portion of their allowance and/or birthday gift money into a savings account, create a budget for a birthday party with their caregiver). It may be beneficial for families to provide an allowance to their child as part of the DLS contract, which then provides experience with spending, saving, and budgeting money based on what the child would like to buy.

- **Young Adults** – Individuals between the ages of 18 and 25 who have struggled to achieve age-appropriate DLS will likely benefit from all of the content in the STRW intervention. It may still be critical to have a caregiver provide support and coaching, but the young adult may also prefer to have a friend, older sibling, or other family member serve in this role. Further, young adults may benefit from a more in-depth discussion of how to apply the content and evidence-based strategies to other DLS. For example, if a young adult is living in a dorm room with others, it may be beneficial to develop a cleaning checklist of the bathroom and/or living room of the dorm room. As another example, if a young adult has a part-time job, they may benefit from additional sessions that allow them to practice how to budget their money based on income and fixed and variable expenses.
- **Children, Teens, and Young Adults with an Intellectual Disability** – The content of the STRW intervention is likely appropriate for many children and teens who have an intellectual disability. It may be necessary to modify the pace (e.g., the laundry session has a lot of content and may need to be broken down into two sessions) and content (e.g., money management sessions may be more applicable for older teens and/or young adults who have a part-time job). Overall, the therapist will need to ensure that they are individualizing the content for both the individual and their caregiver based on their profile of strengths and challenges and their specific DLS goals.
- **In-Person Caregiver Group, Teen Group Sessions, and/or Dyad Sessions** – STRW was previously delivered in the outpatient clinic setting with separate in-person caregiver and teen groups. There are advantages to this delivery modality, including allowing the caregivers and teens to interact with one another while normalizing DLS challenges and practicing new DLS. However, it is important to note that this delivery type requires the adolescent to generalize the skill from the clinic setting to their home environment, which is an extra step that may interfere with the acquisition and mastery of the DLS. Further, delivery of the STRW intervention in the outpatient setting requires significant materials (e.g., cooking supplies, ingredients for recipes, access to a microwave, stove, and oven) and additional staff (e.g., one to two therapists for the teen group and one therapist for the caregiver group if they are being run concurrently).

Research Evidence on the STRW Intervention

- **How was STRW developed?**
    - STRW is the first evidence-based DLS intervention package for autistic adolescents (14–21 years of age) with average or above-average cognitive abilities (full scale IQ ≥ 70). The intervention was created through a 10-year iterative process, and both adolescents and their caregivers were involved in the development and continued refinement. Therapists who delivered the STRW intervention also provided critical feedback on the intervention during the iterative process (Duncan et al., 2021). A range of evidence-based strategies that have been shown to be effective for building daily living skills in autistic

adolescents were incorporated throughout the iterative development of the intervention (Bennett & Dukes, 2014; Cullen & Alber-Morgan, 2015; Gardner & Wolfe, 2013; Hong et al., 2017; Hrabal et al., 2023; Hume et al., 2009; Myles & Simpson, 2001; Palmen et al., 2012; Steinbrenner et al., 2020).

- During the COVID-19 pandemic, the STRW intervention was modified from being delivered in the outpatient setting (i.e., separate, concurrent caregiver and teen group sessions) to being delivered in the adolescent's home via videoconferencing technology (i.e., caregiver group session and individual caregiver/teen dyad sessions). The transition to STRW-telehealth allowed for adolescents to practice DLS in their own home and eliminated the extra step of generalizing DLS from the clinic setting to the home environment. Additional advantages of STRW-telehealth included the dyad session, which allowed for collaboration and cooperation between the caregiver and teen when learning and practicing DLS. Teens were also able to practice DLS in their home environment (e.g., cook in their kitchen, do laundry using their washing machine and dryer), which allowed for individualization of the core STRW content (e.g., choice of recipes to cook, choice of events to practice budgeting for). For additional information about the development of STRW, please see Duncan et al. (2021), and more information is also available on the STRW website (www.strw.org).

♦ **What is the research evidence on STRW?**

- Our team has completed a series of research studies as we sought to develop, refine, and evaluate the efficacy of the STRW intervention. Additional information on methods and results can be found in the peer-reviewed articles that are referred to at the end of each of the following research study summaries (see also "References").
  - **Case Studies** – Our team first sought to understand the profile of DLS strengths and challenges in autistic teens without an intellectual disability (i.e., IQ $\geq$ 70) (Duncan & Bishop, 2015). We then conducted single-subject case studies of autistic adolescents in the school setting (n = 3) and in a clinic setting (n = 2) to identify essential features (e.g., content, structure, treatment ingredients) of a DLS intervention. These studies helped us to identify what skills needed to be targeted based on adolescent and caregiver input and what evidence-based strategies may be best to implement. For example, it became clear that teens were struggling with the various DLS that needed to be completed from the time that they woke up until the time that they needed to leave for school (e.g., brush teeth, put on deodorant, make breakfast, pack backpack, etc.). Caregivers responded positively to the use of a DLS contract to identify specific goals and also provide external rewards to the teen as they practiced DLS. Our team determined that a school setting was not ideal for a DLS intervention because high caregiver involvement appeared to be critical to the teen's success with acquiring new skills (e.g., caregiver provides instruction and support on newly learned DLS). Caregivers and teens also expressed interest in a group outpatient intervention to allow for discussion and normalization of DLS strengths and challenges and to provide opportunities for the teens to learn and practice DLS with other teens. See Duncan et al. (2021) for additional information.

- **Study 1** – In the next study, our team conducted a pre-post study of the STRW intervention (Duncan et al., 2017) to examine the feasibility of implementing it in a group outpatient setting and to assess satisfaction with content and use of evidence-based strategies. The Vineland Adaptive Behavior Scales, 2nd Edition (Sparrow et al., 2005), caregiver interview was used to assess gains in DLS from pre-treatment to post-treatment. Results from the seven autistic adolescents who received the STRW intervention indicated that they made clinically significant improvements such that they gained 2 years of skills over the course of the 12-week intervention. Caregivers and adolescents provided significant feedback that was utilized to further refine the STRW intervention (e.g., added in additional money management sessions, increased interactive activities in the teen group). See Duncan et al. (2017) for additional information.
- **Study 2** – In our next study (Duncan et al., 2022), ten autistic adolescent participants were randomized to either participate in the STRW intervention or a waitlist control group (i.e., did not receive any intervention and were put on the waitlist while the other group received the STRW intervention). Adolescents in the STRW intervention group made significant DLS gains on the Vineland Adaptive Behavior Scales, 3rd Edition (VABS-3; Sparrow et al., 2016), caregiver interview from pre-treatment to post-treatment compared to the control group. Of note, the control group did not make any improvement on DLS while on the waitlist. However, when the control group participants crossed over and completed the STRW intervention, the combined sample of STRW participants demonstrated statistically significant and clinically meaningful gains in personal, domestic, and community DLS. Our team made additional refinements to the STRW intervention based on caregiver and adolescent feedback (e.g., incorporated more apps and technology as evidence-based strategies, increased discussion of individualization of goals in the caregiver group). See Duncan et al. (2022) for additional information.
- **Study 3** – Our team then received funding from the National Institute of Child Health and Human Development (NICHD) to conduct a pilot randomized clinical trial of the STRW intervention for 9th- and 10th-grade high school students (Duncan et al., 2025). A total of 48 autistic adolescents were randomized and completed STRW ($n = 26$) or a social skills control group ($n = 22$). Due to the COVID-19 pandemic, we modified STRW to be delivered via telehealth in June 2020. While STRW content remained the same, the format changed such that the adolescent group sessions were replaced with a dyad session that was attended by both the caregiver and adolescent each week. The format and content of the social skills control group did not change when delivered via telehealth. Approximately 22.9% of our sample completed in-person STRW and the control group, and the remaining 77.1% completed STRW or the control group via telehealth. Data from in-person and telehealth were combined and analyzed together. The VABS-3 caregiver interview was the primary outcome measure. Results revealed that adolescents in STRW made significant gains on overall DLS and domestic DLS (e.g., cleaning, cooking, laundry) compared to adolescents in the control group from pre- to post-treatment. The clinical meaningfulness of this change in DLS is illustrated by an 18-point gain on

the VABS-3 DLS domain standard score as it improved from 64.9 at baseline to 83.1 at post-treatment for teens in STRW, which signifies a narrowing of the gap between DLS and chronological age, as this score approaches being in the "average range" (i.e., 85–115). See Duncan et al. (2025) for additional information.

- **Study 4** – Our team also received funding from the Department of Defense Autism Research Program to conduct a pilot randomized clinical trial of the STRW intervention for 11th- and 12th-grade high school students (Duncan et al., 2023). Approximately 64 autistic adolescents were randomized and completed STRW (n = 34) or the social skills control group (n = 30). As noted in Study 3, STRW was modified to be delivered via telehealth, and 28.1% of the participants completed in-person STRW or the control group, and the remaining 71.9% completed STRW-T or the control group. The VABS-3 caregiver interview was the primary outcome measure. The adolescents in STRW made significantly greater gains on overall DLS and domestic DLS from pre- to post-treatment compared to adolescents in the social skills control group. The clinically meaningful gains on the DLS domain translate into a 20-point increase in their standard score from baseline (56.2) to post-treatment (76.6) and move STRW youth much closer to DLS in the average range of functioning. See Duncan et al. (2023) for additional information.

♦ **What was the inclusion criteria for the research studies conducted on the STRW intervention?**
- A diagnosis of autism – the adolescent was required to have a documented diagnosis from a psychologist, pediatrician, or other medical provider. The diagnosis was confirmed by the administration of the Autism Diagnostic Observation Schedule, 2nd Edition (Lord et al., 2012), and the clinical judgment of the psychologist conducting the assessment.
- IQ > 70 – the teen received a cognitive assessment to confirm their IQ was 70 or above.
- A DLS deficit – this was defined as having DLS that were 15 points below one's IQ. DLS were assessed by the Vineland Adaptive Behavior Scales (Sparrow et al., 2016).
- Between the ages of 14 and 21.
- Having a caregiver who was willing to participate in all intervention sessions.

♦ **In the research studies on STRW, how did you assess whether therapists administered the STRW intervention as it was written in the manual?**
- Research staff completed fidelity checklists on 25% of all STRW caregiver group session and caregiver/teen dyad sessions. These fidelity checklists (see "Therapist Resources") assessed whether therapists were administering all of the sections of the STRW sessions. Our STRW therapists had high rates of fidelity such that 90%–95% of session components were rated as being completed.

♦ **How did you assess how satisfied caregivers and teens were with STRW sessions?**
- At the end of each caregiver group session and each caregiver/teen dyad session, satisfaction forms (see "Therapist Resources") were emailed to

participants to obtain their level of satisfaction and solicit feedback on the session. Both caregivers and teens expressed high levels of satisfaction with the STRW intervention, and the feedback that they provided has been incorporated into the current version of the STRW intervention. For example, caregivers provided consistent feedback about how they wanted to work on money management concepts throughout the STRW intervention, which led to the inclusion of the Guess the Price activity and the money assignment on each Real World Practice.

- **Did the STRW therapists receive any supervision while administering the intervention?**
  - STRW therapists met weekly for supervision to discuss areas such as maintaining fidelity to the manual, building rapport with the caregivers and teens, individualizing content to specific caregiver and teen dyads, and problem solving how to address common challenges (e.g., committing to working on DLS goals each week, building motivation and buy-in from the teen). Supervision was especially helpful for therapists who had not previously facilitated the STRW intervention because they were able to learn from other therapists.

Session Overviews

Surviving & Thriving in the Real World

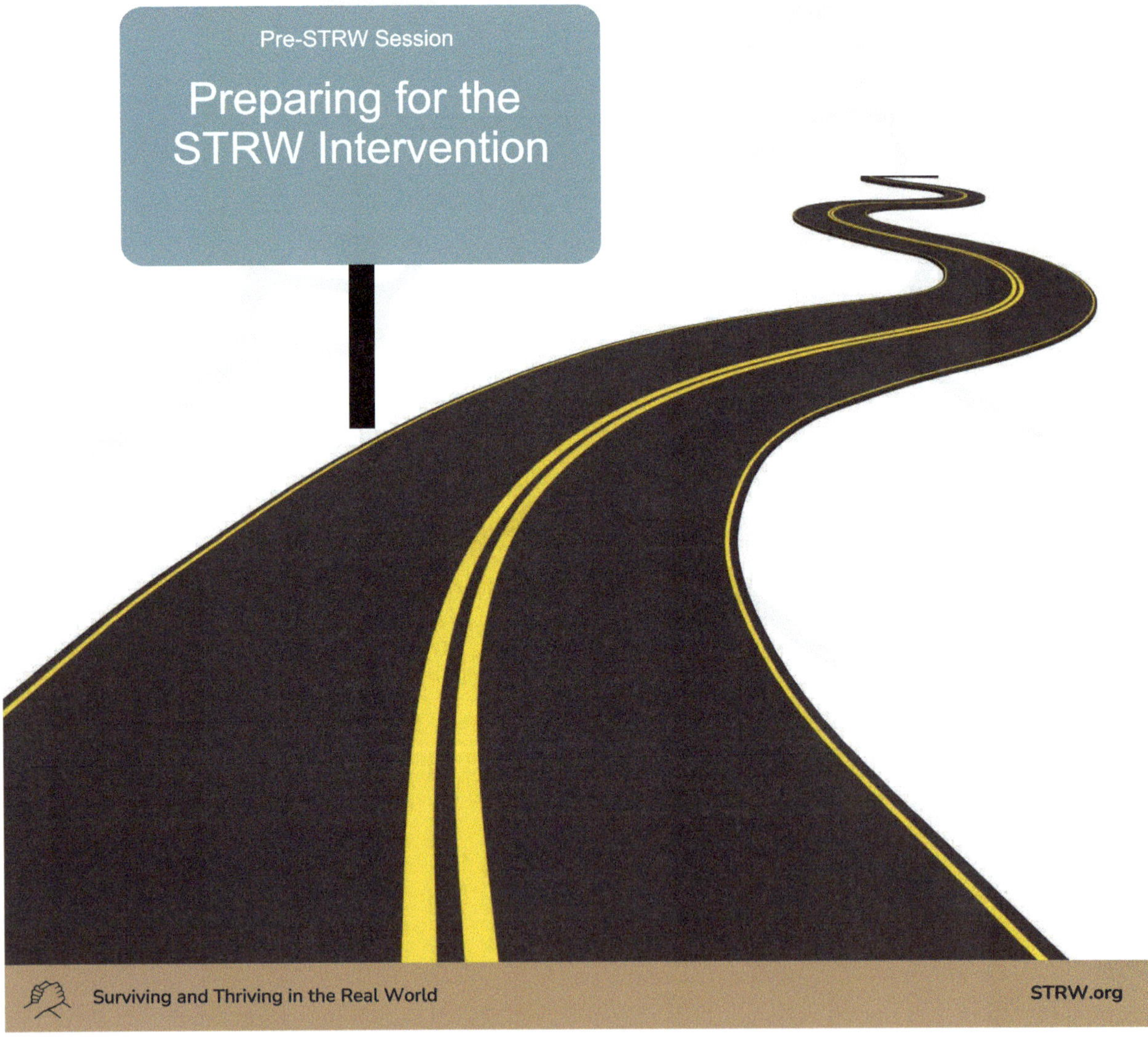

Pre-STRW Session

Preparing for the STRW Intervention

Aims

- Establish rapport between the teen, their parent/caregiver, and therapist
- Describe the purpose of the Surviving and Thriving in the Real World (STRW) intervention
- Discuss the logistics of the STRW intervention
- Discuss the teen's strengths and challenges in the area of daily living skills (DLS)
- Develop individualized DLS goals for the teen based on assessment results and their profile of strengths and challenges

Structure

- Caregiver/teen dyad session via telehealth

Session Supplies

- Handouts
    - DLS Strengths and Challenges
    - Individualized DLS Goals

Caregiver/Teen Preparation for Session

- Both the caregiver and the teen should complete a DLS assessment (see "Therapist Resources" in the STRW Manual) specified by the therapist prior to the session.

Therapist Preparation for Session

- The therapist should review the results of the DLS assessments that the caregiver and teen completed to get an understanding of what DLS strengths and challenges were identified by each. Specifically, the therapist should identify two to three strengths and challenges in the DLS areas of hygiene/self-care, cleaning, laundry, cooking, grocery shopping, and managing money that the caregiver and teen identified.

DOI: 10.4324/9781003458838-3

- It will be beneficial to identify areas of challenge that (1) were agreed upon by both the caregiver and the teen and (2) align with the DLS targeted in STRW.
- While there will often be some disagreement between identified strengths and challenges, it is important for the caregiver and teen to feel heard when setting DLS goals.

- The therapist should have provided a hard copy of the STRW workbook (either in person or via mail) to the caregiver and teen so that they are able to refer to all handouts used in this session and in future STRW sessions (see "Therapist Resources"). The STRW workbooks can also be provided via email – but it is essential that the therapist and teen have hard copies of all handouts so that they can be used during the session.
- The therapist may want to review the Possible Solutions to Common Challenges that Arise for STRW Therapists handout (see appendix), which includes ideas for how STRW therapists can address common challenges that arise when facilitating the caregiver group and dyad sessions including commitment, engagement, inattention, too much prompting, and family factors such as time, use of rewards, and caregiver/teen relationship.

Session Notes

- The DLS Strengths and Challenges and Individualized DLS Goals handouts can also be completed by the therapist during the session to facilitate discussion with the caregiver and teen. A fillable PDF of this handout is available on the STRW website and can be emailed to the family after the session.

Caregiver/Teen Dyad Pre-STRW Session Content (60 mins)

Preparing for STRW Session Schedule (3 mins)

- *Welcome to the first session of the Surviving and Thriving in the Real World intervention or STRW for short! I am excited to start working with you on building daily living skills (or DLS for short) such as hygiene, cleaning, laundry, and cooking. We are going to get to know each other really well during these dyad sessions over the next 15 weeks.*
    - If the therapist has not met the caregiver and teen prior to this first session, they should do some brief introductions.

- *For these sessions, it will be helpful to sit together at a table so that we can all see each other and work together. Please pull out your STRW workbook. Your workbook contains handouts for all of the STRW sessions. At the start of each session, you will see that there is a blank page that can be used to take any additional notes during the dyad session.*
- *This session is called Preparing for STRW. Please turn to that section in your workbook.*
- *At the start of each session, we will go over our session schedule so that you know what we will be doing. Please feel free to ask any questions about our schedule!*
- Briefly go over each item on the Session Schedule.

Overview of Caregiver/Teen Dyad Sessions (2–3 mins)

- *We will meet for the next 15 weeks via video. Let's talk through some important points about these caregiver/teen dyad sessions.*
- Read the bullet points on the slide.
    - *Dyad sessions will start off by meeting together at a table.*
    - *Some dyad sessions will be held in the kitchen, laundry area, and the teen's bedroom, which will allow for us to practice DLS in the actual areas that you need to do them!*
    - *You may need to do some preparation for sessions such as getting ingredients for a recipe.*
    - *You will need to practice the skills that you learn in session throughout the week.*
    - *Please come prepared each session with your STRW workbook and be ready to discuss how things are going!*

- Ask: *Any questions about the dyad sessions?*

Videoconferencing Etiquette and Tips (3–4 mins)

- *You may be familiar with meeting via videoconferencing, but let's just go over some etiquette and tips to make sure our sessions run smoothly!*
- Read the following etiquette and tips from the bullets on the slide.
  - *It is helpful to check your audio and video before each session.*
  - *Set up an intentional space to meet that is free from distractions and noise.*
  - *Please keep your video turned on so that we can see each other and also see what skills are being worked on.*
  - *Please feel free to keep your mic on.*
  - *It may be helpful to wear headphones to ensure that the discussion remains private and confidential.*

- If needed, the therapist can take some time to briefly go over any specific features of the specific videoconferencing platform being used.
- Ask: *Any questions or comments on using videoconferencing during our sessions?*

Session Rules (3–4 mins)

- *Since we will be working together for the next 15 weeks, let's talk about some of the session rules that are meant to set a positive tone for our session and foster collaboration as we work together on building DLS.*
- Read the following session rules from the bullet on the slide:
  - *Be respectful.*
  - *Pay attention to the material.*
  - *Listen to others.*
  - *Work together.*
  - *Stay on topic.*
  - *Do not use your phone or other device during the session.*

- Ask: *Are there any other rules that may be important to add?*
- *As a reminder, we are mandated reporters and required to take action if we believe that either you or your caregiver have any plans or intentions of harming yourself or others.*
- Ask: *Do you have any questions about that?*

Overview and Logistics of STRW (2–3 mins)

- *As a reminder, daily living skills (or DLS for short) are all of the things that you do every day to take care of yourself at home, at school, and in the community. DLS include skills such as taking a shower, putting on deodorant, making snacks and meals, cleaning your room, vacuuming and mopping, doing laundry, and saving up money to buy things.*
- *The STRW intervention is focused on building DLS in teens to increase their independence and help teens when they transition from high school to the adult world of working at a job, going to college, and living on their own. We will discuss STRW in more detail in our next session, but let's go over a few important details.*

- *Parents and caregivers will meet weekly as a group on DAY and TIME.*
- *You and your caregiver will meet weekly with me on* **DAY** *and* **TIME** *to learn new DLS and work on DLS goals in the areas of hygiene and self-care, cleaning, laundry, cooking, grocery shopping, and money management.*

♦ *Over the next 15 weeks, we will be working together as a team to build DLS that will allow you to meet your short-term and long-term goals. For example, if you have the goal of taking college classes and living on your own, you will need to learn, practice, and master DLS such as doing laundry, cooking for yourself, cleaning your room, and setting a monthly budget based on your income and your expenses. We will collaborate to set goals that consider your strengths; your challenges; how you like to learn and remember things; and also your time, energy, and motivation.*

♦ Ask: *Any questions about the STRW intervention?*

Review Results of Daily Living Skills Assessments (20 mins)

♦ Refer to previously completed DLS Assessments by the caregiver and teen.

♦ *Prior to meeting today, you and your caregiver completed an assessment to understand your DLS strengths and challenges. After reviewing the assessments you both completed, we are now going to discuss your strengths in the DLS areas of hygiene and self-care, cleaning, laundry, cooking, grocery shopping, and managing money.*

♦ *It is possible that you and your caregiver may have different opinions of what is a strength vs. what is a challenge. We will discuss this, but the important thing that we will focus on is having you learn and practice DLS that are expected of other teens your age. This includes skills like getting up on your own in the morning and getting ready to go to school, cooking simple meals for yourself, and doing your own laundry.*

♦ *We will also discuss whether you are doing DLS independently – which means without any prompting or reminders from other people. It can take some time to become independent, and we will talk about how to slowly build your independence as we work together over the next 15 weeks.*

♦ Refer to DLS Strengths and Challenges handout.

♦ *Take out your* **DLS Strengths and Challenges** *handout. Let's review some of the strengths and challenges that you both identified in the areas of hygiene/self-care, cleaning, laundry, cooking, grocery shopping, and managing money. Please write them down on the handout in your STRW workbook so that we can then use them to help us set specific goals to work on.*

♦ Review the strengths and challenges in each of the areas using the DLS assessments completed by the caregiver and teen.

- The caregiver and teen can write their responses down on the handout or the therapist can transcribe responses directly onto the slide or onto the fillable PDF of the handout.

- The therapist can start by asking a broad question (e.g., "What strengths do you have in the area of hygiene?") and then incorporate the responses from the assessments completed by the caregiver and teen.
- The therapist can get additional details about certain strengths and challenges (e.g., how often a skill is performed, the teen's level of independence, the strategies that may work for remembering to do a skill). However, there will also be opportunities to get more in-depth information about a teen's skills in future sessions.
- If disagreement arises about identified strengths and challenges, the therapist can briefly discuss why (e.g., needs a prompt to get started, caregiver does not always observe when teen completes the skill, etc.). However, the therapist should note that the teen and caregiver have their own perspective that is valuable and that the goal of this activity is to understand the teen's profile of strengths and challenges and how to build independence.

Individualized Daily Living Skills Goals (20 mins)

- ♦ *We are now going to work together to set six DLS goals based on your specific strengths and challenges and the DLS that you will be learning in STRW. We want both of you to take an active role in setting these goals so that you are committed to working on them over the course of the STRW intervention. I may also sometimes ask questions or make comments to help create goals that are specific, achievable, and realistic.*
- ♦ Ask: *Any questions before we work on developing the DLS goals?*
- ♦ Refer to <u>Individualized DLS Goals</u> handout.
- ♦ *Let's spend the rest of our time together setting DLS goals in the areas of hygiene and self-care, cleaning, laundry, cooking, grocery shopping, and managing money. We will aim to set DLS that are expected of other teens your age and increase your overall independence.*
- ♦ *Some examples of goals that other teens have set include:*
    - *For Hygiene/Self-Care: Brush my teeth, wash my face, and put deodorant on every morning before I eat breakfast.*
    - *For Cleaning: Pick up my belongings in my room and put them where they go every Sunday night by 8 pm.*
    - *For Doing Laundry: Do my laundry from start to finish on Wednesday after school before I go to bed.*
    - *For Cooking: Pack my lunch for school during the week (Monday–Friday).*
    - *For Grocery Shopping: Find items to buy at the grocery store using a list.*
    - *For Managing Money: Check the balance of my checking and savings accounts every Friday night.*

- ♦ *When making goals, we want to be specific about what needs to be done and also when, where, and how often it needs to be done. You should write down the goals we come up with on your <u>Individualized DLS Goals</u> handout.*
    - Discuss and create individualized DLS goals with the teen and their caregiver.
    - The caregiver and teen can write their responses down on the handout or the therapist can transcribe responses directly onto the slide or onto the fillable PDF of the handout.

Preparing for the Next Dyad Session (3 mins)

- ***We will have our next dyad session on DAY and TIME. At this session, we will go over the details of the STRW intervention in more detail as we prepare to begin working on building your DLS.***
- The therapist may want to encourage the family to keep a folder on their computer where they store all STRW documents, including DLS contracts and handouts that are completed within each session (e.g., the Individualized DLS Goals handout from the current session).
- Ask: ***Are there any questions before we end the session?***

Wrap-Up

- Therapists should send a calendar invite with the next dyad session's day/time to the caregiver and teen.
- Therapists should email any documents that were completed during the session to the caregiver and teen.

DLS Strengths and Challenges

Strengths	**Challenges/Areas to Improve**
Hygiene/Self-Care	Hygiene/Self-Care
Cleaning	Cleaning
Doing Laundry	Doing Laundry
Cooking	Cooking
Grocery Shopping	Grocery Shopping
Managing Money	Managing Money
Other	Other

Individualized DLS Goals

- Hygiene/Self-Care:

- Cleaning:

- Doing Laundry:

- Cooking:

- Grocery Shopping:

- Managing Money:

Surviving & Thriving in the Real World

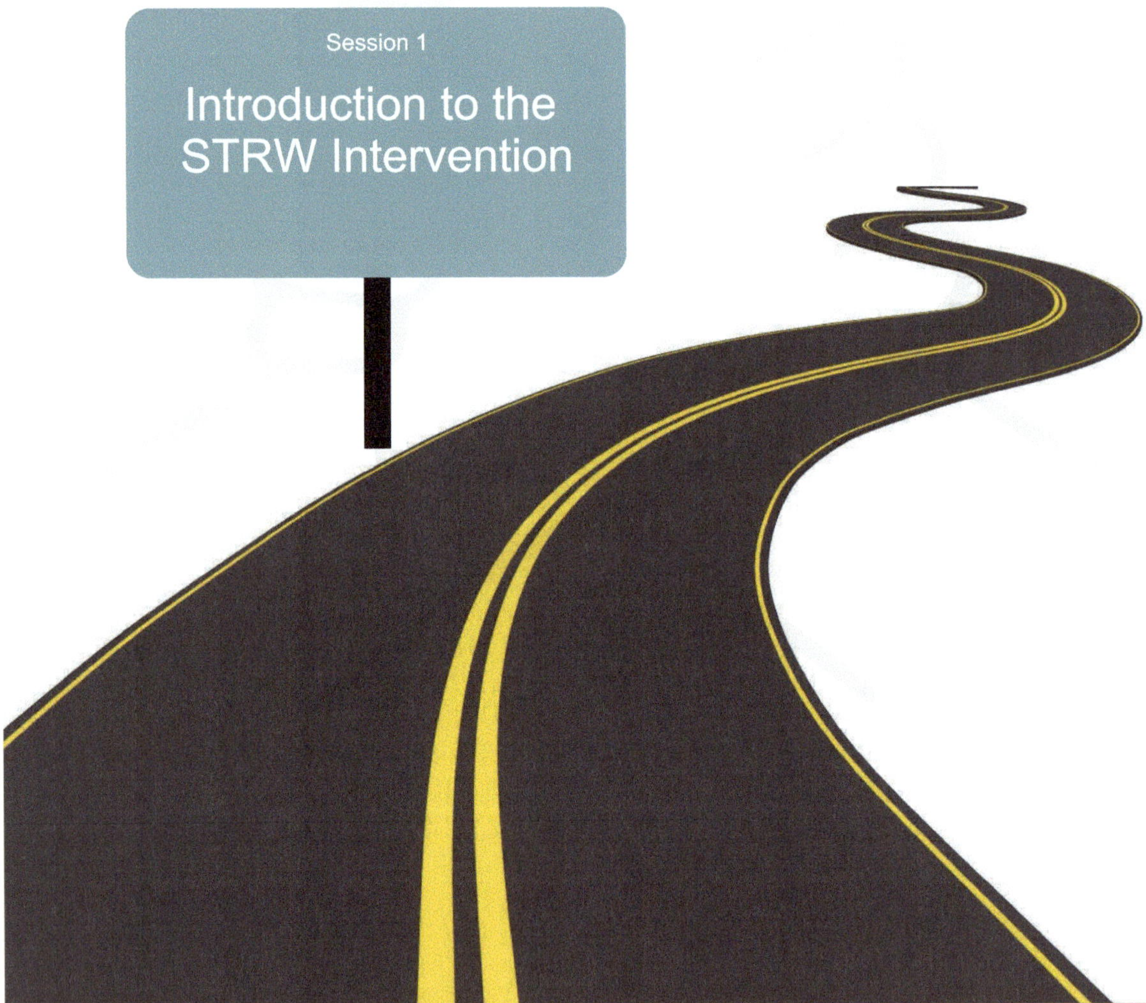

Session 1

Introduction to the Surviving and Thriving in the Real World Intervention

Aims

- Build rapport between caregiver group members and the therapist
- Continue to build rapport between the teen, caregiver, and therapist
- Describe the purpose of the Surviving and Thriving in the Real World (STRW) intervention
- Provide a detailed overview of the STRW intervention
- Identify the daily living skills (DLS) that will be targeted during STRW
- Discuss the commitments that teens and caregivers will make during the STRW intervention
- Identify short-term and long-term goals for the teen
- Describe essential DLS that are needed to meet future goals

Structure

- Caregiver group session via telehealth
- Caregiver/teen dyad session via telehealth

Session Supplies

- Caregiver Group Handouts
    - Essential Life Skills for All Teens
    - STRW Session Overview
    - DLS Contract
    - STRW Resources (to be emailed to caregivers by the therapist)

- Caregiver/Teen Dyad Handouts
    - Essential Daily Living Skills for Meeting Future Goals
    - Essential Life Skills for All Teens
    - STRW Session Overview
    - Session 1 – Real World Practice
    - What Motivates You

DOI: 10.4324/9781003458838-4

Caregiver/Teen Preparation for Session

- None

Therapist Preparation for Session

- The therapist should email all caregivers the STRW Resources handout (see "Therapist Resources"), which has various resources (e.g., websites, books, articles, apps) related to the STRW intervention curriculum. This handout is also available on the STRW website and is regularly updated.
- The therapist may want to review the Possible Solutions to Common Challenges that Arise for STRW Therapists handout (see appendix), which includes ideas for how STRW therapists can address common challenges that arise when facilitating the caregiver group and dyad sessions including commitment; engagement; inattention; too much prompting; and family factors such as time, use of rewards, and caregiver/teen relationship.

Session 1 Notes

- A primary goal of Session 1 is to build rapport and also set the foundation for why age-appropriate DLS may lead to successful adult outcomes in work, college, independent living, and community participation.
- Therapists should be open to addressing questions from caregivers and teens about expectations, logistics, and concerns.
- The term "caregiver" is used to reflect that parents, grandparents, siblings, and other family members may be participating in the STRW intervention with the teen. The therapist can choose to use the term "parent" instead of "caregiver" when appropriate.
- The Essential Daily Living Skills for Meeting Future Goals handout can also be completed by the therapist during the session to facilitate discussion with the caregiver and teen. A fillable PDF of this handout is available on the STRW website and can be emailed to the family after the session.

- Caregiver Group Session
    - Throughout this session and in future sessions, caregivers may have questions about how to identify age-appropriate daily living skills to target. The therapist can refer them to the assessment resources on the STRW Resources handout for additional information or discuss options for identifying daily living skills to target as a group (e.g., identifying skills that the teen is motivated or interested in learning; identifying skills that are needed to increase teen's independence at home, school, or in the community).

- Dyad Session
    - The Essential Daily Living Skills for Meeting Future Goals handout can also be completed by the therapist during the session to facilitate discussion with the caregiver and teen. A fillable PDF of this handout is available on the STRW website and can be emailed to the family after the session.

Caregiver Group Session 1 Content (90 mins)

Surviving and Thriving in the Real World (2–3 mins)

- *Welcome to the first caregiver group session of Surviving and Thriving in the Real World or STRW for short! Before we get started and do some introductions, we ask that you respect others' privacy by keeping all information that is discussed in these sessions confidential. This will allow us to have a level of trust as we work together over the next 14 weeks.*
- *As a reminder, we are mandated reporters and required to take action if we believe that you or your teen have any intentions of harming yourself or others.*
- *STRW is an intervention that aims to help teens learn and master daily living skills (or DLS for short) that will allow them to survive and thrive in the real world – in areas such as college, work, and living on their own. Caregivers will coach teens in acquiring new DLS during the individual dyad sessions and then support teens as they practice these newly learned skills at home and in the community. Teens will commit to learning and mastering DLS in collaboration with their caregiver and the therapist.*
- *We will discuss the details of the group in more detail later in the session and I will be happy to answer any questions.*
- *Let's briefly review some videoconferencing tips and sessions rules before taking some time to get to know one another.*

Videoconferencing Etiquette and Tips (1–2 mins)

- *You may be familiar with videoconferencing, but let's briefly go over some etiquette and tips to make sure our caregiver group sessions and our caregiver/teen dyad sessions run smoothly!*
- Read the following etiquette and tips from the bullets on the slide and demonstrate features as needed.
  - *Please keep your video turned on so that we can see your face. This increases engagement with the group and allows us to all feel more connected to one another.*
  - *For these group sessions, keep your mic muted unless you are speaking. This eliminates any background noise and allows everyone to hear whoever is speaking.*
    - *However, if you need more detail or clarification on something that is being discussed, please feel free to unmute and ask a question or make a comment.*
  - *It is difficult to hear when more than one person speaks at the same time. Some helpful tips include:*
    - *If you have a question or comment, you can use the Chat feature or Raise Hand feature.*

- *You can also raise your actual hand to indicate that you would like to unmute your mic and speak.*
- *You can use reactions to engage with others such as a thumbs up to indicate agreement or clapping hands to celebrate a success.*

Videoconferencing Etiquette and Tips (1–2 mins)

- *Some other helpful tips include:*
  - *It is helpful to check your audio and video before each session to make sure that they are working.*
  - *Set up an intentional space to meet that is free from distractions and noise.*
  - *It may be helpful to wear headphones to ensure that the discussion remains private and confidential.*
  - *Come prepared to the session by bringing your STRW workbook and any other materials you may need such as a pen or pencil.*

- Ask: *Any questions or comments on using videoconferencing during our sessions?*

Group Rules (3–4 mins)

- *These group rules are meant to set the tone for our group sessions and foster a collaborative, engaging, and supportive group as we work together on building DLS over the next 14 weeks.*
- Review the following group rules:
  - *Be respectful.*
    - *This rule also includes keeping information that is discussed in session private. While we cannot enforce this rule, other group members are more likely to openly share if there is a shared understanding that this is a safe and private space to discuss things.*
  - *Listen to others.*
  - *Be attentive. This includes when others are talking and when information is being presented.*
  - *Do not use your phone or other device during the session.*
  - *Stay on topic.*
  - *We will try to reserve the final 5–10 minutes of each session for "off-topic" questions.*

- Ask: *Are there any other rules that may be important to add?*

Getting to Know One Another (15 mins)

- The therapist should give a brief introduction of themself (e.g., name, background, previous experience, etc.) if they have not yet done this.
- *We will be working closely together over the next 14 weeks! Let's all take a turn answering these questions to get to know each other a little bit better.*
- Have caregivers each take a turn to answer the questions on the slide about themselves and their teen.

- The therapist can also answer the questions to start the activity and as a way to build rapport.
- The therapist can choose to edit any of the questions.
- It can be helpful for the therapist to point out commonalities between the caregivers and/or their teens.

STRW Session 1 Goals (1 min)

- *The goal of today's session is to discuss the essential DLS that will facilitate a successful transition from high school to the adult world for your teen. We will also discuss the content and logistics of the STRW intervention in detail.*

Essential Life Skills for All Teens (20 mins)

- *Please pull out your STRW workbook. As a reminder, your workbook contains handouts for all of the STRW sessions. At the start of each session, you will see that there is a blank page that can be used to take any additional notes during the caregiver group session or the dyad session.*
- *This session is called Introduction to the STRW Intervention – Caregiver Group Session. Please turn to that section in your workbook.*
- Refer to the <u>Essential Life Skills for All Teens</u> handout.
- *These are some of the essential life skills that are critical when becoming an adult – if you have these skills, you will be more likely to have a smoother and easier transition from high school to the adult world. You will notice that many of these life skills are DLS and probably include many of the DLS we talked about with you and your teen at the Preparing for STRW dyad session.*
- *Some of the essential life skills that caregivers and teenagers are often working towards developing in high school include skills in the areas of independent living, academics, employment, and navigating the community.*
- *For example, the area of independent living may include learning specific life skills including hygiene and self-care (such as showering), health care (such as taking medications and making appointments for the doctor), at home (such as laundry, cleaning, and cooking), and money management (such as making a budget and keeping track of spending).*
- *While it can be somewhat overwhelming to look at all of these life skills that are needed in adulthood, it will also be helpful in identifying what DLS need to be targeted and then coming up with a plan for learning these DLS.*
- *I am going to ask you a few questions related to these essential life skills, and I want you to take a moment and think about or jot down your answers. You can also refer back to the Strengths and Challenges list that we came up with during our Preparing for STRW session with your teen. We will then share and discuss with the group.*
  - *What are two to three strengths your teen has in the area of DLS?*
  - *What are two to three challenges your teen has in the area of DLS? In other words, what skills do you want them to develop or become more independent in?*

- *Take a minute to think about these questions and then we will share your responses and discuss them as a group.*
- Have the caregivers discuss their teen's strengths and challenges.
  - Try to keep the discussion focused on DLS (not social skills, academic difficulties, family relationship issues).
  - Point out commonalities between the caregivers' responses.
  - It may be helpful to normalize that caregivers may feel overwhelmed as they look at all of the essential life skills that their teen may need to work on.

- *Now that you have shared your teen's DLS strengths and challenges, let's talk more about what DLS they will be working on building during STRW.*

STRW Session Content (10 mins)

- Refer to the Session Overview handout.
- *As all teens get older, it becomes important to start learning all of the DLS that will help them reach their life goals. As we discussed in the Preparing for STRW session with your teen, DLS are life skills that are needed to take care of yourself and include taking a shower, wearing deodorant, taking medications, cleaning up your room, cooking in the microwave or on the stove, doing the laundry, purchasing items at a store, using a debit or credit card, and budgeting your money. These skills become especially important as teens become adults and start thinking about going to college, getting a job, and/or moving out of their family's home and into their own apartment or home.*
- *The name of this intervention is Surviving and Thriving in the Real World because we want to help teens develop the essential DLS that will be important as they transition from high school to the adult world. With the help of their caregivers and everyone else on their support team, we will work on building these life skills in the dyad sessions and then practicing them in the real world, which includes their home, school, and community. While we know that it will take some practice and hard work from both caregivers and teens to learn and practice DLS, we will discuss how to build excitement, motivation, and buy-in while making progress towards goals.*
- *Over the next 14 weeks, STRW sessions will target the acquisition and mastery of DLS in the areas of personal hygiene and self-care, cleaning one's room, doing laundry from start to finish, cooking, grocery shopping, and money management.*
- *While some teens may have already developed some of these DLS, we will also teach these skills using strategies that can be applied to learn a wide range of other DLS such as setting and reaching goals, managing time, prioritizing tasks, meal planning, cooking for others, paying bills, and keeping a household clean. Also, it can be helpful to gain additional practice with a DLS even if you or your teen feels that they already know how to do it. We can also help teens fine-tune or further develop some of their DLS if they have already learned a skill.*
- *Caregivers will play a large and extremely important role as they coach their teens on developing these DLS, which is also very hard work. In order to learn DLS, it will be important for teens and caregivers to be committed because this will help with developing and mastering DLS.*
- Ask: *Any questions about what we will be covering in the upcoming STRW sessions?*

Daily Living Skills Contract (2 mins)

- *Throughout STRW we will introduce you and your teen to many strategies that have been shown to help teens build their DLS.*
- Refer to the DLS Contract handout.
- *One of the main strategies that we will use is the DLS contract. Starting in Session 3, we will use this DLS contract to work on specific DLS that are introduced and practiced in the dyad sessions. Teens will be able to earn a reward if they meet their DLS goal. We will discuss the DLS contract in more detail in the next two caregiver group and dyad sessions.*

Logistics of STRW Sessions (3–4 mins)

- *Let's briefly go over some of the logistics of the caregiver group sessions and the caregiver/teen dyad sessions.*
  - *During the weekly caregiver group sessions, we will discuss your teen's progress as they work towards achieving their DLS goals. This will be an opportunity to brainstorm solutions and get guidance or support on anything you may be encountering at home as your teen works on their DLS goals. We will also discuss the content and activities in each dyad session so that you can be prepared.*
  - *During the dyad sessions, we will be in your home with you via videoconferencing. We will be asking you to hold sessions in areas such as your kitchen, laundry area, and your teen's bedroom to work on specific DLS. Practicing DLS at home has a lot of advantages for your teen compared to learning DLS at school or in a clinic. For example, by learning how to cook a recipe that your teen is motivated to eat in their own kitchen using their specific kitchen equipment such as pots and pans, it actually makes it easier for your teen to start practicing and mastering these skills.*
  - *Having sessions in the home can make some families nervous or self-conscious, but we want to emphasize that we are only focused on helping your teen to learn these skills in the environment that they will actually be doing them.*

- Ask: *Any questions about the logistics of the STRW sessions?*

Committing to the STRW Intervention (3 mins)

- *To get the most out of STRW, we ask that both teens and their parents/caregivers make specific commitments.*
- *For teens, we ask that they commit by:*
  - *Working on DLS with their caregiver in weekly dyad sessions*
  - *Practicing and mastering DLS at home and in the community*
  - *Making an active effort to complete weekly Real World Practice assignments, including the DLS contract*

- *For caregivers, we ask that they commit by:*
  - *Putting in the time and effort to work on DLS with the teen during weekly dyad sessions and throughout the week – both at home and in the community*

   - *We recognize how much time and energy caregivers put into this intervention, and we will work with you to figure out how to build your teen's DLS in your everyday life. For example, a teen can learn a lot of cooking and cleaning skills just by cooking dinner with you in the kitchen 1–2 days per week.*
- *Regularly attending sessions*
- *Participating in the discussion with other caregivers*
- *Assisting teen with completing weekly Real World Practice assignments, including the DLS contract*
- *Rewarding the teen when they meet the goals on their DLS contract*

♦ It may be helpful for therapists to discuss the following:
- Reminder emails will be sent before each session and will include information about any preparation that needs to be done by the caregiver and/or teen
- Information about the videoconferencing invites
- How to communicate any absences
- Information on rescheduling sessions
- Best way to contact the therapist with questions, comments, concerns, etc.

♦ Ask: *Are there any questions about these commitments?*

Review Dyad Session 1 Content (20–22 mins)

♦ ***During each caregiver group session, we will also review the material that will be covered in the upcoming dyad session with your teen. This will allow you to have some time to prepare for the upcoming session. Please feel free to ask any questions as we go over the content of the dyad session.***

♦ The therapist should refer to the PowerPoint presentation slides for Dyad Session 1 while reviewing the content for the session.

♦ The therapist should have also prepared for the session by reviewing the Dyad Session 1 content discussed in the manual, which has detailed information about the content that will be covered. If the therapist reviews all of the slides for Dyad Session 1, the caregiver will be adequately prepared for the upcoming dyad session with their teen.

♦ The important points to make while reviewing the Dyad Session 1 slides and content are:
- The goals of STRW and the specific roles of the teen and their parent/caregiver will be discussed.
- Videoconferencing tips and session rules will be briefly reviewed.
- The teen will identify short-term and long-term goals to get an understanding of how they view their future and also to discuss how DLS are linked to at least some of their future goals. The caregiver will be asked to provide additional details or comments on the teen's goals.
- The teen will list DLS that are essential to learn, practice, and master as they get older.
- The therapist will discuss how developing essential life skills in adolescence will make the transition from high school to the adult world easier.

- The STRW intervention consists of 15-weekly sessions that focus on personal hygiene and self-care, cleaning, laundry, cooking, grocery shopping, and managing money.
- The therapist will review the logistics of STRW sessions and the commitments that need to be made by both the teen and their caregiver.
- The teen and their caregiver will play the Guess the Price game in which they compete against each other to identify the prices of hygiene products.
- A Real World Practice assignment will be assigned each week to help with building DLS at home. It will be important to complete the Real World Practice assignment before the next dyad session.
- The therapist will discuss any preparation that needs to happen before the next session and confirm the date/time of the next dyad session.

♦ Ask: ***Any questions about the content for the upcoming dyad session?***

Prep for the Next Caregiver Session (3 mins)

♦ ***We will have our next caregiver group session on DAY and TIME. At this session, we will discuss several of the strategies that we will be using to help your teen achieve their DLS goals.***

♦ ***After your dyad session with your teen, it will be important to prioritize working on the Real World Practice assignment so that we can celebrate successes and also discuss any challenges or questions that arose in the caregiver group session.***

♦ ***I will also email you a copy of the* STRW Resources *handout after today's session, which has resources including books, websites, videos, and apps that may be helpful as we target DLS during the STRW intervention.***
  - It may be helpful for the therapist to show families the STRW website (www.STRW.org) and direct them to the parent resources and blog articles.

♦ Ask: ***Are there any questions before we end the session?***

Wrap-Up

♦ Therapists should send a calendar invite with the next caregiver group session's day/time to the caregiver.

♦ Therapists should email the caregiver a copy of the STRW Resources handout (see "Therapist Resources") that contains resources and links related to the STRW curriculum. This handout is available on the STRW website (www.strw.org).

Essential Life Skills for Adolescents

HYGIENE/SELF-CARE

Taking a shower; Brushing teeth; Wearing deodorant; Dressing appropriately

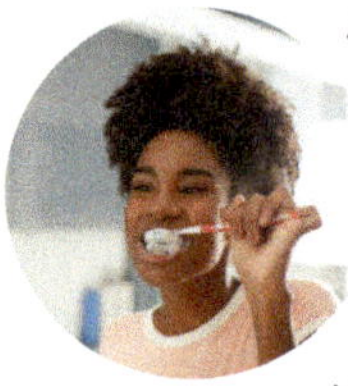

HEALTH CARE

Taking medications, Refilling medications, Making medical appointments

EXERCISE AND NUTRITION

Exercising regularly, Eating a balanced diet

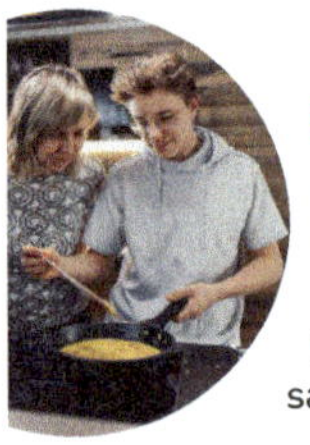

COOKING

Using appliances to cook snacks and meals, Meal planning, Kitchen safety,

AT HOME

Doing laundry, Cleaning one's bedroom, Cleaning a bathroom, Understanding household maintenance tasks

IN THE COMMUNITY

Buying items at a store using a list, Navigating from one place to another, Grocery shopping

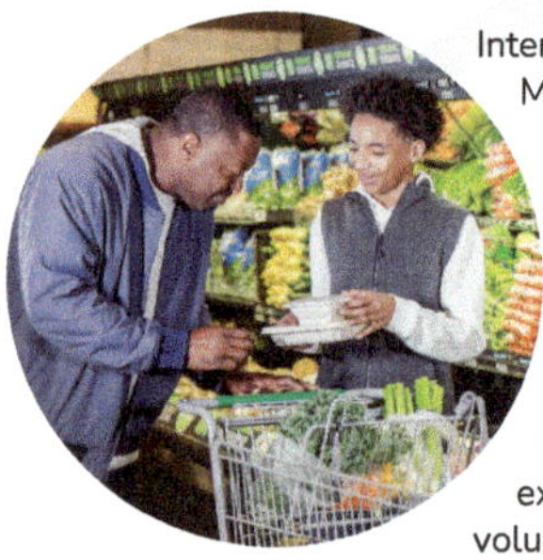

ACADEMIC

Organizing classroom materials, Planning and Prioritizing assignments, Studying effectively for tests

EMPLOYMENT

Applying for a part-time job, Interviewing for a job, Responding to feedback from a supervisor

EXECUTIVE FUNCTIONING

Using a calendar to manage appointments, Using a to-do list, Organizing personal belongings, Setting long-term goals, Time management

SOCIAL RELATIONSHIPS

Interacting with peers, Making and keeping friendships, Dating, Relationships with family

LEISURE

Participating in extracurricular activities, volunteering in the community, engaging in hobbies/ interests

TRANSPORTATION

Getting a driver's license, Using public transportation, Navigating from one place to another

MONEY MANAGEMENT

Budgeting for an event, Saving up money for large purchases, Spending responsibly

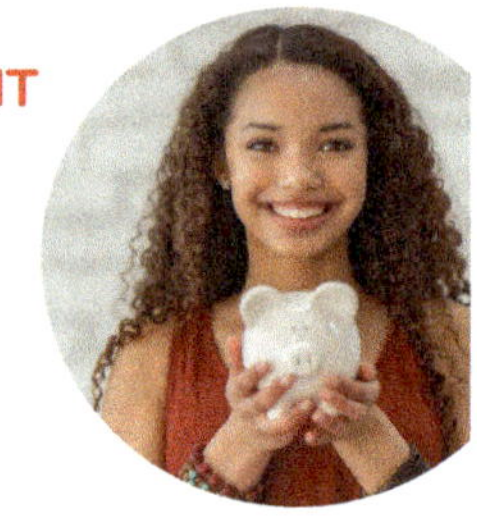

FUTURE PLANNING

Setting goals related to college, work, and/or independent living

SELF-ADVOCACY AND SELF-DETERMINATION

Identifying your strengths and challenges, Asking for help, Advocating for oneself

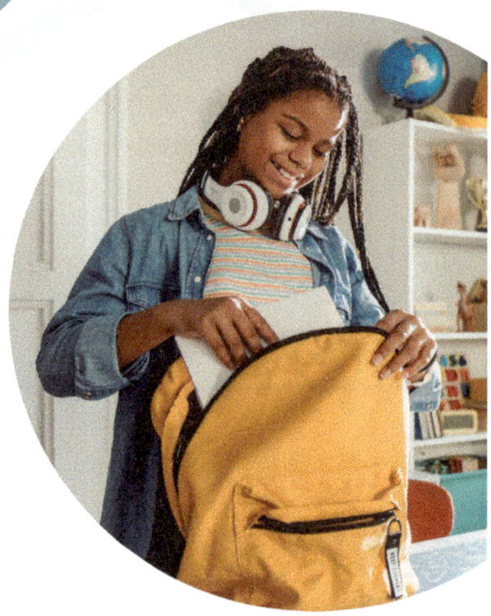

Content of the STRW Intervention Sessions

SESSION	CONTENT
Preparing for STRW	• Setting DLS goals to work on in STRW • Reviewing results of DLS assessment
Session 1	• Overview of STRW
Session 2	• Personal hygiene and self-care skills
Session 3	• Morning routine
Session 4	• Cleaning one's bedroom
Session 5	• Doing laundry
Session 6	• Cooking in the microwave • Kitchen safety
Session 7	• Cooking in the oven • Mixing and measuring ingredients
Session 8	• Cooking on the stove top • Cleaning the kitchen
Session 9	• Grocery shopping
Session 10	• Understanding the cost of items • Purchasing items
Session 11	• Using a checking and savings account
Session 12	• Budgeting for purchases
Session 13	• Budgeting for an event
Session 14	• Graduation • Evaluating whether DLS goals were met • Looking ahead and setting future DLS Goals

Daily Living Skills Contract

Date ____________________

Goal	Expectations	Reward	MONDAY	TUESDAY	WEDNESDAY	THURSDAY	FRIDAY	SATURDAY	SUNDAY

____________________ Teen

____________________ Parent / Caregiver

Caregiver/Teen Dyad Session 1 Content (60 mins)

STRW Session 1 Schedule (1–2 mins)

- The therapist should greet the caregiver and teen.
- *Let's get started! As a reminder, it will be helpful to sit together at a table so that we can all see each other and work together. Please pull out your STRW workbook that contains handouts for all of the STRW sessions. This session is called Session 1 – Introduction to the STRW Intervention. Please turn to that section in your workbook.*
- *Let's go over the session schedule so that you know what we will be doing. Please feel free to ask any questions about our schedule!*
- Briefly go over each item on the Session Schedule.

Overview of STRW (1–2 mins)

- *As a refresher, Surviving and Thriving in the Real World (or STRW for short) is an intervention that aims to help teens learn and master daily living skills (or DLS for short) that will allow them to survive and thrive in the real world – in areas such as college, work, and living on their own.*
- *Parents and caregivers will support and coach teens in acquiring new DLS during individual sessions and then practicing these newly learned skills at home and in the community.*
- *Teens will commit to learning and mastering DLS in collaboration with their parent/caregiver and therapist.*
- *We will discuss the details of the group in more detail later in the session, and I will be happy to answer any questions.*
- Ask: *Any questions?*

Videoconferencing Etiquette and Tips (1–2 mins)

- *Let's briefly review some etiquette and tips to make sure our sessions run smoothly!*
- Briefly review or read the following etiquette and tips from the bullets on the slide.
  - *It is helpful to check your audio and video before each session.*
  - *Set up an intentional space to meet that is free from distractions and noise.*
  - *Please keep your video turned on so that we can see each other and also see what skills are being worked on.*
  - *Please feel free to keep your mic on.*
  - *It may be helpful to wear headphones to ensure that the discussion remains private and confidential.*

- If needed, the therapist can take some time to briefly go over any specific features of the videoconferencing platform.
- Ask: *Any questions or comments on using videoconferencing during our sessions?*

STRW Session Rules (1–2 mins)

- *These group rules are meant to set the tone for our dyad sessions and foster collaboration as we work together on building DLS over the next 14 weeks.*
- Have teen read the STRW Session Rules from the slide:
  - Be respectful.
  - Pay attention to the material.
  - Listen to others.
  - Work together.
  - Stay on topic.
  - Do not use your phone or other device during the session.

- Ask: *Are there any other rules that may be important to add?*

Future Goals (4–5 mins)

- *The main goal of the STRW intervention is to help teenagers develop the life skills that are needed to reach their short-term goals now – such as getting ready for school in the morning and not being late for school – and their long-term goals in the future – such as getting a part-time job, going to college, and living on their own.*
- *There are a lot of DLS that need to be learned and mastered along the way as teens work towards their short-term and long-term goals. For example, if you have the long-term goal of getting a job and living with a roommate in an apartment, you will need to master DLS such as getting up on time, taking your medications, doing your laundry, cooking meals for yourself, and budgeting your money.*
- *Let's take a few minutes to think through some of your short-term and long-term goals.*
- Have the caregiver and teen identify two to three short-term and long-term goals for the future.
  - The teen should be leading the conversation. The therapist should encourage the teen to answer the questions before having their caregiver give their thoughts.
  - Common short-term goals for teens include getting good grades at school; getting a part-time job; getting a driver's license; and having more freedom at home, school, or in the community (e.g., staying home alone, going places with friends).
  - Common long-term goals for teens include going to college (i.e., 2-year, 4-year, or trade school), getting a part-time or full-time job, living independently or semi-independently (e.g., with a roommate, with a family member), being able to travel or navigate the community independently and with confidence, and building friendships and/or romantic relationships.

Essential Daily Living Skills for Meeting Future Goals (12 mins)

- Refer to the Essential Daily Living Skills for Meeting Future Goals handout.
- *Now that we have thought through some of your short-term and long-term life goals, let's list some DLS that are essential for teenagers to learn, practice, and master.*

- *As a reminder, DLS are life skills that are needed to take care of yourself and may include taking a shower, wearing deodorant, taking vitamins or medications, cleaning up your room, cooking in the microwave or on the stove, doing the laundry, purchasing items at a store, using a debit or credit card, and budgeting your money.*
- *These DLS become especially important as teens become adults and start thinking about going to college, getting a job, and/or moving out of their family's home and into their own apartment or home.*
- *It may be helpful to think about yourself, your short-term and long-term goals, and what DLS you might need to learn to accomplish these goals. For example, if you have the goal of getting a part-time job, you might need to learn skills such as filling out job applications and interviewing for jobs. Personal hygiene skills such as wearing deodorant and brushing teeth are also important when applying for a job.*
- *Let's identify DLS that fit into the categories of living independently, attending college, getting and working at a job, and navigating the community. You can also write these down on your handout.*
    - The caregiver and teen can write their responses down on the handout or the therapist can transcribe responses directly onto the slide or onto the fillable PDF of the handout.
    - The therapist should have the caregiver and teen come up with several essential DLS that fit in each of the categories. The therapist can assist as needed by reframing questions (e.g., "How would you make sure your apartment or house was clean if you were living on your own?") or asking the caregiver to help with filling out the first few responses. The caregiver and teen can also take turns coming up with responses for each of the categories.
    - Encourage the teen to participate as much as possible.

Essential Life Skills for All Teens (6–8 mins)

- Refer to the Essential Life Skills for All Teens handout.
- *Let's take a look at this handout. Similar to what we just discussed, these are some of the essential life skills, which include DLS, that are necessary in adulthood. If you have these skills, you will be more likely to have a smoother and easier transition from high school to college, work, or living on your own.*
- *Let's spend some time getting an understanding of what DLS you have been working on and what has been successful and what has been challenging as you learn new DLS.*
- Ask the caregiver/teen dyads the following questions and discuss their responses:
    - *What DLS have you been working on at home or in the community?*
    - *What has worked to help you learn and master new DLS?*
    - *What has been challenging about learning and mastering new DLS?*

STRW Session Content (8 mins)

- Refer to the Session Overview handout.
- *As all teens get older, it becomes important to start learning all of the DLS that will help them reach their life goals.*

- *The name of this intervention is Surviving and Thriving in the Real World because we want to help teens develop the essential DLS that will be important as they transition from high school to the adult world.*
- *With the help of your caregiver and everyone else on their support team, you will work on building these DLS in the dyad sessions and then practicing them in the real world. While we know that it may take some practice and hard work (on the part of both you and your caregiver) to learn these DLS, you will earn rewards for learning these skills at home and will likely feel excited about and motivated by the progress you are making each week.*
- *Over the next 14 weeks, STRW sessions will target the development of DLS in the areas of personal hygiene and self-care, cleaning one's room, doing laundry from start to finish, cooking, grocery shopping, and money management.*
- *While you may have already developed some of these DLS, we will also teach these skills using strategies that can be applied to learn a wide range of other skills such as setting and reaching goals, managing time, prioritizing tasks, meal planning, cooking for others, paying bills, and keeping a household clean. Also, it can be helpful to gain additional practice with a DLS even if you feel that you already know how to do it. We can also help you fine-tune or further develop some of the DLS you have already learned.*
- *Your caregiver will play a large and extremely important role as they coach you on developing these DLS, which is also very hard work. In order to learn DLS, it will be important for both of you to be committed to putting in the time and energy needed.*
- Ask: *Any questions about what we will be covering in the upcoming STRW sessions?*

Logistics of STRW Sessions (3–4 mins)

- *Let's briefly go over some of the logistics of the caregiver/teen dyad sessions.*
  - *During the dyad sessions, we will be in your home and will be asking you to hold sessions in areas such as your kitchen, laundry area, and bedroom to work on specific DLS. This can make some teens or caregivers nervous or self-conscious, but we want to emphasize that we are only focused on helping you to learn these skills in the place that you will actually be doing them. Learning these skills in your home has a lot of advantages compared to learning DLS at school or in a clinic. For example, by learning how to cook a recipe that you are excited to eat in your own kitchen using your own pots and pans, it actually makes it easier for you to start practicing and mastering these skills outside of STRW sessions.*
  - *In each session, we will do the following:*
    - *Review the activities that we will be doing at the start of each session*
    - *Discuss any DLS that you worked on over the last week*
    - *Learn and practice a new DLS*
    - *Update your DLS contract with new goals, expectations, and rewards*
    - *Plan for the next session if needed*
  - *It is important that you come prepared to each dyad session by practicing any DLS and completing any Real World Practice assignments.*

- Ask: *Any questions about the logistics of the STRW sessions?*

Committing to the STRW Intervention (3 mins)

- *To get the most out of STRW, we ask that both teens and their parents/caregivers make specific commitments.*
- Have the teen read the following commitments aloud from the bullet points on the slide:
  - Working on DLS with my caregiver in weekly dyad sessions
  - Practicing and mastering DLS at home and in the community
  - Making an active effort to complete weekly Real World Practice assignments

- Ask: *Any questions about these teen commitments?*
- Have the parent/caregiver read the following commitments aloud from the bullet points on the slide:
  - Putting in the time and effort to work on DLS with the teen during dyad sessions and throughout the week – both at home and in the community
  - Regularly attending sessions
  - Participating in the discussion with other caregivers
  - Assisting the teen with completing weekly Real World Practice assignments
  - Rewarding the teen when they meet the goals on their DLS contract

- Ask: *Are there any questions about these parent/caregiver commitments?*

Guess the Price (6–7 mins) – OPTIONAL

- *We will often end each session by playing a Guess the Price game, which is just meant to be a fun way to build up your understanding of how much things cost.*
- *Money concepts such as knowing what things cost and purchasing items at the store can sometimes be overwhelming for teens, which is why we are going to focus on building these skills gradually in each session. We will then spend the last four STRW sessions going over money concepts like spending, saving, and budgeting in detail. Let's see if you know the prices of some common personal hygiene items even if they are not necessarily items that you use!*
- The therapist can have just the teen guess the price or have the caregiver and teen compete against each other.
- The therapist should click through the next four slides that contain examples of common personal hygiene items. Prior to the session, the therapist will need to look up the prices to ensure that they are accurate.
  - Therapists can change the personal hygiene items for the Guess the Price game.
  - This activity is meant to be fun and engaging! If the teen is averse to playing the game, it can be skipped. However, it would be helpful for the caregiver and teen to find other ways to build up an understanding of what things cost (e.g., compare the cost of products at the grocery store, involve the teen when purchasing personal hygiene items).

Real World Practice (3 mins)

- Refer to the Real World Practice handout and the What Motivates You? handout.
- *Each week you will have a Real World Practice assignment to help with building your DLS at home. Let's go over your first Real World Practice assignment.*

- The therapist should review the instructions for the Real World Practice assignment:
  - Refer to the What Motivates You? handout.
  - *You will have the opportunity to earn rewards when you work on learning and mastering DLS. Using this handout, identify rewards that you are interested in earning and feel free to add in any rewards that are not on the handout. It may be helpful to do this with your caregiver.*
  - *Each Real World Practice will always include a task related to understanding how to use and manage money. We will work on practicing skills like understanding what things cost and purchasing items at the store before we discuss money management concepts in later STRW sessions. For this week's assignment, while you are at the store with your caregiver, locate some of the items you may use in your morning routine such as toothpaste, deodorant, or shampoo to get an idea of how much things cost. There is flexibility for this money assignment each week and our goal is to make sure you are getting practice with understanding what things cost and spending money. For example, for this week's assignment, you could also look up the prices of personal hygiene products you buy online or help your caregiver with grocery shopping this week.*

- Ask: *Any questions about your Real World Practice assignment?*

Preparing for the Next Dyad Session (2 mins)

- *We will have our next caregiver/teen dyad session on DAY and TIME. At this session, we will discuss personal hygiene and self-care in detail and go over some strategies to help make sure you complete the necessary personal hygiene activities each day.*
- *It will be important to complete your Real World Practice assignment before our next dyad session and come prepared to discuss it.*
- Ask: *Are there any questions before we end the session?*

Wrap-Up

- Therapists should send a calendar invite with the next caregiver/teen dyad session's day/time to the caregiver and teen.
- Therapists should email any documents that were completed during the session to the caregiver and teen.

Essential Daily Living Skills for Meeting Future Goals

Living Independently	Attending College	Getting and Working at a Job	Navigating the Community	Other

Essential Life Skills for Adolescents

HYGIENE/SELF-CARE

Taking a shower; Brushing teeth; Wearing deodorant; Dressing appropriately

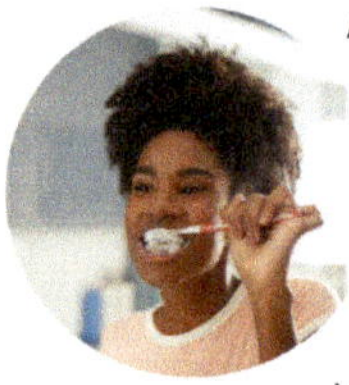

HEALTH CARE

Taking medications, Refilling medications, Making medical appointments

EXERCISE AND NUTRITION

Exercising regularly, Eating a balanced diet

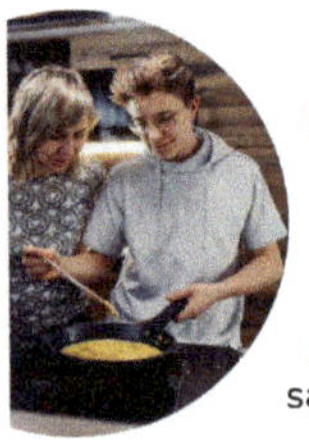

COOKING

Using appliances to cook snacks and meals, Meal planning, Kitchen safety,

AT HOME

Doing laundry, Cleaning one's bedroom, Cleaning a bathroom, Understanding household maintenance tasks

IN THE COMMUNITY

Buying items at a store using a list, Navigating from one place to another, Grocery shopping

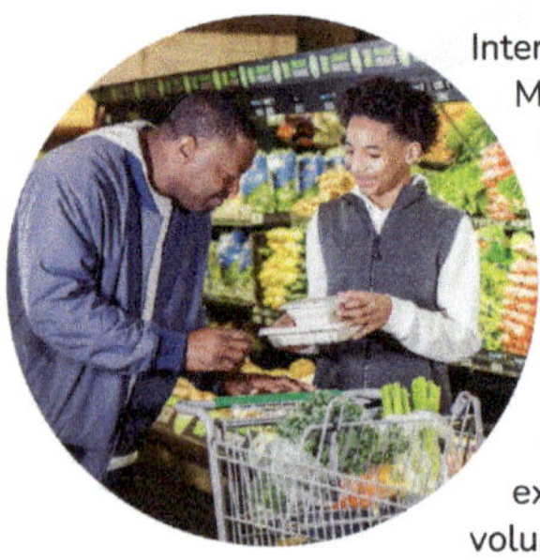

ACADEMIC

Organizing classroom materials, Planning and Prioritizing assignments, Studying effectively for tests

EMPLOYMENT

Applying for a part-time job, Interviewing for a job, Responding to feedback from a supervisor

EXECUTIVE FUNCTIONING

Using a calendar to manage appointments, Using a to-do list, Organizing personal belongings, Setting long-term goals, Time management

SOCIAL RELATIONSHIPS

Interacting with peers, Making and keeping friendships, Dating, Relationships with family

LEISURE

Participating in extracurricular activities, volunteering in the community, engaging in hobbies/interests

TRANSPORTATION

Getting a driver's license, Using public transportation, Navigating from one place to another

MONEY MANAGEMENT

Budgeting for an event, Saving up money for large purchases, Spending responsibly

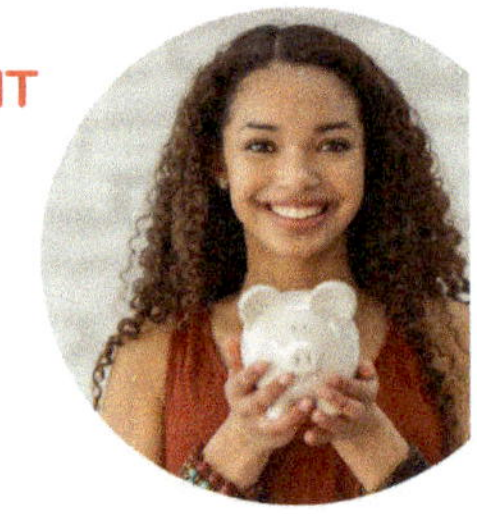

FUTURE PLANNING

Setting goals related to college, work, and/or independent living

SELF-ADVOCACY AND SELF-DETERMINATION

Identifying your strengths and challenges, Asking for help, Advocating for oneself

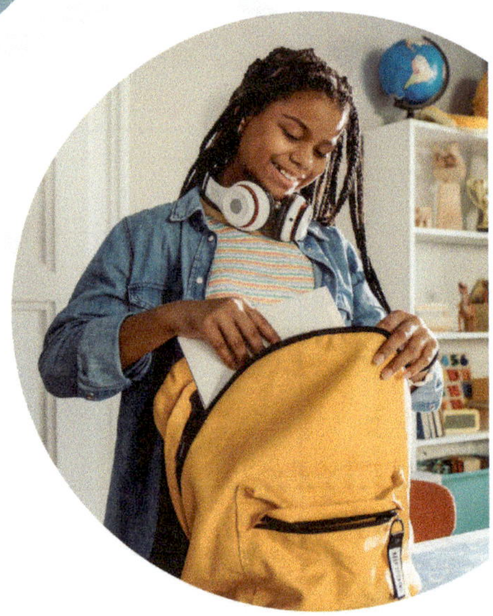

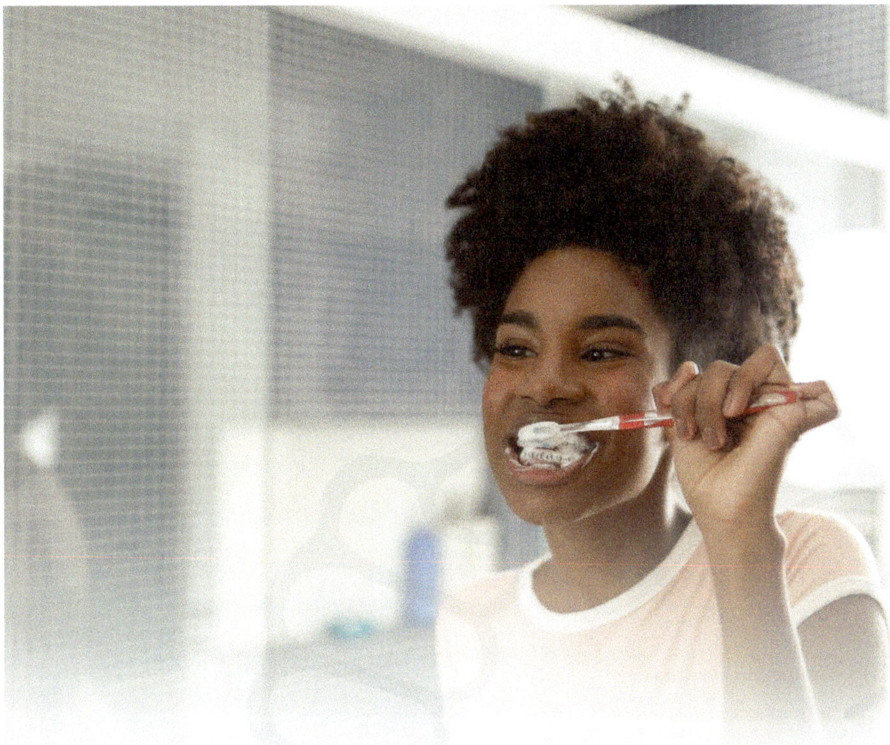

Guidelines for Good Personal Hygiene

- Take a shower at least every other day.
- Use shampoo and conditioner each time you take a shower.
- Wash your face every morning and night, using warm water and mild soap or facewash.
- Brush your hair before leaving the house.
- If you have body hair, it is a good idea to shave several times per week (face for men, legs and underarms for women).
- Put on deodorant every day before you leave the house. You may need to re-apply after you exercise or do any activity that makes you sweat.
- Brush your teeth twice a day (in the morning and at night).
- If something gets stuck in your teeth, excuse yourself and go to the bathroom. Use floss, not your fingers, to get it out.
- It's a good idea to look in the mirror after you eat to make sure you don't have food on your face or in your teeth.
- Keep your fingernails and toenails clean, and trim them every 1-2 weeks.
- Change your clothes every day.
- Check to make sure that your clothing is not stained and is not on backwards or inside out before leaving the house.
- Always wash your hands after you use the restroom and before eating.
- If you have to cough or sneeze, cough or sneeze into your elbow and say, "excuse me."'
- Blow your nose discreetly and try not to be loud.

NOTE: These guidelines may need to be modified based on personal preferences or individual characteristics.

Content of the STRW Intervention Sessions

SESSION	CONTENT
Preparing for STRW	• Setting DLS goals to work on in STRW • Reviewing results of DLS assessment
Session 1	• Overview of STRW
Session 2	• Personal hygiene and self-care skills
Session 3	• Morning routine
Session 4	• Cleaning one's bedroom
Session 5	• Doing laundry
Session 6	• Cooking in the microwave • Kitchen safety
Session 7	• Cooking in the oven • Mixing and measuring ingredients
Session 8	• Cooking on the stove top • Cleaning the kitchen
Session 9	• Grocery shopping
Session 10	• Understanding the cost of items • Purchasing items
Session 11	• Using a checking and savings account
Session 12	• Budgeting for purchases
Session 13	• Budgeting for an event
Session 14	• Graduation • Evaluating whether DLS goals were met • Looking ahead and setting future DLS Goals

Surviving and Thriving in the Real World (STRW) Session 1 – Real World Practice

- Using the What Motivates You? handout, identify the rewards that would be motivating to you as you work on building your daily living skills. Try to identify at least eight to ten rewards.
- While at the store, check out the prices of some common products that you may buy for your morning routine. Examples of products include shampoo, conditioner, body wash, deodorant, and toothpaste. It is a good idea to start learning the prices of products so that you can become a savvy shopper!

What Motivates You?

Directions: With your parent/caregiver, circle the items that are rewarding for you and may motivate you to work on your daily living skills goals. If there are things that motivate you that are not listed here, write them in the blank boxes. Please be detailed and specific about the things that motivate you!

Video and computer games	Watching YouTube videos
Dessert or favorite snacks	Watching/renting/streaming a movie
Money	Extra screen time
Time or an activity with a family member or sibling	Sleeping in on the weekends
Going out to eat at a restaurant	Having a family member cook your favorite meal
Buying a new book	Going to a favorite store
Saving up for large purchase	Buy a clothing item of choice
Music	Buying something for hobby (e.g., Legos)
Spending time with a friend	Going to a special event
Outdoor activities (e.g., basketball)	Going to the library

Surviving & Thriving in the Real World

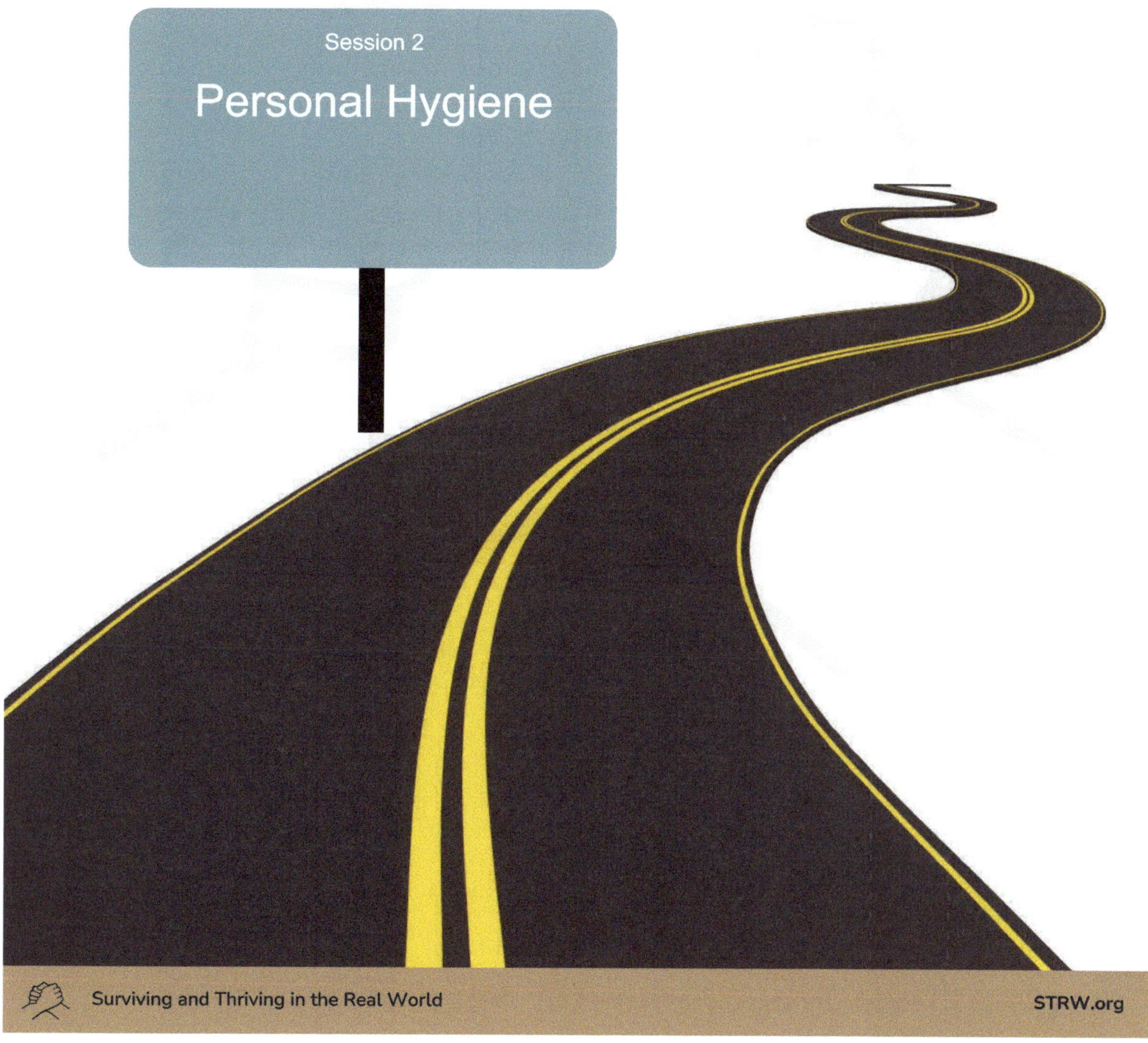

Session 2

Personal Hygiene

Aims

- Continue to build rapport between caregiver group members and the therapist
- Continue to build rapport between the teen, caregiver, and therapist
- Understand the importance of personal hygiene
- Identify personal hygiene and self-care tasks that need to be completed regularly
- Increase ability to use a task analysis to break down specific DLS into smaller steps
- Develop an understanding of the four elements for developing an effective system to achieve DLS goals

Structure

- Caregiver group session via telehealth
- Caregiver/teen dyad session via telehealth

Session Supplies

- Caregiver Group Handouts
  - Elements of an Effective System for Achieving DLS Goals
- Caregiver/Teen Dyad Handouts
  - Guidelines for Good Personal Hygiene
  - Personal Hygiene and Self-Care Tasks
  - Elements of an Effective System for Achieving DLS Goals
  - Task Analysis Steps (2 copies)
  - Session 2 – Real World Practice
  - Task Analysis Worksheet

Caregiver/Teen Preparation for Session

- None

DOI: 10.4324/9781003458838-5

Therapist Preparation for Session

- The therapist may want to review the Possible Solutions to Common Challenges that Arise for STRW Therapists handout (see appendix), which includes ideas for how STRW therapists can address common challenges that arise when facilitating the caregiver group and dyad sessions, including commitment; engagement; inattention; too much prompting; and family factors such as time, use of rewards, and caregiver/teen relationship.
- The therapist may want to review the Motivating Rewards Identified by Teens in the STRW Intervention handout (see appendix), which includes a list of rewards that were identified by teens in categories including food, money, spending time with family, spending time with friends, screen time, shopping, outings, and privileges.

Session 2 Notes

- The therapist can choose to skip the sections on Video Conferencing Etiquette and Tips and Group Rules. However, these should be reviewed as needed for the caregivers or teens.
- The Personal Hygiene and Self-Care Tasks and Task Analysis handouts can also be completed by the therapist during the session to facilitate discussion with the caregiver and teen. A fillable PDF of each of these handouts are available on the STRW website and can be emailed to the family after the session.

- Caregiver Group Session
  - The caregiver group session is highly didactic, so it will be important for therapists to check in with caregivers as they discuss critical concepts to ensure they are paying attention to and understanding the content.
  - The therapist will need to be particularly mindful of how much time they spend on each section of the session to ensure that they are able to cover all of the content, which sets a critical foundation for targeting DLS. The therapist can always make a note to come back to discuss a particular topic in more detail at a future caregiver group session or can send out additional resources on a particular topic of interest.

- Dyad Session
  - If a teen has mastered their morning routine such that they are consistently and independently completing all of the steps, the therapist can work with the dyad to identify another routine (e.g., nighttime routine, after-school routine) to target.

Caregiver Group Session 2 Content (90 mins)

Videoconferencing Etiquette and Tips (1–2 mins) – OPTIONAL

- The therapist should greet the caregivers and welcome them to the session.
- *You may be familiar with videoconferencing, but let's just go over some etiquette and tips to make sure our sessions run smoothly!*
- Read the following etiquette and tips from the bullets on the slide and demonstrate features as needed.
    - *Please keep your video turned on so that we can see your face. This increases engagement with the group and allows us to all feel more connected to one another.*
    - *For these group sessions, keep your mic muted unless you are speaking. This eliminates any background noise and allows everyone to hear whoever is speaking.*
    - *It is difficult to hear when more than one person speaks at the same time. Some helpful tips include:*
        - *If you have a question or comment, you can use the Chat feature or Raise Hand feature.*
        - *You can also raise your actual hand to indicate that you would like to unmute your mic and speak.*
        - *You can use reactions to engage with others such as a thumbs up to indicate agreement or clapping hands to celebrate a success.*

Videoconferencing Etiquette and Tips (1–2 mins) – OPTIONAL

- *Some other tips are:*
    - *It is helpful to check your audio and video before each session to make sure that they are working.*
    - *Set up an intentional space to meet that is free from distractions and noise.*
    - *It may be helpful to wear headphones to ensure that the discussion remains private and confidential.*
    - *Come prepared to the session by bringing your STRW workbook and any other materials you may need such as a pen or pencil.*

- Ask: *Any questions or comments on using videoconferencing during our sessions?*

Group Rules (1–2 mins) – OPTIONAL

- *These group rules are meant to set the tone for our group sessions and foster a collaborative, engaging, and supportive group as we work together on building daily living skills (or DLS for short).*

- Review the following group rules:
  - Be respectful.
    - This rule also includes keeping information that is discussed in each session private. While we cannot enforce this rule, other group members are more likely to openly share if there is a shared understanding that this is a safe and private space to discuss things.
  - Listen to others.
  - Be attentive. This includes when others are talking and when information is being presented.
  - Do not use your phone or other device during the session.
  - Stay on topic.
  - We will try to reserve the final 5–10 minutes of each session for "off-topic" questions.

Review – Real World Practice Assignment (10 mins)

- The therapist should greet the caregivers and welcome them to the session if they have not yet done this.
- ***During our sessions, we will briefly review Real World Practice assignments, and this is an opportunity to discuss issues that may be important to review outside of dyad sessions with your teen and hear from other caregivers. For example, it may be helpful for other caregivers to hear what other teens identified as rewards so that they can get additional ideas for how to reward their teen for working towards and achieving DLS goals.***
- Discuss the Real World Practice assignment by briefly going through each assignment. Have a few caregivers discuss how their teen did with the assignment. It may also be helpful to discuss challenges with completing the assignment that can also be problem-solved in the caregiver/teen dyad session.
- Therapists may want to encourage caregivers to use the chat feature of the video conferencing platform when going over the Real World Practice assignments (e.g., listing out the rewards that their teen identified as motivating, suggesting an idea to build money skills while shopping at the grocery store).
- Points of discussion may include the following:
  - Rewards
    - ***It is important to identify a range of rewards that motivate teens. Ideally, you want to have eight to ten rewards identified that can be classified as low – such as extra screen time or staying up later on the weekend, medium – such as renting a video game or choosing a restaurant to eat at, and high – such as a King's Island season pass or money towards a new laptop.***
    - ***Rewards can be monetary based, but can also be activity based – such as going to a store, going to a restaurant, practicing driving with a parent, or a ticket for an event or concert. Rewards can also be privilege based – such as earning more screen time or staying up later on the weekend.***
    - ***Caregivers sometimes have to rework the system for earning rewards and privileges. For example, if a teen is very motivated by playing video games and previously was allowed to play video games during free time on the***

    weekends, the caregiver may rework the system such that the teen needs to earn some or all of their video game time by doing chores such as cleaning their room, doing laundry, and helping with dinner.
    - *Some teens may also be interested in earning points, tokens, or tickets that can be used to trade in for a reward. This can be a precursor to earning money that can then be deposited into a checking or savings account.*
  - Money Assignment – *STRW was developed with input from many caregivers, and they consistently stated that it was critical to expose teens to money and financial concepts before we address it in STRW. These small assignments are meant to increase awareness of what things cost and how to pay for things, which will allow teens to feel more comfortable with spending, saving, and budgeting.*

- Ask: *Any questions about the Real World Practice assignment?*

STRW Session 2 Goals (1 min)

- *The goal of today's session is to go over why we are targeting building DLS in adolescents, what factors we need to consider when setting and working towards DLS goals, and how to build an effective system to help you and your teen achieve their DLS goals now and in the future.*
- *We will be discussing a lot of content in this session that may be helpful in the future, so it may be beneficial to take notes.*

Demands in Adolescence (10 mins)

- *It is important to be aware that the teenage years are very difficult for just about every teen due to factors such as puberty; trying to figure out and establish their identity; increased demands at home, school, and with peers; and anxiety about the future. While we were all teens once too, it is sometimes easy to forget about all of the demands that teens may be experiencing! Some common challenges that teens face include:*
  - *Identity development – figuring out who they are, how to become independent, and how to advocate for themselves*
  - *Demands of high school – managing classes and homework, teacher expectations, extracurricular activities, and social stressors*
  - *Family relationships – getting along with caregivers and siblings*
  - *Demands at home – pressure or expectations from caregivers and juggling home responsibilities*
  - *Puberty and sexuality – going through puberty, understanding their sexual identity, wanting to date, and dating*
  - *Navigating the social world – initiating and maintaining friendships, working with peers on small group projects at school, asking for help, and building social and emotional insight*
  - *DLS – building and mastering the necessary DLS to meet expectations at home and to also be successful in the future*

- *Planning for the future – figuring out what they want to do after high school, finding and getting a part-time job, and applying for and preparing for college*
- *Executive functioning – organizing their materials, managing their time, prioritizing tasks, initiating tasks, and sustaining and completing tasks*
- *Mental health – managing symptoms of anxiety and depression and using effective coping strategies*

♦ *Teens may feel like they are juggling all of these areas at once and may struggle to understand how to manage and prioritize the competing demands.*
♦ Ask and Discuss: *What has been particularly difficult about the teen years thus far?*

Link Between DLS and Adult Outcomes (5 mins)

♦ *Both neurotypical teens and neurodivergent teens with diagnoses such as autism and ADHD are more likely to have better adult outcomes in areas such as living on their own, getting and maintaining a part-time or full-time job, attending and graduating from college, having a group of friends, and reporting a higher quality of life if they have age-appropriate DLS. This makes practical sense. If you are able to wake yourself up in the morning, cook your own meals, clean your home, and stick to a budget, you are more likely to get to work or class on time, live on your own, and feel better about yourself. So, if you have better-developed DLS, you really are more likely to survive and thrive in the real world as an adult.*
♦ *This link between age-appropriate DLS and better adult outcomes is important because we can absolutely teach the necessary DLS to teens. DLS are often easier to learn than some of other challenges that teens may have. However, it does take time, effort, and commitment from both the caregiver and the teen to learn DLS such as doing laundry, cooking, and budgeting for expenses.*
♦ Ask and Discuss: *Does anyone have any thoughts or questions about the link between DLS and adult outcomes?*

Targeting DLS Goals in STRW (4–5 mins)

♦ *Our goal in STRW is not only to develop age-appropriate DLS in your teens but also to develop a system that teens can utilize now and throughout their life to learn and master DLS.*
♦ *There has been a ton of work done on understanding how to effectively develop and meet one's goals. Here is a quote from James Clear, who wrote the bestselling book* Atomic Habits *on how to reach your goals using evidence-based and proven strategies.*
  - *"Goals are good for setting a direction, but systems are best for making progress. You fall to the level of your systems." In essence, this quote is saying that goals give us a direction, but we need effective systems to really make progress in achieving our goals and making our progress last.*

♦ *In the Preparing for STRW session, we set goals with your teen that align with the specific DLS that we will be targeting in STRW sessions. However, a major focus in STRW sessions will be building the systems that will help your teen reach their specific DLS goals.*

- *Let's go through an example to illustrate this point about building a system. If your teen set a goal to do their own laundry from start to finish, then if they meet their goal, they will have clean laundry for just that one day. However, what your teen actually needs is a system to do laundry consistently, completely, and independently – which may include how to remember to do all of the steps of laundry, how to remember to get started on doing laundry, how to remember to switch clothing from the washer to the dryer, and how to put clothes away in an organized way. We want them to have clean laundry for the rest of their life!*
- *In STRW sessions, we will work on creating an effective system that takes into account your teen, your role as a caregiver, your household and environment, and also the strategies and tools that we know lead to achieving DLS goals.*
- Ask and Discuss: *Any questions or comments?*

Targeting DLS Goals in STRW: Some Initial Points (3–4 mins)

- *As we get ready to start targeting your teen's DLS, here are some initial points to keep in mind:*
  - *Some DLS are very simple. For example, putting dirty clothes in a hamper, bringing the hamper to the washing machine, and putting the dirty clothes into the washing machine are all very simple on their own. However, the part that is challenging for many teens is putting many "simple" DLS together to form the more complex skills – such as doing laundry from start to finish.*
  - *While many of the DLS we are going to teach are somewhat complex, such as cleaning the bedroom and going grocery shopping, we are going to teach them using strategies that we know work for adolescents. Once a strategy works for a teen, it can be used again and again to learn other DLS in the future.*
  - *DLS do need to be taught in various environments, including at home, at school, and throughout the community. Most of the skills we are teaching in STRW will need to be practiced at home, such as cooking and cleaning, but some will need to be practiced outside of the home such as grocery shopping. For example, a teen may learn how to make a grilled cheese on their stove at home and will eventually need to be able to also apply this skill to other environments such as cooking a grilled cheese at a family member's house or cooking a grilled cheese in their apartment or dorm room.*

- Ask and Discuss: *Any questions or comments about these points?*

Targeting DLS Goals in STRW: Role of the Teen (4–5 mins)

- *Over the next several weeks, we will strive to teach age-appropriate DLS to your teen so that their skills are more similar to same-aged peers. For example, if your teen is 16 years old, we want them to be able to do the DLS that most 16-year-olds are expected to do, which will then make the goals that they have in adulthood easier to achieve.*

- *Knowing your teen is a key component that will allow you to be more successful at helping them to build their DLS. Specifically, it is important to:*
    - *Understand how your teen's specific strengths and difficulties may affect their ability to learn and apply DLS. For example, if your teen has executive functioning challenges such as planning and prioritizing, keeping track of all of the steps in their morning routine may be extremely difficult.*
    - *Understand what may motivate your teen to learn DLS. For example, if your teen enjoys baking cookies and brownies, they may be more motivated and interested in learning how to cook. DLS are NOT always intrinsically fun or rewarding (at first!), so they will likely need to be rewarded in some way.*
    - *Understand your teen's preferred learning style and what strategies help them learn best. For example, some teens really like to use their phone to set alarms or reminders, while for other teens, this use of technology is overwhelming, and they may prefer to use an alarm clock to wake up or a whiteboard to remember the steps of a task.*
    - *Understand how to increase your teen's buy-in and motivation to work on these DLS to make it more likely that they will be successful. This is linked to motivation, but it could also be talking through how skills such as laundry and cooking are critical to living on their own one day.*

- Ask and Discuss: *What do you think is an important thing to consider as you begin to work on DLS with your teen?*

Targeting DLS Goal in STRW: Impact of the Parent/Caregiver (6–7 mins)

- *We have considered your teen's strengths and challenges, but it is also important to think about how you and other caregivers and/or siblings in your household may impact your teen's ability to learn and master DLS. In the same way we want to make this doable for your teen, we want to make this doable for you and your family. Here are a few things to think about for yourself as we get ready to work on DLS with your teen:*
    - *Time – how much time do you have daily and/or weekly to dedicate to helping your teen? We want to be realistic in determining how much time you may have to dedicate to working on building these skills. We also want to think through how you can bring your teen in to learn skills during tasks you already have to do. For example, you could have your teen observe you as you start a load of laundry, have them help with prepping dinner, or have them pay bills with you.*
    - *Energy – how much energy do you have to devote to working on DLS with your teen? Would it be better to tackle skills on the weekend or weekdays? Would it be better to carve out a specific time every week to devote to this? Taking the time to think through your energy level increases your likelihood of successfully supporting your teen.*
    - *Stress – it is essential to think through how teaching new skills to your teen may increase your stress level. We can talk about this openly in this group, too, to help with navigating this and hearing how other caregivers are addressing*

this. I also want to point out that many caregivers who have completed the STRW intervention talk about how their stress level actually decreased once their teen started doing more on their own. If we can give the teens more responsibility and increase their independence, it often lightens the load of caregivers. For example, one parent talked about how much easier her morning was once her teen started packing his lunch and doing his morning routine independently.

- *Motivation – what is your overall motivation to help your teen build these skills? Are there others who could help with teaching skills to your teen? While we will have a group of caregivers through these STRW group sessions that will help with keeping motivation up and holding caregivers accountable as they work on helping their teens achieve their DLS goals, it can also be helpful to surround yourself with others who are actively supporting you and acting as an accountability partner.*
- *Commitment – are you committed to working on building these DLS in your teen? This includes being present in the caregiver and dyad sessions, setting aside time to work on DLS with teens, and problem-solving when things are not working or going according to plan. Your commitment is a critical ingredient to supporting your teen with building DLS.*

- Ask and Discuss: *What comments or questions do you have about the role you play in building your teen's DLS?*
- *At the beginning of each caregiver group session for STRW, we will review how the Real World Practice assignments are going, and this is a great opportunity to of course talk about the successes but also to discuss any challenges. We have a great group of caregivers who have a lot of experience raising teens, and we can openly listen to challenges and help with brainstorming possible solutions.*
- Ask and Discuss: *Any questions or comments?*

Targeting DLS Goals in STRW: Parenting Styles (6 mins)

- *Another aspect that may affect your teen's ability to achieve DLS goals is your parenting style, which may have changed over time depending on your child's age, their needs, and their goals. While your parenting style has likely influenced many of your child's successes, it often needs to be adjusted for teens so that they can become increasingly independent. We are going to discuss a parenting style that may be particularly helpful as we begin teaching your teen DLS.*
- *Let's briefly talk through three parenting styles and we may come back to these throughout STRW as we work on DLS goals.*
  - *Adaptive protection – this occurs when a child presents with challenges and a caregiver "consciously titrates" the child's exposure to challenging environmental events to create successful experiences. In other words, this is a caregiving response that encourages independent behaviors but provides appropriate protection while taking the child's unique strengths and difficulties into account. This is where you want to aim to be most of the time when you are parenting.*

        - *For example, a caregiver who is using adaptive protection will assist their teen with developing their skills of cooking in the oven by using strategies such as letting them observe how to cook in the oven, providing oven mitts to decrease any anxiety about burning oneself, and rehearsing and going over the steps of cooking in the oven. The caregiver provides support but also appropriately "pushes" their child to learn a new skill.*
    - *Excessive protection – this occurs when a caregiver may limit a child's exposure to anxiety-provoking situations through avoidant behavior, even when the child possesses the necessary skills for success. Caregivers who allow their child to avoid specific situations or do not expose them to new situations can limit the opportunities to develop and master new skills. In recent years, terms such as helicopter parenting or lawnmower parenting have been used to describe a parenting style in which caregivers may do things for the child to increase their likelihood of a successful experience.*
        - *For example, a caregiver who is using excessive protection may not allow their child to cook their own snack or meal on the stove because they are worried that they may hurt themselves on the burner.*
    - *Passive protection – this occurs when a caregiver does not encourage a child to acquire and master new skills because of the amount of time or effort required, resistance from the child, or decreased motivation from the child. Caregivers who engage in passive protection may complete activities for their child because it is easier than attempting to teach the child a new skill.*
        - *For example, a caregiver who is engaging in passive protection may do their child's laundry and put it away because it is "easier" and "less time consuming" than teaching the child or having to provide prompting to complete the steps of these tasks.*

- *We likely all have used these different parenting styles, but when teaching DLS, the adaptive protection style will increase the likelihood of learning, mastering, and continuing to use age-appropriate DLS. The goal is to increase your teen's independence and decrease their dependence on you.*
- Ask and Discuss:
    - *Any questions or comments about these parenting styles?*
    - *What style do you predominantly use?*
    - *Are there situations where you may use passive or excessive protection?*

Targeting DLS Goals in STRW: Evidence-Based Strategies (1–2 mins)

- *Throughout STRW, we will introduce various evidence-based teaching strategies that have been shown to lead to teens acquiring age-appropriate DLS. These strategies will be used to develop an effective system to target DLS goals. During the upcoming dyad session with your teen, we will talk about using a Task Analysis to begin to work on increasing independence with your teen's morning routine.*
- Ask: *Any questions about the use of evidence-based strategies?*

Targeting DLS Goals in STRW: The Four Laws of Behavior Change (5 mins)

- *To sum up what we have discussed so far today, we went over the importance of targeting DLS in adolescence to be better prepared for the transition to adulthood. We also discussed how critical it is to understand (1) the strengths and challenges of your teen, (2) how you as a caregiver may impact your teen's ability to meet their DLS goals, and (3) that evidence-based strategies and tools will be used to teach and master DLS.*
- *The final element of developing an effective system to achieve DLS goals is to use the Four Laws of Behavior Change, which you can find more information about in the book* Atomic Habits *by James Clear. These are laws that will make it more likely that you will achieve your goals. You do not need to include all four laws to be successful, but you are even more likely to be successful if you include all of them. As we set DLS goals and build an effective system to meet our goals, we will consider the Four Laws of Behavior Change.*
  - *Obvious – the cues to get started on your goal should be as obvious as possible. You can usually do this by modifying your environment to make it more likely you will meet your goals. For example, you can put all of the items you need for your morning hygiene routine in the same place in the bathroom. You can also make the cue to get started more obvious by linking it to time or location. For example, after I get home from piano lessons every Wednesday, I will start my laundry.*
  - *Attractive – the goal should be appealing to increase the teen's motivation and follow-through. It can be tricky to make a DLS goal attractive – but we will discuss some ideas about how to do this in each session! For example, you can do one of your favorite things at the same time as a DLS goal, such as listening to music while folding and putting your laundry away.*
  - *Easy – make achieving the goal as simple as possible. This is a critical one because we want the teens to have success with meeting goals. Thus, we may break a complex DLS goal into simple, achievable goals to make it more likely that they will work on building this DLS.*
  - *Satisfying – it is critical to make achieving DLS goals satisfying and rewarding for teens because it increases the likelihood that they will continue to work on meeting their goals. This can be done with rewards or verbal praise but also by pointing out how it can feel good inside to be independent with DLS goals.*

- Ask: *Any questions about the Four Laws of Behavior Change?*
- *Let's go through a few examples of setting goals using the Four Laws of Behavior Change.*

Targeting DLS Goals in STRW: Example #1 of The Four Laws of Behavior Change (3–4 mins)

- *Here is an example of how we might utilize the Four Laws of Behavior Change to develop an effective system to meet the DLS goal of doing all of the steps of a teen's morning routine independently. You do not necessarily need to do all of these things, but even doing one of them makes it more likely you will meet your goal!*

- The therapist should have a few caregivers take turns reading through the following bullet points on the slide for Obvious, Attractive, Easy, and Satisfying.
  - Goal – Do all steps of the morning routine independently.
    - Obvious
      - Calendar reminder or alarm to get started on morning routine at 8 am
      - Post a task analysis of steps for morning routine in bedroom and/or in bathroom
    - Attractive
      - Listen to music for 10 mins while in the shower
      - Have favorite breakfast options available to make
    - Easy
      - Post a checklist with all steps so that expectations are clear
      - Start by targeting a few steps and gradually increasing expectations
      - Set up an easy system (e.g., basket with all morning routine hygiene items in the bathroom) on
    - Satisfying
      - Making progress and becoming independent is satisfying in itself
      - Provide verbal praise (e.g., "Great job getting ready for school today!")
      - Provide a reward (e.g., extra screen time until school starts, preferred snack in lunch box)

- Ask and Discuss: ***Any questions about how the Four Laws of Behavior Change were used to target the morning routine goal?***

Targeting DLS Goals in STRW: Example #2 of The Four Laws of Behavior Change (3–4 mins)

- ***Here is an example of how we might utilize the Four Laws of Behavior Change to develop an effective system to meet the DLS goal of making dinner one day per week.***
- The therapist should have a few caregivers take turns reading through the following bullet points on the slide for Obvious, Attractive, Easy, and Satisfying.
  - Goal – Make dinner one time per week.
    - Obvious
      - Calendar reminder the night before making dinner to set expectations and make a plan
      - Alarm at 5 pm to get started on making dinner
    - Attractive
      - Cook a recipe that teen loves to eat and/or enjoys making
    - Easy
      - Only do a few steps of the recipe until the teen can do all the steps
      - Choose a recipe with simple steps
      - Choose a recipe that a caregiver has provided instruction or modeling on
    - Satisfying
      - Making progress is satisfying in itself (e.g., ask teen how they feel after cooking dinner!)

- Eating a preferred recipe is naturally satisfying
- Provide verbal praise (e.g., "This dinner is delicious! Thanks so much for cooking tonight.")
- Provide a reward (e.g., dessert, do the dishes, extra screen time, stay up 30 mins late)

- Ask and Discuss: *Any questions about how the Four Laws of Behavior Change were used to target the cooking goal?*

Elements of an Effective System for Achieving DLS Goals (2–3 mins)

- Refer to the Elements of Effective System for Achieving DLS Goals handout.
- *As we work together to help teens achieve their DLS goals in STRW, we will consider the qualities of the teen and the caregiver; use evidence-based strategies to teach and master DLS; and use the Four Laws of Behavior Change to make sure that goals are obvious, attractive, easy, and satisfying. We will revisit this framework each session to make sure that we are considering all of the factors needed to increase the likelihood of achieving DLS goals by developing the best system!*
- Ask: *Any questions or comments?*

Review Dyad Session 2 Content (15–17 mins)

- *Let's review the material that will be covered in the upcoming dyad session with your teen. This will allow you to prepare for the upcoming session. Please feel free to ask any questions as we go over the content of the dyad session.*
- The therapist should refer to the PowerPoint presentation slides for Dyad Session 2 while reviewing the content for the session.
- The therapist should have also prepared for the session by reviewing the Dyad Session 2 content discussed in the manual, which has detailed information about the content that will be covered.
- The important points to make while reviewing the Dyad Session 2 Content are:
  - Good personal hygiene means keeping your body looking, smelling, and feeling clean and healthy.
  - Maintaining good hygiene affects our health, social acceptance, body image, and mental well-being.
  - It can be helpful to review the guidelines and unspoken rules about taking care of your body.
  - Making a list of personal hygiene activities clearly defines what tasks need to be completed and how often they need to be completed by the teen.
  - Task analysis is a strategy that breaks a complex task down into manageable steps. It can then be used as a checklist!
  - The elements of an effective system for achieving DLS goals will be discussed with the teens.

- Ask: *Any questions about the content for the upcoming dyad session?*

Prep for the Next Caregiver Session (1–2 mins)

- *We will have our next caregiver group session on DAY and TIME. At this session, we will discuss how to use a DLS contract to begin working on your teen's morning routine.*
- *After your dyad session with your teen, it will be important to prioritize working on the Real World Practice assignment so that we can celebrate successes and also discuss any challenges or questions that arose in the caregiver group session.*
- Ask: *Are there any questions before we end the session?*

Wrap-Up

- The therapist should send a calendar invite with the next caregiver group session's day/time to the caregiver.

Elements of an Effective System for Achieving DLS Goals

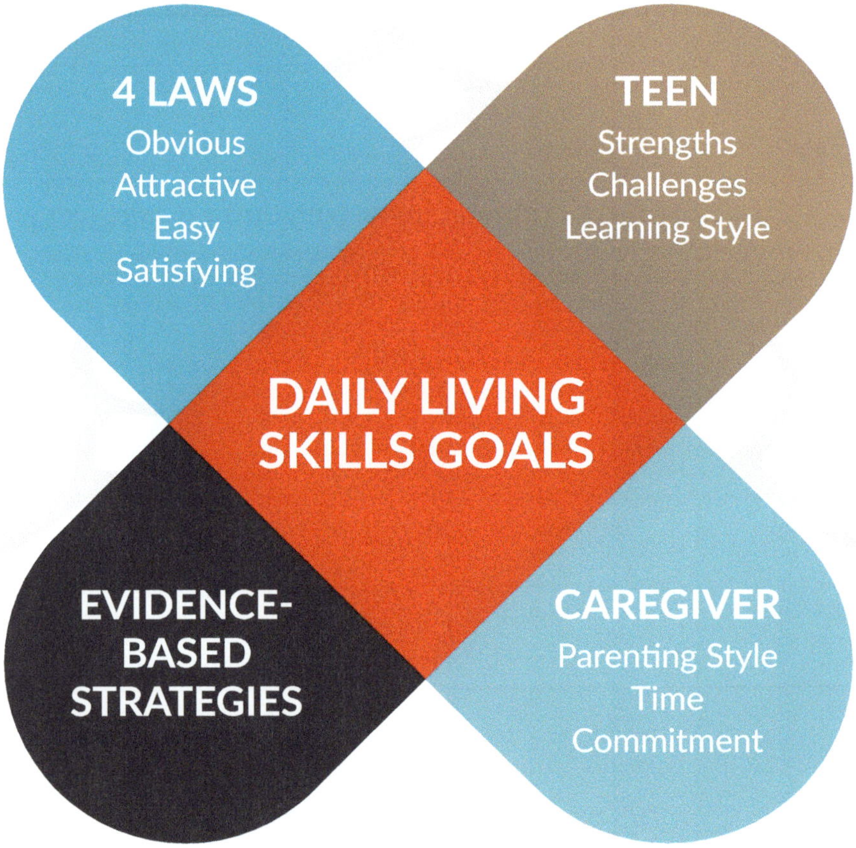

Caregiver/Teen Dyad Session 2 Content (60 mins)

STRW Session 2 Schedule (1 min)

- The therapist should greet the caregiver and teen.
- *Let's get started! As a reminder, it will be helpful to sit together at a table so that we can all see each other and work together. Please pull out your STRW workbook that contains the handouts for all STRW sessions. This session is called Session 2 – Personal Hygiene. Please turn to that section in your workbook.*
- *Let's go over the session schedule so that you know what we will be doing. Please feel free to ask any questions about our schedule!*
- Briefly go over each item on the Session Schedule.

STRW Session Rules (1 min) – OPTIONAL

- *Let's briefly review the group rules, which are meant to set the tone for our dyad sessions and foster collaboration as we work together on building DLS.*
- Have teen read the STRW Session Rules from the slide:
  - Be respectful.
  - Pay attention to the material.
  - Listen to others.
  - Work together.
  - Stay on topic.
  - Do not use your phone or other device during the session.

- Ask: *Are there any other rules that may be important to add?*

Real World Practice Check-In (8–10 mins)

- Refer to the What Motivates You? handout.
- Discuss the Real World Practice assignment with an emphasis on the following points:
  - What Motivates You? handout
    - Ideally, caregiver/teen dyads should have identified eight to ten rewards that vary so that they can be utilized for earning low-, medium-, and high-end rewards.
    - If needed, help dyads brainstorm additional rewards, and this can be assigned as part of their Real World Practice assignment for this week again if needed. It is critical to have rewards identified before the DLS contract is implemented in Session 3.

- Money assignment
    - Review the prices of the hygiene products that the dyad identified at the store.
    - As a reminder, there is flexibility with the money assignment for each session and the goal is to increase the teen's skills in areas such as spending, saving, and budgeting money.

- If the caregiver/teen dyad struggled to complete the Real World Practice assignments, the therapist should spend some time discussing how to identify days/times that they could designate to commit to working on the assignments.
- If the therapist used a fillable PDF of the DLS Contract handout in the previous session, it may be helpful to share this on the screen so that the goal, expectations, and reward can be easily discussed.

Importance of Hygiene (5 mins)

- *For the next two sessions we are going to talk a lot about personal hygiene and self-care and how to make sure that you are doing all of these activities regularly.*
- Ask teen: *What is personal hygiene?*
    - Discuss as needed: *Good personal hygiene means keeping your body looking, smelling, and feeling clean and healthy.*

- Ask teen: *Why is hygiene important?*
    - Discuss the following points as needed depending on teen's responses:
        - *Health: Poor hygiene affects a teen's health in a negative way. For example, if you don't regularly brush your teeth, floss, and use mouthwash, you may have bad breath and may also have dental problems such as cavities and gum disease.*
        - *Social Acceptance: Poor hygiene can increase the likelihood that you may be bullied or teased by others at school. For example, if you have body odor, have oily or greasy hair, or wear clothes with stains or dirt on them to school, this may make you a target for being bullied or ostracized by others. The way we look and smell can change the way other people think or feel about us. For example, good hygiene may influence the first impression you make when meeting others or when interviewing for a job.*
        - *Positive Body Image: Body image is a person's opinions, thoughts, and feelings about their own body and physical appearance. Having a positive body image means feeling satisfied with the way you look, appreciating your body for its capabilities, and accepting your body's imperfections.*
        - *Mental Well Being: Being clean; smelling nice; and having clear skin, clean hair, and healthy teeth help boost confidence. If you know that you look your best, you are likely to feel better about yourself.*

Guidelines for Good Personal Hygiene (4 mins)

- Refer to the Guidelines for Good Personal Hygiene handout.
- *Hygiene rules are not always communicated clearly. Many teens find it helpful to clearly define hygiene rules or guidelines so that they know what they need to do. Let's go over some common guidelines and discuss if and how they may apply to you.*

- Have the caregiver and teen take turns reading the Guidelines for Good Personal Hygiene handout and discuss any comments/questions as needed.
    - Some of the rules may not be applicable or may be different for some teens. It is important to acknowledge this and discuss this with the teen and caregiver. For example, some teens may only wash their hair one to two times per week and some teens may not want to shave their legs.

Personal Hygiene and Self-Care Tasks Activity (10 mins)

- Refer to the Personal Hygiene and Self-Care Tasks handout.
- The caregiver and teen can write their responses down on the handout or the therapist can transcribe responses directly onto the slide or onto the fillable PDF of the handout.
- Ask the dyad: ***What personal hygiene activities should you be doing regularly?***
    - Activities to possibly include in the list if not generated by the caregiver/teen: shower/bathe, brush teeth, brush/comb hair, wash face, wash hands, put on lotion, use acne face wash/medicine, change clothing, put on deodorant, put on make-up, put on perfume/body spray, shave, trim nails, trim toenails, use mouthwash, clean glasses, and put in contact lenses.

- After a list has been generated, ask the dyad: ***How often should you be doing each of these activities?***
    - The therapist should help with determining guidelines for how often and should defer to the discussion on the Guidelines for Good Personal Hygiene as needed.

- The following points should be discussed if not brought up by the dyad:
    - ***It is a good idea to shower every day or every other day.***
    - ***You should change your clothes and wear deodorant every day.***
    - ***Many personal care activities will require you to pay attention to how things look, smell, or feel. This might mean that you need to take a moment to look in the mirror to check your hair, face, or clothing. You may also need to pause to think about how your body feels after you eat or get dressed. For example, you may want to look in the mirror to make sure your shirt is buttoned correctly or that you do not have pizza sauce on your face.***

- Ask: ***Do you have any difficulties, challenges, or preferences that might impact hygiene activities?***
    - Discuss any of the following points as needed or indicated by the caregiver/teen:
        - ***Common challenges for teens may include fine or gross motor difficulties, anxieties, or sensory aversions. For example, some teens report not liking the feel of water on their face, aversion to the feel of a razor on their skin, not liking the smell of minty toothpaste, and having fine motor difficulties that make washing hair difficult.***
        - ***If it is difficult to complete personal hygiene tasks for any reason, it will be helpful to talk about this with your caregiver so that they can help you identify a solution.***

- *Possible solutions to common challenges may include using a showerhead to control the flow of water on your face and head, using a facial wipe to wash your face, or choosing a non-scented toothpaste or deodorant.*

♦ *So how can you make sure you complete necessary hygiene tasks? Make it part of your daily routine! By making it part of a routine, you will be less likely to forget to complete hygiene tasks, and they will just become a normal part of your daily life.*

What Is a Task Analysis? (2 mins)

♦ Refer to the Task Analysis Steps handout
♦ *One of the first DLS goals you are going to work on is becoming independent with your morning routine, which often includes hygiene tasks. We will use an evidence-based strategy called task analysis to increase the likelihood that you will more successfully make specific personal hygiene tasks part of your regular routine.*
♦ *Task analysis is a strategy that breaks a complex or difficult skill into more manageable steps.*
♦ Ask teen: *Have you ever used a task analysis?*
  - *You have likely used a task analysis and did not even realize it! One common task analysis is a recipe, which breaks down all of the steps for cooking. For example, it may be difficult if someone told you to "Bake a dozen chocolate chip cookies," but it is much easier to use a recipe that breaks down all of the steps you need to complete to make chocolate chip cookies.*

Example Task Analysis (2 mins)

♦ *Here is an example of a task analysis for the skill of taking a shower, which breaks the complex task down into ten simple and more manageable steps.*
♦ *A task analysis is often individualized. Some people may include fewer steps on their task analysis, and some may include more detailed steps. You want to create a task analysis that works for you!*
♦ Ask: *Any questions before we create a task analysis?*

Task Analysis for Making a Sandwich (8 mins)

♦ Refer to the Task Analysis Steps handout.
♦ *Let's take a few minutes to come up with a task analysis for breaking down the steps of making a peanut butter-and-jelly sandwich. We want to make the steps as detailed as needed for you to be able to complete this task.*
  - NOTE: The therapist can choose to do another option for this activity, including skills such as making breakfast, packing a lunch, packing a backpack before school, or washing hands.
  - NOTE: This activity can also be skipped if necessary (e.g., running out of time, teen has experience creating a task analysis). The therapist could assign it to the caregiver and teen to complete as part of the Real World Practice assignment.

- The caregiver and teen can write their responses down on the handout or the therapist can transcribe responses directly onto the slide or onto the fillable PDF of the handout.
- Ask: ***Any questions about the task analysis strategy?***

Task Analysis of a Teen's Morning Routine (1 min)

- ***So, you may be wondering how a task analysis and hygiene are related. The answer is that a task analysis is an evidence-based strategy or tool that can be used to remember each step in your morning routine, which may then lead to better hygiene.***

Elements of an Effective System for Achieving DLS Goals (2 mins)

- Refer to the Elements of Effective System for Achieving DLS Goals handout.
- ***As we work towards achieving your DLS goals in STRW, we will not only think through what evidence-based strategies to use, like a task analysis, but we will also consider:***
  - ***Your unique qualities and characteristics – what are your strengths? How do you learn best?***
  - ***Your caregiver's qualities and characteristics – are they committed to supporting you build DLS? Do they have the time and energy to help you?***
  - ***Evidence-based strategies – we will use tools like a task analysis to help with learning and mastering DLS***
  - ***Use the Four Laws of Behavior Change – you may not be familiar with these, but these are four laws that make it more likely you will meet your goals by making them obvious, attractive, easy, and satisfying.***

- Ask and Discuss: ***Any questions or comments?***

Targeting DLS Goals in STRW: Four Laws of Behavior Change (3 mins)

- ***Let's briefly talk through what the Four Laws of Behavior Change are and how they relate to building an effective system to target DLS goals in STRW.***
- ***There are four laws to building an effective system to target DLS goals like doing your morning routine steps independently or doing your own laundry. You do not need all four laws to be successful, but if you include all four, you are even more likely to be successful. These are also laws that will help you to achieve any goal, not just DLS goals. However, during STRW, we will focus on DLS goals. Let's discuss the Four Laws of Behavior Change:***
  - ***Make It Obvious – the cues to get started on your goal should be as obvious as possible. You can usually do this by modifying your environment to make it more likely you will meet your goals. For example, you could put all of your morning routine hygiene routine items in the same spot in the bathroom to make it more obvious what the steps in your morning routine are.***

- *Make It Attractive – the goal should be appealing to increase your motivation and follow-through. It can be tricky to make DLS goals attractive – but we will discuss some ideas about how to do this each session!*
- *Make It Easy – make achieving the goal as simple as possible. This is a critical one because we want you to have success with meeting goals. Thus, we may break a complex DLS goal, such as doing the laundry, into a simple, achievable goal, such as loading the washing machine, to make it more likely that you will reach your goal.*
- *Make It Satisfying – make achieving goals satisfying. Building DLS and becoming independent is often inherently satisfying, but we still need to consider how to make sure that you are being rewarded for learning a new skill so that you feel good about continuing to work on meeting your goal.*

♦ *Let's go through one example of working on a DLS goal using the Four Laws of Behavior Change.*

Targeting DLS Goals in STRW: Four Laws of Behavior Change Example (3 mins)

♦ *Here is an example of how we might utilize the Four Laws of Behavior Change to develop an effective system to meet the goal of doing all of the steps of a teen's morning routine independently.*

♦ Have the caregiver and teen take turns reading how the Four Laws of Behavior Change were used to target the goal of a teen's morning routine by reading through the following bullet points on the slide for Obvious, Attractive, Easy, and Satisfying.

- Goal – Do all steps of the morning routine independently.
  - Obvious
    - Calendar reminder or alarm to get started on morning routine at 8 am
    - Post a task analysis of steps for morning routine in bedroom and/or in bathroom
  - Attractive
    - Listen to music for 10 mins while in the shower
    - Have favorite breakfast options available to make
  - Easy
    - Post a checklist with all steps so that expectations are clear
    - Start by targeting a few steps and gradually increasing expectations
    - Set up an easy system (e.g., basket with all morning routine hygiene items in the bathroom) on
  - Satisfying
    - Making progress and becoming independent is satisfying in itself
    - Provide verbal praise (e.g., "Great job getting ready for school today!")
    - Provide a reward (e.g., extra screen time until school starts, preferred snack in lunch box)

♦ Ask and Discuss: *Any questions about how the Four Laws of Behavior Change were used to target the morning routine goal?*

Task Analysis of a Teen's Morning Routine (1 min)

- *Going back to a task analysis – this is a strategy that we can use to make achieving our goal more likely, and it relates back to two of the Four Laws of Behavior Change.*
  - *Make it EASY – a task analysis makes achieving our goals easier because all of the steps are clearly defined in sequential order.*
  - *Make it OBVIOUS – the task analysis helps us figure out how to make things more obvious. For example, a teen could set their alarm to go off every Monday–Friday at 6:15 am to ensure that they are getting started on their morning routine on time.*

- Ask and Discuss: *Any questions?*

Elements of an Effective System for Achieving DLS Goals (1 min)

- *To sum it up, during STRW, we will consider all of these important elements when targeting your DLS goals, and we will revisit this framework in each session to increase the likelihood that you will achieve your DLS goals by developing the best possible system!*
- Ask and Discuss: *Any questions or comments?*

Real World Practice (3 mins)

- Refer to the Real World Practice handout and the Task Analysis Worksheet handout.
- Discuss the details of the Real World Practice assignment.
- *The first DLS goal that we will target at next week's session is the morning routine, which may consist of tasks such as waking up, getting dressed, brushing teeth, taking medications, packing lunch, and packing your backpack. It is typically the best idea to start working on the morning routine because the steps tend to be the same each weekday and need to be completed before you go to school.*
  - *Practice trying to do your morning routine independently two to three times this week so that you know what steps you might need help with, including reminders from others; help from others; or using an alarm clock, a timer, or a checklist. With the help of your caregiver, discuss (1) the steps of your morning routine that you need help with and (2) the steps of your morning routine that you are able to do independently and completely on your own.*
  - *With the help of your caregiver, complete a task analysis of the morning routine that you are going to be working on using the Task Analysis Worksheet handout:*
    - *List the steps of the routine.*
    - *Determine if you can do the step independently or if you need help, such as a reminder or assistance with a part of a step.*
    - *Think about what you could do to become more independent. For example, if you have trouble remembering to take vitamins or medications, you could put them in a pill box on the kitchen table.*

- *Last, purchase a personal hygiene item using cash or debit/credit card. It may be helpful to have your caregiver help you if you have never used a debit/credit card or have never purchased an item.*
- *We will begin working on actually doing your morning routine AFTER next week's session, but let's hold off on until then!*

♦ Ask: *Any questions about your Real World Practice assignment?*

Guess the Price (3 mins) – OPTIONAL

♦ *Let's play a quick round of Guess the Price, which is just meant to be a fun way to build up your understanding of how much things cost.*
♦ *Let's see if you know the prices of some common personal hygiene items even if they are not necessarily items that you use!*
♦ The therapist can have just the teen guess the price or have the caregiver and teen compete against each other.
♦ The therapist should click through the next four slides that contain examples of common personal hygiene items. Prior to the session, the therapist will need to look up the prices to ensure that they are accurate.
  - Therapists can change the personal hygiene items for the Guess the Price game.
  - This activity is meant to be fun and engaging! If the teen is averse to playing the game, it can be skipped. However, it would be helpful for the caregiver and teen to find other ways to build up an understanding of what things cost (e.g., compare the cost of products at the grocery store, involve the teen when purchasing personal hygiene items).

Preparing for the Next Dyad Session (1 min)

♦ *We will have our next caregiver/teen dyad session on DAY and TIME. At this session, we will discuss how to use a contract to begin working on your first DLS goal of completing your morning routine.*
♦ *It will be important to complete your Real World Practice assignment before our next dyad session and come prepared to discuss it.*
♦ *It may also be helpful to gather some of the supplies you use for your morning routine so that we can practice how to do your morning routine.*
♦ Ask: *Are there any questions before we end the session?*

Wrap-Up

♦ The therapist should send a calendar invite with the next caregiver/teen dyad session's day/time to the caregiver and teen.
♦ Therapists should email any documents that were completed during the session to the caregiver and teen.

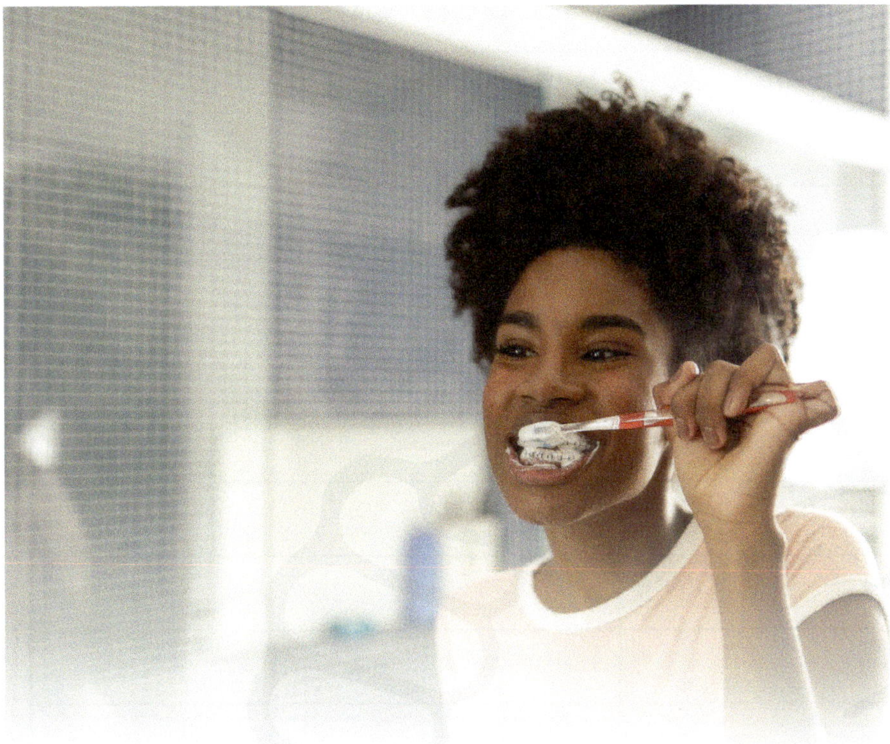

Guidelines for Good Personal Hygiene

- Take a shower at least every other day.
- Use shampoo and conditioner each time you take a shower.
- Wash your face every morning and night, using warm water and mild soap or facewash.
- Brush your hair before leaving the house.
- If you have body hair, it is a good idea to shave several times per week (face for men, legs and underarms for women).
- Put on deodorant every day before you leave the house. You may need to re-apply after you exercise or do any activity that makes you sweat.
- Brush your teeth twice a day (in the morning and at night).
- If something gets stuck in your teeth, excuse yourself and go to the bathroom. Use floss, not your fingers, to get it out.
- It's a good idea to look in the mirror after you eat to make sure you don't have food on your face or in your teeth.
- Keep your fingernails and toenails clean, and trim them every 1-2 weeks.
- Change your clothes every day.
- Check to make sure that your clothing is not stained and is not on backwards or inside out before leaving the house.
- Always wash your hands after you use the restroom and before eating.
- If you have to cough or sneeze, cough or sneeze into your elbow and say, "excuse me."'
- Blow your nose discreetly and try not to be loud.

Personal Hygiene and Self-Care Tasks

Personal Hygiene or Self-Care Task	How Often?

Elements of an Effective System for Achieving DLS Goals

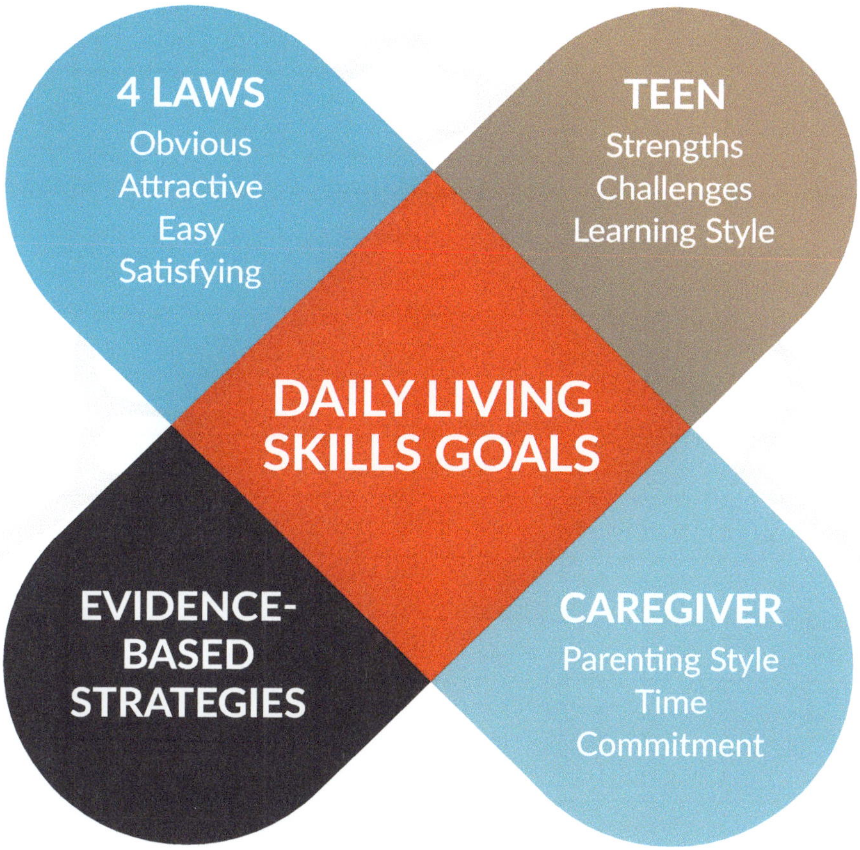

Task Analysis Steps

Task Analysis

Skill: ______________________________

Steps:

____

____

____

____

____

____

____

____

____

____

____

____

____

____

____

____

____

____

____

Task Analysis Steps

Task Analysis

Skill:

Steps:

Surviving and Thriving in the Real World
Session 2 – Real World Practice

- Practice trying to do your morning routine independently two to three times this week so that you know what steps you might need help with (e.g., reminders from others, an alarm clock, a checklist of steps).
- With the help of your caregiver, complete a task analysis of your morning routine that you are going to be working on. Use the Task Analysis Worksheet handout.
  - First, list the steps for the routine.
  - Second, determine if you can do this step independently or if you need help from a caregiver (e.g., a reminder to get started, help with the entire step, or assistance with part of the step).
  - Third, think about what you could do to become more independent. For example, if you have trouble remembering to take vitamins or medications, you could put them in a pill box on the kitchen table.

- Purchase a personal hygiene item at the store using cash or a debit/credit card. It may be helpful to have your caregiver help you.

Task Analysis Worksheet

Task Analysis

Skill ______________________________

Step	Can you do this step independently?	What could you do to become more independent?

Surviving & Thriving
in the Real World

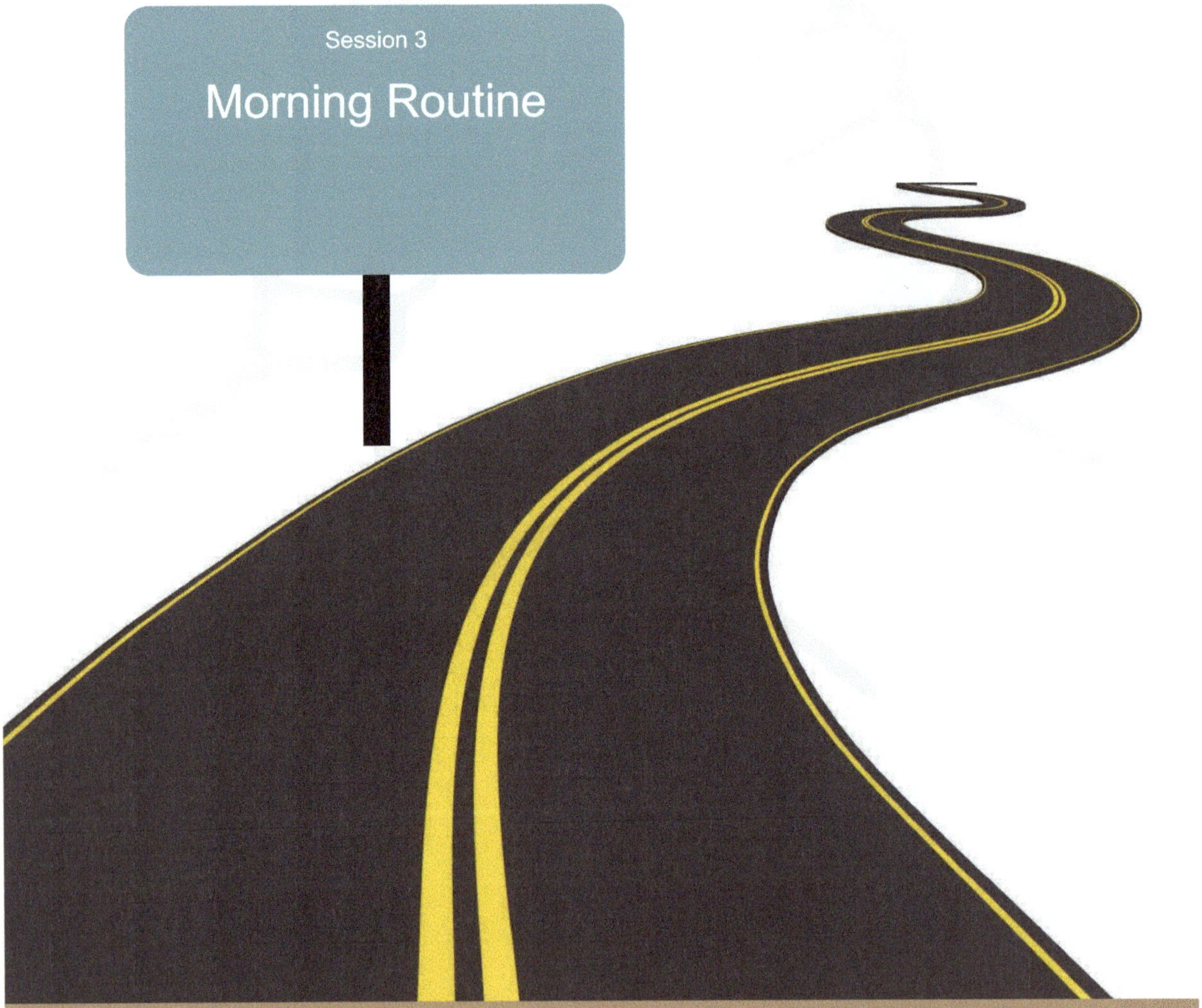

Session 3

Morning Routine

Aims

- Continue to build rapport between caregiver group members and the therapist
- Continue to build rapport between the teen, caregiver, and therapist
- Develop an understanding of the steps of the teen's morning routine and what steps are independently completed
- Review the four elements for developing an effective system to achieve the teen's DLS goals
- Use a task analysis to identify a goal and define the expectations for the teen's morning routine
- Understand how to create and implement a DLS contract to target the morning routine goal

Structure

- Caregiver group session via telehealth
- Caregiver/teen dyad session via telehealth

Session Supplies

- Caregiver Group Handouts
  - DLS Contract
  - Simplified DLS Contract

- Caregiver/Teen Dyad Handouts
  - DLS Contract
  - DLS Contract Example
  - Matthew's Task Analysis
  - Matthew's DLS Contract
  - Task Analysis Worksheet
  - Session 3 – Real World Practice

- Videos (links available on the STRW website and the STRW Resources handout)
  - Example DLS Contract

DOI: 10.4324/9781003458838-6

Caregiver/Teen Preparation for Session

- Optional: Caregiver and teen can gather personal hygiene supplies to practice the teen's morning routine during the dyad session as a way to rehearse the steps and identify strategies that may increase the likelihood of meeting this goal.

Therapist Preparation for Session

- The therapist may want to review the Example DLS Contracts handout (see appendix), which includes examples of DLS contracts from previous STRW teen participants. These may be helpful to get an understanding of how to individualize goals, expectations, use of evidence-based strategies and supports, and rewards.
- The therapist may want to review the Example Task Analyses handout (see appendix), which includes examples of how STRW teen participants broke down the steps for the tasks of morning routine, nighttime routine, cleaning the bedroom, and laundry. These may be helpful to get an understanding of how detailed to get when creating task analyses with caregiver and teen participants.
- The therapist may want to review the Strategies Commonly Used to Target Goals on the DLS Contract handout (see appendix), which includes the evidence-based strategies, supports, and tools that teens utilize as they work on their DLS goals of morning routine, cleaning the bedroom, laundry, cooking, grocery shopping, and money management. It may be beneficial for therapists to review these prior to facilitating these sessions and developing the DLS contract with the caregiver/teen dyads.

Session 3 Notes

- The therapist can choose to skip the Group Rules section. However, these should be reviewed if it may be beneficial for the caregivers or teens.
- The content in both the caregiver group and caregiver/teen dyad sessions sets the foundation for how to use a contract for targeting DLS for the remainder of the intervention, so it will be important for the therapist to check in to assess the caregiver and teen's understanding of how to set it up and begin implementing the DLS contract for the teen's morning routine goal.
- The DLS Contract, Simplified DLS Contract, and Task Analysis Worksheet handouts can also be completed by the therapist during the session to facilitate discussion with the caregiver and teen. A fillable PDF of each of these handouts are available on the STRW website and can be emailed to the family after the session.

- Caregiver Group Session
  - The DLS Contract handout will be used in this session and in all STRW sessions moving forward. However, there is also a Simplified DLS Contract handout that some caregivers and teens may also find helpful to use. The Simplified DLS Contract is included in Session 3 handouts only and is also available on the STRW website.

- Dyad Session
  - When developing the DLS contract at the end of the dyad session, the therapist should incorporate information from the past two sessions (e.g., discussion of the teen's morning routine task analysis, essential elements of an effective system for achieving DLS goals, identifying rewards, etc.). The therapist should also consider the goals that the caregiver and teen collaboratively developed during the Preparing for STRW session.
  - It will be important to make sure that the goal and expectations on the DLS contract are realistic and doable for the teen. For example, if the teen is only able to complete two out of eight steps independently, they may want to work towards doing three to four steps independently with the necessary strategies and supports in place (e.g., alarm clock to get up, checklist of all steps posted in the bathroom, etc.). Alternatively, the teen may benefit from just working on one step of their morning routine (e.g., getting up and out of bed by 6:45 am).
  - It is critical that the therapist and caregiver set the teen up for success for all of their goals on the DLS contract by ensuring that the teen knows what they need to be doing (i.e., clearly defining the goal and expectations) and has the necessary strategies and supports in place to be successful. For example, many teens benefit from having reminders to start a task and also a check-in from a caregiver after the task is completed to ensure that it was done correctly and thoroughly.
  - It is just as critical that the teen be motivated by the reward because this makes it more likely that they will work towards the goal. It may be beneficial to refer to the What Motivates You? handout that was completed by the teen in Session 1 when discussing rewards in this and upcoming sessions.
  - Many therapists find it helpful to modify/complete the DLS contract with the caregiver and teen at the end of each dyad session using an editable PDF of the DLS Contract handout. The therapist can then email a copy of the DLS contract to the caregiver and teen. This may save time and also provide information about the goals, expectations, and rewards that the teen is working on. Further, the therapist can quickly incorporate any changes to the DLS contract in future sessions.

Caregiver Group Session 3 Content (90 mins)

Group Rules (1 min) – OPTIONAL

- *These group rules are meant to set the tone for our group sessions and foster a collaborative, engaging, and supportive group as we work together on building DLS.*
- Review the following group rules:
    - *Be respectful.*
        - *This rule also includes keeping information that is discussed in session private. While we cannot enforce this rule, other group members are more likely to openly share if there is a shared understanding that this is a safe and private space to discuss things.*
    - *Listen to others.*
    - *Be attentive. This includes when others are talking and when information is being presented.*
    - *Do not use your phone or other device during the session.*
    - *Stay on topic.*
    - *We will try to reserve the final 5–10 minutes of each session for "off-topic" questions*

Review – Real World Practice Assignment (24 mins)

- The therapist should greet the caregivers and welcome them to the session if they have not yet done this.
- Discuss the Real World Practice assignment by briefly going through each assignment. Have at least one to two caregivers discuss how their teen did with each assignment. Points of discussion or questions to ask include the following:
    - Practice trying to do your morning routine independently.
        - *What did you notice as your teen did this?*
        - *What steps did your teen need help with?*
        - *What strategies might be helpful to increase your teen's independence with their morning routine steps?*
    - Task Analysis
        - *Was it easy/hard to list the steps of your teen's morning routine?*
        - *Was your teen able to understand if they were doing a step independently?*
        - *How did it go discussing how to become more independent with some of their morning routine steps?*
    - Money Management
        - *Was your teen able to purchase an item at the store?*
        - *What went well?*
        - *What skills still need to be practiced?*

- Ask: *Any questions about the Real World Practice assignment?*

STRW Session 3 Goals (1 min)

- *The goal of today's session is to review how to build an effective system to help you and your teen achieve their DLS goals now and in the future. We will also discuss how we will be targeting the first DLS goal of completing one's morning routine using a DLS contract and other evidence-based strategies.*
- *We will be discussing a lot of content in this session, so you may want to take notes.*

Targeting DLS Goals in STRW (1 min)

- *Our goal in STRW is to not only build age-appropriate DLS in your teens but also to develop a system that they can utilize now and throughout their life to learn and master DLS. As we discussed last week, developing an effective system makes it more likely that your teen will be able to reach their DLS goals now and in the future.*

Elements of an Effective System for Achieving DLS Goals (2 mins)

- *In order to help teens achieve their DLS goals in STRW, we will (1) consider the qualities of the teen and the caregiver; (2) use evidence-based strategies to teach and master DLS; and (3) use the Four Laws of Behavior Change to make sure that goals are obvious, attractive, easy, and satisfying.*
- *We will revisit this framework each session to make sure that we are considering all of the factors needed to increase the likelihood of achieving goals by developing the best possible system!*
- Ask and Discuss*: Any questions or comments?*

Targeting DLS Goals in STRW: Example of the Four Laws of Behavior Change (4 mins)

- *Last week, we went through this example of how we might utilize the Four Laws of Behavior Change to develop an effective system to meet the DLS goal of doing all of the steps of a teen's morning routine independently.*
- The therapist should briefly review each point on the slide for using the Four Laws of Behavior Change to target a morning routine goal by reading through the following bullet points on the slide for Obvious, Attractive, Easy, and Satisfying.
  - *Goal – Do all steps of the morning routine independently.*
    - *Obvious*
      - *Calendar reminder or alarm to get started on morning routine at 8 am*
      - *Post a task analysis of steps for morning routine in bedroom and/or in bathroom*
    - *Attractive*
      - *Listen to music for 10 mins while in the shower*
      - *Have favorite breakfast options available to make*
    - *Easy*
      - *Post a checklist with all steps so that expectations are clear*
      - *Start by targeting a few steps and gradually increasing expectations*

- ❍ *Set up an easy system (e.g., basket with all morning routine hygiene items in the bathroom) on*
- ■ *Satisfying*
  - ❍ *Making progress and becoming independent is satisfying in itself*
  - ❍ *Provide verbal praise (e.g., "Great job getting ready for school today!")*
  - ❍ *Provide a reward (e.g., extra screen time until school starts, preferred snack in lunch box)*

- Ask and Discuss: *Any questions about how the Four Laws of Behavior Change were used to target the morning routine goal?*

Using a DLS Contract: The Basics (3–4 mins)

- Refer to the DLS Contract handout.
- *We are going to start using a contract, which is an evidence-based strategy for clearly outlining goals, expectations, and rewards. As you will see, a contract also relates back to one of the Four Laws of Behavior Change, "make it satisfying," by specifying a reward and allowing for the tracking of progress.*
- *A contract is a written set of expectations between two people. A contract typically includes basic rules, expectations, consequences, and rewards.*
- *We are going to be using a DLS contract to hold teens accountable for practicing DLS at home, and in return, caregivers will provide support as needed and deliver rewards when goals are met. The DLS contract will lead to increased independence as the teen begins to achieve their DLS goals.*
- The therapist should read the following bullet points on the slide.
- *A Contract:*
  - *Clearly outlines the behaviors each person needs to do*
    - *Teen works on the DLS goal(s)*
    - *Caregiver provides support (as needed) and a reward*
  - *Clearly defines the expectations of the behavior*
  - *States what can be earned by performing a specific behavior*
  - *Is mutually agreed upon after negotiation*
  - *Can be renegotiated*
  - *Leads to increased independence over time*

- Ask and Discuss: *Any questions about using a contract?*
- Refer to the Simplified DLS Contract handout.
- *We will be using the DLS Contract in all STRW sessions. There is also a Simplified DLS Contract handout in your caregiver workbook that you may find helpful to use now or in the future. Both of the DLS Contract handouts are available on the STRW website.*

Using a DLS Contract: Rewards (7–8 mins)

- *When you are rewarded for a specific behavior, it makes it more likely that you will do it again.*
- Ask and Discuss: *What are some examples of rewards that you may receive for specific behaviors?*

- Examples to discuss may include the following: you receive a paycheck for going to work; you are rewarded with a delicious dessert after you spend time baking it; your neighbor says "thank you" after you shovel snow from their driveway; you lose 2 pounds after regularly working out for 2 weeks.

♦ *One key part of the DLS contract is that your teen will earn a reward for working on and achieving their DLS goals. We will use rewards in STRW, as opposed to punishment, because it is more positive, naturally motivating, and more effective. For example, when discussing the DLS contract with teens, we will say "You will earn extra screen time if you meet your morning routine goal" instead of "You will NOT get any extra screen time if you do NOT meet your morning routine goal."*

♦ *Let's go over some important components of using rewards:*
- *Consistent – a reward should be given every time a specific behavior is demonstrated*
  - *This leads to the teen trusting that they will be rewarded, which in turn leads to the teen engaging in the behavior more often.*
  - *For example, teens are more likely to cut the grass if they earn $5 every time they do it.*
- *Meaningful – a reward should be strong enough to motivate the teen to complete the behavior*
  - *Teens are more likely to do their own laundry if they earn 30 minutes of extra screen time as opposed to 30 minutes of extra math homework.*
  - *Teens are more likely to do their laundry if they earn $2 rather than 2 cents.*
  - *Many DLS have natural rewards, and it is ideal to use these as rewards when possible. For example, cooking brownies involves a lot of skills such as mixing, measuring ingredients, operating the oven, and cleaning up the kitchen – and a natural reward is being able to eat a brownie or maybe even an extra brownie.*
  - *It can be helpful to encourage teens to find ways to reward themselves after they complete a task based on what drives them. These self-rewards may work better for teens who are highly motivated to be independent.*
  - *Some teens may benefit from caregivers discussing the concept of "First Work, Then Play." This just means that sometimes you have to get your work done (e.g., get ready for school in the morning) and then you can have some time to play (e.g., read a book or listen to music before leaving for school).*
- *Individualized – rewards should be personalized for the teen. Some things to think about include:*
  - *Rewards may include earning money and/or earning privileges such as extra time to practice learning how to drive on the weekend, choosing the movie for movie night, staying up later, extra screen time, or having a friend over.*
  - *Teens may have a lot of ideas for what rewards they would like to earn, and caregivers should discuss this regularly to ensure that a reward continues to be motivating.*
  - *Many teens prefer a monetary reward, which can also help with building their money management skills such as spending, saving, and budgeting. For example, if teens are now earning money as a part of their DLS contract, caregivers can emphasize things such as (1) the need to save up their money*

to go see a movie at the movie theater, (2) how to budget for an expensive purchase, and (3) how to save their money and put it in a savings account.
        - *Many parents also begin having their teen pay for their own expenses if they are now earning money as part of their DLS contract. For example, teens may now need to use their own money to purchase an extra snack at lunch or buy something that they want at the store.*
    - *Fade over time – rewards are needed when learning a new DLS to encourage the teen to practice and master it as it becomes a part of their everyday life. However, we will eventually fade back these rewards so that the teens are just expected to do these DLS. For example, many caregivers may have given stickers, candy, or verbal praise as rewards when their child was being toilet trained. However, these rewards were quickly faded as the child mastered this skill and it became part of their daily routine. We will talk more about fading rewards in later STRW sessions.*

- Ask and Discuss: *Any questions about the use of rewards?*

Using a DLS Contract: Targeting Multiple Goals (3–4 mins)

- Refer to the <u>DLS Contract</u> handout.
- *Each week during the dyad session, you will work with your teen to develop, modify, and then agree to a new DLS contract that goes along with the new DLS that was taught during the session. We will build upon the skills to be targeted on the DLS contract such that teens may eventually be working on multiple goals, including their morning routine, doing laundry once per week, cleaning their room, cooking a recipe in the kitchen, and building their money management skills. However, we will be mindful of ensuring that goals are feasible for both you and your teen to increase the likelihood of successfully meeting DLS goals each week.*
- *Your role with the DLS contract is to:*
    - *Help your teen create specific, measurable, and realistic DLS goals to help them build their independence.*
    - *Identify and then provide a reward if the goal is met.*
    - *Commit to devoting time and effort to practicing and mastering DLS goals in collaboration with your teen.*

- Ask and Discuss: *Do you have any questions or concerns about developing the DLS contract with your teen?*

Review Dyad Session 3 Content (40 mins)

- *Now we will briefly review the material that will be covered in the upcoming dyad session with your teen. This will allow you to have some time to prepare for the upcoming session. Please feel free to ask any questions as we go over the content of the dyad session.*
- The therapist should refer to the PowerPoint presentation slides for Dyad Session 3 while reviewing the content for the session.

- The therapist should have also prepared for the session by reviewing the Dyad Session 3 content discussed in the manual, which has detailed information about the content that will be covered.
- The important points to make while reviewing the Dyad Session 3 Content are:
  - The elements of an effective system for achieving DLS goals will be reviewed.
  - A task analysis can be used to make it more likely that a teen will complete all of the steps of their morning routine.
  - A contract will be used to increase cooperation between the caregiver and teen as they work together to define specific DLS goals that will be targeted and identify the strategies and supports that will increase independence.
  - By signing the DLS contract, teens agree to work on the DLS goal and caregivers agree to provide the reward specified.
  - A DLS contract will incorporate the elements of an effective system for achieving DLS goals.
  - The teens will see an example of how a teen used their task analysis of a morning routine to develop a DLS contract with their caregiver.
  - The caregiver, teen, and therapist will work together to use a task analysis of the teen's morning routine to create the first goal to be targeted on the DLS contract over the next week.

- Ask and Discuss:
  - ***Any questions about the content for the upcoming dyad session?***
  - ***Any additional questions about how you will be targeting your teen's morning routine goal on the DLS contract?***

Prep for the Next Caregiver Session (2 mins)

- ***We will have our next caregiver group session on DAY and TIME. At this session, we will discuss how setting up and implementing the DLS contract went. We will also discuss how to add the goal of cleaning the bedroom to your teen's DLS contract.***
- ***After your dyad session with your teen, it will be important to prioritize working on the goals on the DLS contract and the Real World Practice assignment so that we can celebrate successes and also discuss any challenges or questions that arose in the caregiver group session.***
- Ask: ***Are there any questions before we end the session?***

Wrap-Up

- The therapist should send a calendar invite with the next caregiver group session's day/time to the caregiver.
- The therapist may also want to email the caregiver and teen the DLS Contract and the Simplified DLS Contract handouts or refer them to the STRW website.

Daily Living Skills Contract

Date ____________________

Goal	Expectations	Reward	MONDAY	TUESDAY	WEDNESDAY	THURSDAY	FRIDAY	SATURDAY	SUNDAY

____
Teen

____
Parent / Caregiver

Daily Living Skills Contract

Date: ____________________

Goal	Expectations	Reward	M	T	W	Th	F	Sa	Sun

____________________ Teen

____________________ Parent/Caregiver

Caregiver/Teen Dyad Session 3 Content (60 mins)

STRW Session 3 Schedule (1 min)

- The therapist should greet the caregiver and teen.
- *Let's get started! As a reminder, it will be helpful to sit together at a table so that we can all see each other and work together. Please pull out your STRW workbook that contains the handouts for all STRW sessions. This session is called Session 3 – Morning Routine. Please turn to that section in your workbook.*
- *Let's go over the session schedule so that you know what we will be doing. Please feel free to ask any questions about our schedule!*
- Briefly go over each item on the Session Schedule.

STRW Session Rules (1 min) – OPTIONAL

- *Let's briefly review the group rules, which are meant to set the tone for our dyad sessions and foster collaboration as we work together on building DLS.*
- Have teen read the STRW Session Rules from the slide:
  - Be respectful.
  - Pay attention to the material.
  - Listen to others.
  - Work together.
  - Stay on topic.
  - Do not use your phone or other device during the session.
- Ask: *Are there any other rules that may be important to add?*

Real World Practice Check-In (8 mins)

- Refer to the Session 2 Real World Practice handout and the Task Analysis Worksheet handout.
- Discuss the Real World Practice assignments with an emphasis on the following points:
  - Practicing morning routine steps
    - *What were the steps that you did independently?*
    - *What were the steps that you needed help with?*
    - *Did you use any tools or strategies to help you remember to do the steps?*
  - Task Analysis of Morning Routine
    - Review the steps of the morning routine that were identified in detail and discuss (1) if the teen can do the step independently and (2) what strategy/support would help the teen become more independent with a specific step.

  - It is particularly important that the morning routine steps be described in detail and that the caregiver and teen understand what steps can be done independently so that a specific and appropriate morning routine goal can be added to the DLS contract at the end of the session.
- Money assignment
  - Discuss how the teen did with purchasing a personal hygiene item at the store.

- If the caregiver/teen dyad struggled to complete the Real World Practice assignments, the therapist should spend some time discussing how to identify days/times that they could designate to commit to working on the assignments.
- If the therapist used a fillable PDF of the DLS Contract handout in the previous session, it may be helpful to share this on the screen so that the goal, expectations, and reward can be easily discussed.

Elements of an Effective System for Achieving DLS Goals (1 min)

- *Last session, we talked about how in order to help teens achieve their DLS goals in STRW. We will (1) consider the qualities of the teen and their caregiver; (2) use evidence-based strategies to teach and master DLS; and (3) identify how to make sure that goals are obvious, attractive, easy, and satisfying. We will revisit this framework each session to make sure that we are considering all of the factors needed to increase the likelihood of achieving goals by developing the best system!*

Targeting DLS Goals in STRW: Four Laws of Behavior Change (2 mins)

- *Last session, we also talked about how there are Four Laws of Behavior Change to help you build an effective system to target DLS goals like doing your morning routine steps independently.*
- *These laws are Obvious, Attractive, Easy, and Satisfying. You do not need all Four Laws of Behavior Change to be successful, but if you include all four, you are even more likely to be successful.*
- *Here is an example of how you might apply these laws to a morning routine goal.*
- Briefly read through each of the following bullet points on the slide.
  - *Goal – Do all steps of the morning routine independently.*
    - *Obvious*
      - *Calendar reminder or alarm to get started on morning routine at 8 am*
      - *Post a task analysis of steps for morning routine in bedroom and/or in bathroom*
    - *Attractive*
      - *Listen to music for 10 mins while in the shower*
      - *Have favorite breakfast options available to make*
    - *Easy*
      - *Post a checklist with all steps so that expectations are clear*
      - *Start by targeting a few steps and gradually increasing expectations*

        - *Set up an easy system (e.g., basket with all morning routine hygiene items in the bathroom) on*
    - *Satisfying*
        - *Making progress and becoming independent is satisfying in itself*
        - *Provide verbal praise (e.g., "Great job getting ready for school today!")*
        - *Provide a reward (e.g., extra screen time until school starts, preferred snack in lunch box)*

- Ask and Discuss: *Any questions about how the Four Laws of Behavior Change were used to target the morning routine goal?*

Task Analysis (1 min)

- *For your Real World Practice Assignment, you created a task analysis of your morning routine. A task analysis is a strategy that we will use to make it more likely that you will achieve your morning routine goal because it makes the goal Easy because all of the steps are clearly defined. A task analysis also helps us to understand how to make the steps of the goal more Obvious. For example, if you set your alarm to go off Monday–Friday at 6:15 am, you do not need to remember to set your alarm every day, which then makes it more likely you will get out of bed when your alarm goes off!*

What is a DLS Contract? (3 mins)

- Refer to the DLS Contract handout and the DLS Contract Example handout.
- *This is the first week that you will begin targeting a new DLS goal and earning a reward using a DLS contract that you will develop with the help of your caregiver. The first skill you will include on your DLS contract is completing your morning routine independently, and you will earn a reward if you are able to meet the expectations and the goal that you set with your caregiver.*
- Ask and Discuss: *What is a contract?*
    - *A contract is a written set of expectations between two people. A contract typically includes basic rules, consequences, rewards, and privileges. Contracts are used for everything from buying a house to driving a car. For example, many teens have a contract with their caregiver that outlines the rules for driving a car once they get their license, and it may include rules such as wearing a seatbelt, not using a phone while driving, and letting their caregivers know when they arrive somewhere.*

- *One of the goals of today's session is that you both leave feeling confident that you can (1) set up and use a DLS contract to work on your morning routine goal and (2) understand what strategies and supports could help you complete the steps of your morning routine independently (without any reminding or help from your caregiver). Here is an example of the DLS contract that we will be using over the course of the next several weeks to work on building your DLS.*
- Ask: *Any questions about the DLS contract?*

Why Use a DLS Contract? (2 mins)

- Ask: *Why are we going to use a contract to target your DLS goals?*
  - ***Overall, the main goal of the DLS contract is to work together to define the specific goal, the expectations, and the reward. A DLS contract is also a way to build an effective system to achieve DLS goals because it makes the goal Easy, Obvious, and Satisfying.***

- Have the teen and caregiver take turns reading and discussing the following bullet points on the slide. This may also be a natural opportunity for the therapist discuss any issues that come up about how the caregiver/teen dyad work together and interact with one another.
  - Cooperate and work together towards the goal of building daily living skills in order to increase independence.
  - Clearly define what both the teen and caregiver are expected to do.
  - Increase teen's understanding of what they need to do by making the goal and expectations EASY and OBVIOUS
  - States what reward will be earned, which makes achieving the goal SATISFYING.
  - Allows for teen to track their progress on meeting goals.

- Ask: *Any questions or comments about using a DLS contract?*

Using a Task Analysis to Develop a DLS Contract (3 mins)

- Refer to the Matthew's Task Analysis handout.
- *We are going to go through an example of how to create a DLS contract for the goal of becoming independent with your morning routine. The first step is use a task analysis to break up the complex skill of a morning routine into more doable steps.*
- *As you can see, Matthew is a teen who has eight steps in his morning routine. For example, the first step on his morning routine is to "Wake up on his own." Matthew is able to wake up on his own on about two out of five days of the week. He and his mom decided that they could set an alarm on his phone to automatically go off at 6 am on Monday–Friday. The phone will be on Matthew's desk so that he has to get out of bed to turn the alarm off.*
- *The task analysis is a really useful tool for figuring out how to make sure we can meet our DLS goals by incorporating any helpful strategies or supports that may be needed for each step!*
- Ask: *Any questions?*

How to Develop a DLS Contract (2 mins)

- Refer to the Matthew's DLS Contract handout.
- *After the task analysis has been completed for the goal you want to work on, you will then use the DLS contract to write down the specific goal, expectations, and reward.*
- *As you can see, Matthew's goal is to complete his morning routine independently.*

- *The expectations for his goal are that: (1) he needs to complete the entire morning routine on Monday–Friday mornings, (2) he needs to complete six of the eight steps independently without anyone's help, and (3) his mom will check to make sure that he did each step.*
- *The reward for meeting the goal is that he will receive 30 extra minutes of computer or video game time when he completes his goal.*
- Ask: *Any questions?*

Example DLS Contract Negotiation (8 mins)

- *Let's watch a video of Matthew and his mom using a task analysis of his morning routine to develop a DLS contract.*
- Watch the 6-minute Example DLS Contract video (link is available on the STRW Resources handout on the STRW website and in the Session 3 Dyad PowerPoint presentation).
- *As you saw, the expectations were clear for Matthew such that he knew what he needed to do each morning for his morning routine.*
- *The expectations were also clear for his mom such that she knew what reward Matthew would receive for successfully completing his morning routine.*
- *They also worked together to incorporate a system that would make it more likely that Matthew would achieve his goal. For example, he is making the goal easy by putting all of the hygiene items he uses in the bathroom in one place.*
- Ask: *Any questions?*

Getting Ready to Develop the DLS Contract (4 mins)

- Refer to the DLS Contract handout.
- *We are going to work on developing a DLS contract to target your morning routine. But first, let's just touch base about any feelings, thoughts, or questions you may be having about working with your caregiver on creating a DLS contract.*
- Ask caregiver/teen dyads the following questions and discuss their responses:
  - *How are you feeling about working on building your morning routine using a DLS contract?*
  - *What steps in your morning routine do you need to work on?*
  - *Do you know what rewards might motivate you to work on this goal?*
  - *Do you have any concerns or questions about negotiating the DLS contract with your caregiver?*
  - *Any other questions or concerns about the DLS contract?*

Common Challenges for Morning Routine Goal (3 mins)

- *Before we develop your DLS contract, let's talk through some common challenges teens have and how we can address these challenges by using proven strategies to build an effective system to target DLS goals.*
- Ask the following questions and discuss the solutions that are presented on the slide for waking up and getting out of bed:
  - *Is waking up and getting out of bed challenging for you?*

- *Which of these solutions might be helpful to include as you start working on your morning routine goal?*

- Ask the following questions and discuss the solutions that are presented on the slide for remembering the steps of the morning routine:
  - *Is remembering the steps of your morning routine challenging for you?*
  - *Which of these solutions might be helpful to include as you start working on your morning routine goal?*

- Ask the following questions and discuss the solutions that are presented on the slide for getting started:
  - *Is getting started on the steps of your morning routine challenging for you?*
  - *Would any of the solutions listed be helpful for you?*

- Ask the following questions and discuss the solutions that are presented on the slide for learning/mastering a new DLS:
  - *Are there skills or steps in your morning routine that you have not yet learned how to do on your own?*
  - *Would either of the solutions be helpful for you?*

- *Remember that the Four Laws of Behavior Change, which are meant to help with building an effective system to achieve DLS goals, are to make the goal Obvious, Easy, Attractive, and Satisfying. Strategies such as an alarm or a reminder make it obvious when you need to start a specific step. Strategies such as a checklist or a rehearsal make the goal easy because you know exactly what you need to do for each step.*
- Ask: *Are there any other challenges you want to discuss?*

Elements of an Effective System for Achieving DLS Goals (6 mins)

- The therapist should briefly ask the teen and caregiver about each of the elements and then incorporate their responses into the discussion on developing the DLS contract.
- *As we add your morning routine to the DLS contract, let's make sure we are thinking about the following elements to build an effective system for achieving DLS goals:*
  - *Teen – are we considering your strengths, challenges, preferred learning style, and commitment?*
  - *Caregiver – are we considering your parenting style, time and effort, and commitment?*
  - *Are we using evidence-based strategies?*
    - *We are using a task analysis to break the skill down into simple steps.*
  - *Are we making sure that the morning routine goal is obvious, attractive, easy, and satisfying?*
    - *Obvious – some ideas might be to put all morning routine items in the same place in the bathroom or post the task analysis in the bathroom or bedroom.*
    - *Attractive – some ideas might be to listen to music while getting ready or think about how getting your morning routine done efficiently will lead to more free time in the morning.*

    - *Easy – some ideas might be to set your alarm at the same time every weekday, give yourself plenty of time to get all of the steps done, identify two to three options for breakfast to make deciding and preparing it easy, or put all vitamins and medications in a pill box.*
    - *Satisfying – some ideas might include to identify a reward that you will earn or track your daily progress on the DLS contract.*
  - Ask and Discuss: *Any questions or comments?*

- *Let's apply all of this information to creating your first DLS contract!*

Developing Your DLS Contract (10 mins)

- Refer to the DLS Contract handout
- *We will spend the remainder of our time in today's session creating your first DLS contract to target your morning routine goal. We will use your* Task Analysis Worksheet *that you did for your Real World Practice assignment and a blank copy of the* **DLS Contract.** *The DLS contract will define your goal and can be used to track your progress. You will also define a reward to earn, which makes working on the goal satisfying!*
- The therapist should support the caregiver/teen dyad in creating the DLS contract by doing the following:
  - Incorporate all of the information from the last two sessions (e.g., rewards that are motivating for the teen, use of strategies and supports to build independence with certain steps) to create the DLS contract. The therapist should also consider the goals that the caregiver and teen collaboratively developed during the Preparing for STRW session.
  - Use the Task Analysis Worksheet handout to outline the steps of the morning routine that will be worked on (e.g., what is the step, level of independence, strategies they may benefit from).
  - Use the DLS Contract handout to specify the (1) goal, (2) expectations, and (3) reward.
    - It will be important to make sure that the goal and expectations are realistic and doable for the teen. For example, if they are only able to complete two out of eight steps independently, they may want to work towards doing three to four steps independently with the necessary strategies and supports in place (e.g., alarm clock to get up, checklist of all steps posted in the bathroom, etc.).
  - Encourage the caregiver/teen dyad to work together and model appropriate and supportive coaching as they develop the DLS contract.
  - OPTIONAL – It may be helpful to use actual supplies from the teen's morning routine and/or practice their morning routine in the actual setting (e.g., bathroom). If this cannot be done in session, the caregiver and teen could practice this together before they start targeting the morning routine goal on the DLS contract.

- Possible discussion questions that may be helpful to ask and discuss when creating the DLS contract include:
  - *How often are you going to need to do the routine – every day, every weekday?*
  - *What steps of your morning routine do you need help with?*
  - *What steps do you not know how to do?*

  - *What steps of your morning routine are you doing independently?*
  - *How easy/hard do you think it will be to meet your morning routine goal?*
  - *What reward would you like to earn?*
  - *Does the reward fit the goal? For example, earning 1 hour of screen time for doing your morning routine goal each day is a lot, but maybe earning 15–20 extra minutes of screen time each day would be a better fit.*
  - *How will you check in about your goal daily to discuss if goal was met?*
  - *Where can you post your contract so that you can track goals daily and remember to get your reward if it was earned?*

- The caregiver and teen should write each goal, expectation, and reward on the DLS Contract handout. It may be helpful for the therapist to share their screen and add/modify the goals, expectations, and rewards on a fillable PDF of the DLS Contract handout. The therapist can then email it to the caregiver and teen after the session.
- When the DLS contract has been completed, encourage the dyad to sign it and post it somewhere where they can easily see it so that the goals can be tracked.

Real World Practice (2 mins)

- Refer to the Real World Practice handout.
- Discuss the details of the Real World Practice assignment.
  - *Work on your morning routine goal for the remainder of the week using your DLS contract.*
    - *It may be helpful to do a sort of rehearsal of your morning routine so that you can practice it before you officially start tracking your goal on the DLS contract. This may make it more likely that you earn your reward because you will figure out if there are areas that are challenging and if there is a strategy that you can put into place to help!*
    - *Set aside a specific time such on the way to school or after dinner to discuss how the morning routine went and how to problem-solve for the next day.*
    - *Make sure that if the teen earns the reward, they receive it immediately! This makes it more likely that they will continue to be motivated to meet their goal!*
  - *While at the store, choose a personal hygiene product and purchase it using cash. You will want to make sure you get the right amount of change back.*

- Ask: *Any questions about your Real World Practice assignment?*

Guess the Price (3 mins) – OPTIONAL

- *Let's play a quick round of Guess the Price, which is just meant to be a fun way to build up your understanding of how much things cost.*
- *Let's see if you know the prices of some common personal hygiene items even if they are not necessarily items that you use!*
- The therapist can have the teen guess the price or have the caregiver and teen compete against each other.

- The therapist should click through the next four slides that contain examples of common personal hygiene items. Prior to the session, the therapist will need to look up the prices to ensure that they are accurate.
  - Therapists can change the personal hygiene items for the Guess the Price game.
  - This activity is meant to be fun and engaging! If the teen is averse to playing the game, it can be skipped. However, it would be helpful for the caregiver and teen to find other ways to build up an understanding of what things cost (e.g., compare the cost of products at the grocery store, involve the teen when purchasing personal hygiene items).

Roadmap for Future STRW Sessions (1 min)

- *Over the next several months, you will add goals to your DLS contract that focus on your morning routine, cleaning your room, doing laundry, cooking, grocery shopping, and managing your money. Your contract at the end of STRW may look similar to what is shown here.*
- *While it can feel like a lot to work on all of these goals at once, we will work together to ensure that they are doable. By committing time and energy to meeting the goals on your DLS contract, you will increase the skills that you can do independently and also learn what strategies can be used to learn more DLS in the future.*
- Ask: *Are there any questions about the goals we will be working on over the next several weeks?*

Preparing for the Next Dyad Session (1 min)

- *We will have our next caregiver/teen dyad session on DAY and TIME. At this session, we will discuss how to clean your bedroom and will add that as the second goal on your DLS contract.*
- *It will be important to complete your Real World Practice assignment before our next dyad session and come prepared to discuss it. We will spend a lot of time next session talking about how the DLS contract went!*
- Ask: *Are there any questions before we end the session?*

Wrap-Up

- The therapist should send a calendar invite with the next caregiver/teen dyad session's day/time to the caregiver and teen. The therapist may also want to send the caregiver/teen a copy of the DLS contract if they completed it using a fillable PDF.

Daily Living Skills Contract

Date ______________________

Goal	Expectations	Reward	MONDAY	TUESDAY	WEDNESDAY	THURSDAY	FRIDAY	SATURDAY	SUNDAY

______________________ Teen

______________________ Parent / Caregiver

Daily Living Skills Contract

Date ____________________

Goal	Expectations	Reward	MONDAY	TUESDAY	WEDNESDAY	THURSDAY	FRIDAY	SATURDAY	SUNDAY
Morning Routine	Complete 10 of 11 steps without a reminder on 4/5 weekdays. Post checklist in room and bathroom. Check in with mom when done.	Choice of dinner on the weekend							
Cleaning Bedroom	Clean bedroom on Sunday using checklist. Check with mom when done.	1 hour of extra screen time							
Laundry	Do 1 load from start to finish. Set alarm for starting and switching loads.	30 minutes of extra screen time							
Cooking	Help mom/dad cook dinner from start to finish on Wednesday nights.	Choice of dinner to cook and then eat							
Grocery Shopping & Money	Assist with finding items on the family's grocery list. Pay for items with mom's debit card.	Choice of item at the grocery store							

____________________ Teen

____________________ Parent / Caregiver

Task Analysis

Skill Morning Routine

Step	Can you do this step independently?	What could you do to become more independent?
Wake up on my own	Sometimes - 2 out of 5 days	Set my phone alarm; Put an alarm on my desk so I have to get out of bed
Get dressed	Yes	
Wash face	Sometimes - 3 out of 5 days	Put all of my morning routine supplies in a basket by the sink; Put checklist in bathroom
Brush teeth	Sometimes - 3 out of 5 days	Put all of my morning routine supplies in a basket by the sink; Put checklist in bathroom
Put deodorant and body spray on	Rarely - 1 out of 5 days	Put all of my morning routine supplies in a basket by the sink; Put checklist in bathroom
Comb hair	Rarely - 1 out of 5 days	Put all of my morning routine supplies in a basket by the sink; Put checklist in bathroom
Pack backpack (laptop, wallet, phone)	Sometimes - 3 out of 5 days	Put a checklist of supplies for my backpack by the hook near back door
Take medication and vitamin	Yes	Continue to use my pillbox

Daily Living Skills Contract

Date ____________________

Goal	Expectations	Reward	MONDAY	TUESDAY	WEDNESDAY	THURSDAY	FRIDAY	SATURDAY	SUNDAY
Morning Routine	Complete 6 out of 8 steps independently on Monday-Friday. Check in with Mom to make sure I completed each step.	30 minutes of extra screen time each day I meet my goal.							

____
Teen

____
Parent / Caregiver

Task Analysis

Skill ______________________

Step	Can you do this step independently?	What could you do to become more independent?

Daily Living Skills Contract

Date ______________________

Goal	Expectations	Reward	MONDAY	TUESDAY	WEDNESDAY	THURSDAY	FRIDAY	SATURDAY	SUNDAY

______________________ Teen

______________________ Parent / Caregiver

Surviving and Thriving in the Real World
Session 3 – Real World Practice

- Work on your morning routine goal for the remainder of the week using your DLS contract.
  - Set aside a specific time (e.g., on the way to school, after dinner) to discuss how the morning routine went and how to problem-solve for the next day.
  - Make sure that if a reward is earned, it is provided immediately!

- While at the store, choose a hygiene product and purchase it using cash. You will want to make sure you get the right amount of change back.
  - Schedule a day/time to complete the money assignment.

Surviving & Thriving in the Real World

Session 4

Cleaning the Bedroom

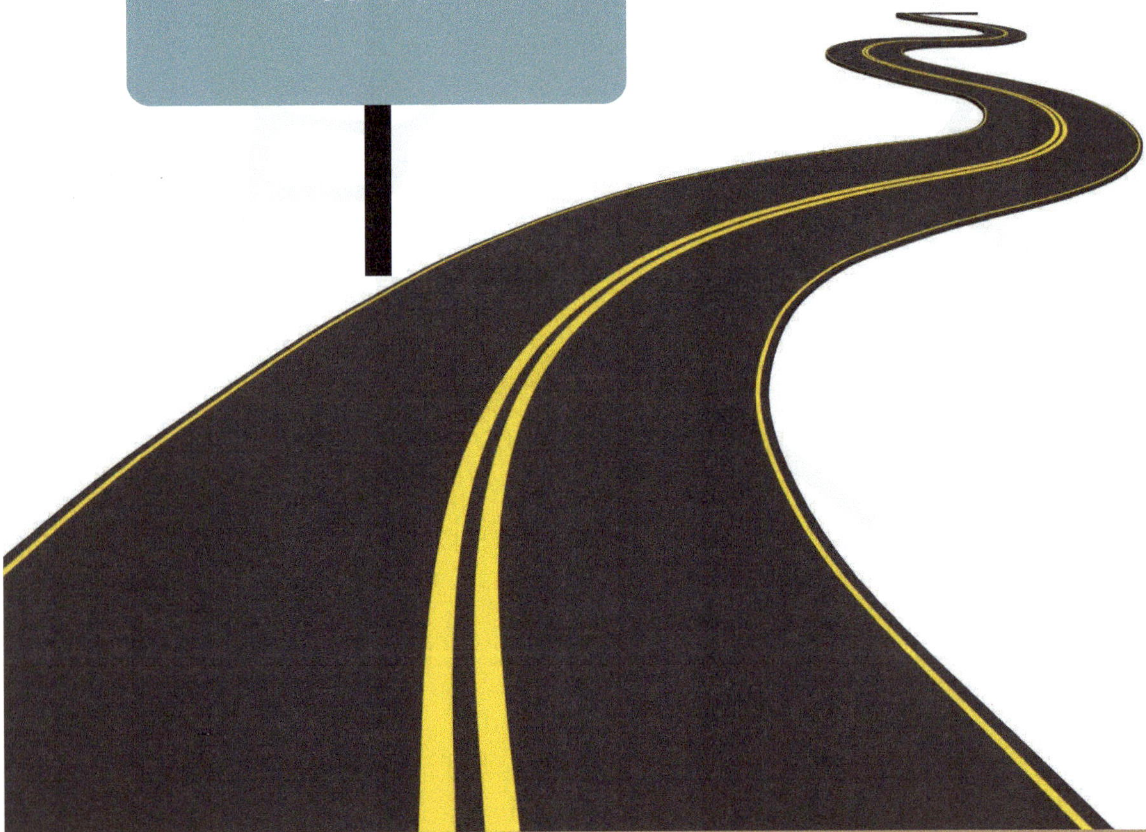

Session 4

Cleaning the Bedroom

Aims

- Continue to build rapport between caregiver group members and the therapist
- Continue to build rapport between the teen, caregiver, and therapist
- Further develop ability to use a DLS contract to set a DLS goal, define expectations, and identify a reward for meeting the goal
- Review the four elements for developing an effective system to achieve the teen's DLS goals
- Discuss the rationale for keeping one's bedroom clean
- Identify the steps for cleaning a bedroom using a task analysis
- Understand how to use the DLS Teaching Method to learn a new DLS
- Create and implement a DLS contract to target the goals of morning routine and cleaning the bedroom

Structure

- Caregiver group session via telehealth
- Caregiver/teen dyad session via telehealth

Session Supplies

- Caregiver Group Handouts
  - Tips for Creating a Successful DLS Contract
  - DLS Contract

- Caregiver/Teen Dyad Handouts
  - Task Analysis Steps
  - DLS Teaching Method for Cleaning Your Bedroom
  - DLS Contract
  - Session 4 – Real World Practice

- Videos
  - None

DOI: 10.4324/9781003458838-7

Caregiver/Teen Preparation for Session

- None

Therapist Preparation for Session

- The therapist may want to review the Example Task Analyses handout (see appendix), which includes examples of how STRW teen participants broke down the steps for the tasks of morning routine, nighttime routine, cleaning the bedroom, and laundry. These may be helpful to get an understanding of how detailed to get when creating task analyses with caregiver and teen participants.
- The therapist may want to review the Strategies Commonly Used to Target Goals on the DLS Contract handout (see appendix), which includes the evidence-based strategies, supports, and tools that teens utilize as they work on their DLS goals of morning routine, cleaning the bedroom, laundry, cooking, grocery shopping, and money management. It may be beneficial for therapists to review these prior to facilitating these sessions and developing the DLS contract with the caregiver/teen dyads.
- The therapist should use the Real World Practice Tracking Sheet (see "Therapist Resources") for each caregiver/teen dyad in all subsequent STRW sessions to track progress on their DLS contract goals.
- The therapist should consider reviewing the Tips for STRW Therapists: How to Facilitate Achievement of DLS Goals handout prior to each caregiver group session or dyad session for tips and strategies on how to help teens achieve the goals on their DLS contract. Tips that may be beneficial for Session 4 include:
  - *Affirm the teen's progress towards DLS goals.* During the Real World Practice Check-In, the therapist should actively recognize and acknowledge any positive change or progress made by the teen with the support of their caregiver. Affirming not only communicates that the therapist understands the caregiver and the teen but also may facilitate continued growth.
  - *Be curious.* As another way to strengthen the collaborative relationship with the caregiver and teen, the therapist should ask questions that will increase their insight and understanding as they target DLS goals. Questions to ask might include "What strategy do you think might work for targeting this goal?", "What do you see as potential obstacles?", or "What ideas do you have?"

Session 4 Notes

- The therapist can choose to go over group rules whenever it is beneficial for the caregivers or teens. However, it will no longer be included in the PowerPoint slides for this and subsequent sessions.

- Caregiver Group Session
  - The therapist should plan on devoting the majority of the caregiver group session to reviewing how the DLS contract is progressing for each caregiver. This is an opportunity to identify any issues and brainstorm solutions prior to the dyad session.

- Therapists should share their expertise about how to target goals using the DLS contract and give direct guidance, instruction, and feedback to caregivers. This is particularly important as caregivers develop an understanding and comfort level with using the contract.
- It is also essential that therapists demonstrate curiosity about the teen's progress towards their goals by asking the caregiver questions (e.g., "What strategy do you think would work best for your teen?" or "Were you surprised by the teen's choice of reward?") and making comments (e.g., "I wonder how we could fade back the reminders that your teen needs in the morning").
- The therapist should refer to the Tips for Creating a Successful DLS Contract handout as needed in this session and in future sessions. This handout reviews some of the important points to keep in mind when working towards a goal on the DLS contract (e.g., clearly defining expectations, re-evaluating rewards regularly to ensure they are motivating, etc.).
- It is important for all caregivers to actively participate and share their experiences during the weekly caregiver group session. This normalizes challenges that they may be experiencing (e.g., teen is not motivated to complete DLS, caregiver is feeling overwhelmed by having to prompt and remind teen about completing DLS). By actively sharing challenges, this also allows for the therapist to understand what is going on outside of the dyad session, which may increase the likelihood of identifying possible solutions. Further, other caregivers will then be able to not only offer support but also suggest ideas for challenges.
- The therapist should make an active effort to ask the other caregivers if they have any ideas about the challenges that other caregivers are experiencing when implementing the DLS contract (e.g., how to identify additional motivators, use of specific strategies to remember to do certain steps of the morning routine, etc.). This will foster additional collaboration and support between the group members.
- The therapist should discuss with caregivers that most teens will not start cleaning their room in Session 4. The main goal is to create a task analysis of the steps to identify what steps the teens need to learn, watch, or practice. Most teens will then add a goal to their DLS Contract that involves a step or multiple steps for cleaning their room. Caregivers are often involved as they provide instruction, support, or feedback.

♦ Dyad Session

- It may be helpful to use a fillable PDF of the DLS Contract handout (available on the STRW website) when reviewing progress during the Real World Practice Review in the dyad session. This may also streamline the discussion when developing the new DLS Contract at the end of the session (e.g., modifying goals, changing rewards, etc.). Further, the DLS Contract handout can then document the progress the teen is making on their goals over the course of the STRW intervention (e.g., how the morning routine goal changed from Session 3 to Session 14). The DLS Contract handout can then be emailed to the caregiver and teen after the dyad session.

- Some teens may benefit from using tracking tools that specifically indicate their daily or weekly progress towards meeting the DLS contract goals and earning a reward. Checklists are the most common tracking tools (e.g., posting the DLS contract and checking off when goals have been met, using a whiteboard to check off when a teen has successfully completed the steps of their morning routine). Tracking tools are helpful because they (1) clearly document progress towards a goal, (2) provide a visual reminder to teens about the goal, (3) may remind caregivers about the teen's progress and success, and (4) increase accountability of the caregiver to provide the reward.
- It can be helpful to cluster DLS tasks that are completed in the same location together. For example, when completing their morning routine before going to school, a teen could cluster the steps by location, including bedroom (e.g., get dressed, put pajamas in hamper, pack backpack) and bathroom (e.g., brush teeth, wash face, put deodorant on), before progressing to other steps in other locations (e.g., eating breakfast in the kitchen).
- If a teen is very skilled and/or is averse to being taught specific skills (e.g., what cleaning products to use), the therapists can allow them to take the lead (e.g., come up with the steps that they need for cleaning their room).
- It can be helpful for the therapist to ask open-ended questions when getting an understanding of the teen's skills so that they get practice with coming up with possible solutions to challenges (e.g., "What ideas do you have for storing your books in your room?").
- When developing the DLS contract at the end of the caregiver/teen dyad session, the therapist should continue to incorporate all of the information and knowledge gained from the past several sessions (e.g., issues that were brought up during the caregiver group session, task analysis steps, discussing how to incorporate the essential elements of an effective system for achieving DLS goals, identifying appropriate rewards, etc.).
- It may be beneficial to refer to the What Motivates You? handout that was completed by the teen in Session 1 when discussing rewards in this and upcoming sessions.

Caregiver Group Session 4 Content (90 mins)

Review – Real World Practice Assignment (55 mins)

- The therapist should greet the caregivers and welcome them to the session.
- Discuss the Real World Practice assignment in detail by having all caregivers share how the first week of using the DLS contract went with their teen. Encourage caregivers to jot down any notes on a blank copy of the DLS Contract handout that they may want to discuss or incorporate into their teen's DLS contract at the next dyad session.
- This first review of the Real World Practice Assignment sets the foundation for future sessions. Therapists should actively encourage caregivers to discuss any questions or comments that they have, and therapists should strive to get a thorough understanding of successes, challenges, and any other issues that may impact the goals on the teen's DLS contract.
- Refer to the Tips for Creating a Successful DLS Contract handout as needed (see next slide) and encourage families to refer to this handout throughout the intervention.
- ***We will have everyone share how the first week of using the DLS contract to target their teen's morning routine goal went. This is an opportunity to celebrate successes and also problem-solve any challenges or obstacles that occurred so that they can be addressed in the upcoming dyad session with your teen.***
- ***We will spend the majority of our session discussing each teen's progress with the DLS contract. I will ask each of you some questions as we go through your teen's contract in detail, and everyone should feel free to offer ideas or suggestions.***
- ***You may want to jot down questions or notes on a copy of the DLS Contract handout, and feel free to ask questions or add to the discussion.***
- ***Last, it may also be helpful to refer to the Tips for Creating a Successful DLS Contract handout today and in future sessions as we discuss your teen's DLS contract.***
- Points of discussion or questions to ask each caregiver include the following:
  - DLS contract
    - ***Did the teen make progress at becoming more independent with their goal?***
    - ***What went well?***
    - ***What was difficult?***
    - ***Did they receive a reward?***
    - ***Did they use any strategies to help them to learn the skill or become more independent?***
    - ***Any obstacles or barriers?***
    - ***Do you plan on modifying any goals on the current DLS contract?***

- Purchasing an item
  - *Was your teen able to purchase an item at the store?*
  - *What went well?*
  - *What skills still need to be practiced?*

♦ Ask: *Any questions about the Real World Practice assignment?*

Tips for Creating a Successful DLS Contract – OPTIONAL

♦ This slide can be used to discuss the Tips for Creating a Successful DLS Contract handout as needed while reviewing the DLS contract with caregivers as a group. Encourage families to refer to this handout throughout the intervention.

STRW Session 4 Goals (1 min)

♦ *The goal of today's session is to discuss how we will be targeting the second DLS goal of cleaning one's bedroom using a DLS contract and other evidence-based strategies. We will also review how to build an effective system to help you and your teen achieve their DLS goals now and in the future.*

♦ Ask: *Any questions about your teen practicing the skill of cleaning their bedroom at the upcoming dyad session?*

Review Dyad Session 4 Content (32 mins)

♦ *Now we will briefly review the material that will be covered in the upcoming dyad session with your teen. This will allow you to have some time to prepare for the upcoming session. Please feel free to ask any questions as we go over the content of the dyad session.*

♦ Ask: *Any questions about your teen practicing the skill of cleaning their bedroom at the upcoming dyad session?*

♦ *Before we review the dyad session content, let's have each caregiver briefly share their teen's experience with cleaning their bedroom, which may include steps such as picking up things on the floor, making their bed, organizing their belongings, bringing dishes or cups to the kitchen, and vacuuming. This is also a time to discuss any issues – such as sharing their room with a sibling – that may impact your teen cleaning their bedroom.*

♦ After each caregiver has shared their teen's experience with cleaning their bedroom, the therapist should refer to the PowerPoint presentation slides for Dyad Session 4 while reviewing the content for the session.

♦ The therapist should have also prepared for the session by reviewing the Dyad Session 4 content discussed in the manual, which has detailed information about the content that will be covered.

♦ The important points to make while reviewing the Dyad Session 4 Content are:

- This will be the first week that we do a Real World Practice Check-In, which will ask you and your teen specific questions about the goals on the DLS contract.

This will be an opportunity to problem-solve any challenges and celebrate successes.
- The elements of an effective system for achieving DLS goals will be reviewed with the teens as it relates to the goals on the DLS contract.
- It is important to keep your room clean so that you can easily find your belongings and have an orderly and tidy space to sleep and live in.
- A task analysis will be used to identify the steps for cleaning one's room including products that might be used when cleaning it.
- The DLS Teaching Method is a process that includes the steps of (1) Learn, (2) Watch, (3) Practice, and (4) Do It Independently. This method is particularly beneficial for learning a new skill because it ensures that the teen has learned, watched, and practiced the DLS before doing it independently.
- The caregiver, teen, and therapist will work together to use a task analysis of how to clean the teen's bedroom to create the second goal to be targeted on the DLS contract over the next week. Teens will also continue to work on their morning routine goal.

- Ask: *Any questions about the content for the upcoming dyad session?*

Prep for the Next Caregiver Session (2 mins)

- *We will have our next caregiver group session on DAY and TIME. At this session, we will discuss how setting up and implementing the DLS contract went. We will also discuss how to add the goal of doing laundry to your teen's DLS contract.*
- *After your dyad session with your teen, it will be important to prioritize working on the goals on the DLS contract and the Real World Practice assignment so that we can celebrate successes and also discuss any challenges or questions that arose in the caregiver group session.*
- Ask: *Are there any questions before we end the session?*

Wrap-Up

- The therapist should send a calendar invite with the next caregiver group session's day/time to the caregiver.
- The therapist may also want to email caregivers a blank copy of the DLS contract or refer them to the STRW website.

Tips for Creating a Successful DLS Contract

- **Create a goal that:**
  - Involves collaboration between you and your teen
  - Will allow the teen to be successful
  - Is doable
  - Has clearly defined expectations
  - Will motivate the teen
  - Will make the teen's life easier
  - Will build the teen's independence

- **Use of Strategies**
  - Actively involve your teen when identifying strategies to use when working towards DLS goals (e.g., calendar reminder, alarm, smart speaker, etc.).
  - Once a strategy works for your teen (e.g., checklist), it can be used again and again as they learn new DLS.
  - Teens should be highly encouraged to try out a new strategy before deciding it does not work or they do not like it.
  - Be mindful of the prompts and reminders that you are providing to your teen and try to minimize these as they work on their goal.
  - Choose the simplest strategy or environmental modification whenever possible (e.g., post DLS contract goal and expectations, send a text message to remind teen to start making dinner, create a calendar reminder for starting laundry, etc.)
  - Try to communicate indirectly when possible (e.g., text, Post-It note reminder).

- **Rewards**
  - Involve the teen in identifying a highly motivating reward that is also in line with the goal.
  - Re-evaluate whether a reward is motivating on a regular basis (e.g., weekly).
  - Praise the teen when they make progress towards and/or meet their goal.
  - Provide constructive and positive feedback and praise to increase the teen's motivation to continue to work towards goal.

- **Expect some resistance from the teen as they work on DLS goals and become increasingly independent.**
  - Discuss how DLS are relevant to both short-term and long-term goals.
  - Discuss the natural rewards and external rewards that the teen is earning.
  - Note that DLS are needed as they transition from adolescence to adulthood.
  - You may need to sometimes ignore complaining or whining from your teen and instead praise and compliment their initiative and independence.

- **Engage in active problem-solving with your teen as issues arise, which will increase their ability to do this on their own as they enter adulthood and need to learn new DLS.**

Daily Living Skills Contract

Date ______________________

Goal	Expectations	Reward	MONDAY	TUESDAY	WEDNESDAY	THURSDAY	FRIDAY	SATURDAY	SUNDAY

______________________ Teen

______________________ Parent / Caregiver

Caregiver/Teen Dyad Session 4 Content (60 mins)

STRW Session 4 Schedule (1 min)

- The therapist should greet the caregiver and teen.
- *Let's get started! As a reminder, it will be helpful to sit together at a table so that we can all see each other and work together. Please pull out your STRW workbook that contains the handouts for all STRW sessions. This session is called Session 4 – Cleaning the Bedroom. Please turn to that section in your workbook.*
- *Let's go over the session schedule so that you know what we will be doing. Please feel free to ask any questions about our schedule!*
- Briefly go over each item on the Session Schedule.

Real World Practice Check-In: Contract and Morning Routine (10 mins)

- Refer to the Session 3 Real World Practice handout and the DLS Contract handout.
- *At the beginning of each session, we will briefly check in on how you are doing with each goal on your DLS contract. Please be honest, as this is an opportunity to talk about what is working and what is not working and do some brainstorming to address any challenges.*
- The following questions should be asked (if applicable), and the responses and any relevant notes should be entered into the Real World Practice Tracking Sheet:
  - *Did you use your DLS contract this week?*
  - *Did you work on your morning routine goal during the week?*
    - *What went well?*
    - *What was challenging?*
    - *How many days did you work on your morning routine goal?*
    - *Did you earn a reward for your morning routine goal?*
    - *How many days did you earn a reward?*
- The therapist may need to spend more time this session modifying the DLS contract and problem solving how to make a more effective system to target the DLS goal (e.g., make expectations more specific, change reward, increase/decrease number of prompts, modify the strategies being used to help with goals).
- If the therapist used a fillable PDF of the DLS Contract handout in the previous session, it may be helpful to share this on the screen so that the goal, expectations, and reward can be easily discussed.

Real World Practice Check-In: Money (2 mins)

- The following questions should be asked (if applicable), and the responses and any relevant notes should be entered into the Real World Practice Tracking Sheet:
  - *For your Real World Practice, you were also given a money assignment.*
    - *Did you work on or complete a money assignment?*
    - *What did you do?*
    - *What went well?*
    - *What was challenging?*

- Ask: *Any questions or comments about your Real World Practice assignments?*
- If the caregiver/teen dyad struggled to complete the Real World Practice assignments, the therapist should spend some time discussing how to identify days/times that they could designate to commit to working on the assignments.
  - If the therapist used a fillable PDF of the DLS Contract handout in the previous session, it may be helpful to share this on the screen so that the goal, expectations, and reward can be easily discussed.

Elements of an Effective System for Achieving DLS Goals (2–3 mins)

- Ask: *Are there any issues you want to discuss or troubleshoot related to the DLS contract?*
- Ask and Discuss: *Are we considering all of the important elements to increase the likelihood of you achieving your DLS goals by developing the most effective system?*
- If applicable, discuss how to modify any DLS goals to address (1) qualities of the teen and their caregiver; (2) use of evidence-based strategies to teach and master DLS; and (3) ensuring that goals are obvious, attractive, easy, and satisfying.

Cleaning the Bedroom (1 min)

- *Today we are going to talk about how to break down the steps for cleaning your bedroom so that you can easily transform it from being messy to being clean and organized!*
- *Cleaning your bedroom will be the second goal that you will work on using your DLS contract. We will first discuss the basics of cleaning your room and the products and supplies you may need to clean your room and then use a task analysis to break down the steps for cleaning your room. We will then work together to add it as a goal on your DLS contract.*

Basics of Cleaning the Bedroom (4–5 mins)

- Ask and Discuss: *Why should you keep your bedroom clean?*
  - *It helps you keep track of your belongings! When your room is clean and tidy, you won't have to waste time looking for things like your favorite pair of pants, your study guide for History class, or your deodorant.*

- *Having a tidy space is relaxing and puts your mind at ease – which is especially important since you need to sleep in your bedroom!*
- *It impacts your health. Taking time to clean your bedroom can decrease the amount of dust, germs, or bacteria that could be on your floor, dresser, desk, or bedding.*
- *It also prepares you for living on your own in the future because you will have to get into a good routine of cleaning your space when you live in a dorm, apartment, or house.*

♦ Ask the teen the following questions with input from the caregiver to get an understanding of the teen's current process, challenges, and use of strategies for cleaning their bedroom:
  - *Do you currently clean your bedroom?*
  - *What are the steps for cleaning your bedroom?*
  - *How often do you do it?*
  - *How long does it take?*
  - *What is challenging about keeping your bedroom clean?*
  - *What strategies work well for keeping your bedroom clean?*

♦ NOTE: If a teen has mastered the skill of cleaning their bedroom, discuss if there are ways to refine their skills (e.g., becoming more independent, cleaning or organizing their room on a more regular basis, helping out with cleaning another room such as the family room).

Basics of Cleaning the Bedroom: Using a Task Analysis (1 min)

♦ Refer to the Task Analysis Steps handout
♦ *As a reminder, a task analysis is a strategy that breaks a complex or difficult task into more manageable steps. We used a task analysis to break down the steps of your morning routine in the last session.*
♦ *Before we talk about the steps for cleaning your bedroom, let's briefly go over some common steps to include when cleaning your room and cleaning products and supplies you may use. We will then finalize the task analysis for cleaning your room so that you can add it to your DLS contract!*

Possible Steps for Cleaning the Bedroom (3 mins)

♦ Have teen read the steps for cleaning the bedroom from the PowerPoint slide:
  - Put any belongings (e.g., books, backpack, clothes) in the appropriate place.
  - Make bed.
  - Take sheets off bed and put clean sheets on bed.
  - Hang/fold clean clothes.
  - Put dirty laundry in the hamper.
  - Wipe down any surfaces (e.g., table, dresser).
  - Sweep and/or vacuum the floor.
  - Empty the trash and replace the trash bag.

- There will be some variability in the steps – so it will be helpful to ask and discuss the following questions:
  - ***Are these the same steps that you use to clean your bedroom?***
  - ***Do you need to include any additional steps such as:***
    - ***Tidying up your desk?***
    - ***Taking out any dirty dishes or food items?***
    - ***Mopping the floor?***
    - ***Spraying air freshener?***
    - ***Other tasks?***

Cleaning Products and Supplies (3 mins)

- Ask and Discuss: ***What kind of cleaning products or supplies do you use to clean your bedroom?***
  - Discuss common supplies that are needed to clean one's bedroom such as trash bags, vacuum, broom, mop, floor cleaner, dusting rags, dusting spray, air freshener, or multi-purpose cleaning spray.

- Ask: ***Do you use any organizational strategies to keep your bedroom tidy such as bins under your bed to store extra sheets or clothing, hooks on your door to hang up your sweatshirts or coats, or a trash can to throw away papers?***
  - Discuss if additional organizational strategies are needed (e.g., additional hangers to hang up clothing, bins to hold belongings, etc.)

- ***It can be helpful to incorporate cleaning supplies and any organizational strategies that you use when developing the task analysis for cleaning your room.***
- Ask: ***Any questions before we create the task analysis for cleaning your bedroom?***

Task Analysis (7–8 mins)

- Refer to the Task Analysis Steps handout.
- ***Let's take a minute to transition to having the session in your bedroom so that we can get a better understanding of what steps need to be included on the task analysis for cleaning your bedroom. As a reminder, we are not judging how clean or dirty your bedroom is, and we really just want to get an understanding of what steps need to be completed to clean your room and how you can do this independently!***
- Allow time for the caregiver and teen to transition to the teen's bedroom.
- ***Now that we are in your bedroom, let's talk through the steps for cleaning your room using a task analysis. Remember, task analysis is a strategy that we can use to make it more likely we will achieve our goal and it relates back to the Four Laws of Behavior Change for building an effective system.***
  - ***Make it EASY – A task analysis makes achieving our goals easier because all of the steps are clearly defined.***

- *Make it OBVIOUS – The task analysis helps us figure out how to make things more obvious when doing each step. For example, you could set a reminder to clean your room on Sunday nights at 6 pm, or you could put a hamper in your room to keep all of the dirty clothes off of the floor.*

- *You should write the steps for cleaning your room on the Task Analysis Steps handout so that you can use it as a checklist or to make sure you have done all of the steps.*
- Discuss the teen's steps for cleaning their room and have them write it down on their Task Analysis Steps handout. The caregiver and teen can write their responses down on the Task Analysis Steps handout or the therapist can transcribe responses directly onto the slide or onto the fillable PDF of the handout.
  - The therapist should also consider what has already been discussed thus far related to cleaning supplies and organizational strategies.

Evidence-Based Strategy: DLS Teaching Method (4 mins)

- Refer to DLS Teaching Method for Cleaning Your Bedroom handout.
- *Another evidence-based strategy that we will use is the DLS Teaching Method, which shows that we often move through the 4 steps of Learn – Watch – Practice – Do It Independently when learning a new skill.*
- *During STRW sessions, we will often use a task analysis to assist you with the Learn step before progressing to the steps of watching, practicing, and doing it independently. Depending on your experience with a new skill, you may spend less time watching and may skip right to practicing it with some feedback or help from your caregiver.*
- *Let's talk about how we will use the DLS Teaching Method to increase the likelihood that you will be able to independently clean your bedroom. This is a strategy that is helpful for many teens as they start working on cleaning their room – especially if they are not used to thoroughly cleaning it or if their caregivers often help them with cleaning their room. Let's walk through it together.*
- Read through each step of the DLS Teaching Method and go through the corresponding example of how it would be used when cleaning their room.
  - *Learn – You create a task analysis and then read through the steps for cleaning your bedroom.*
  - *Watch – Your caregiver demonstrates how to clean your bedroom by going through all of the steps and using all of the necessary cleaning products. Your caregiver may demonstrate all steps or some of the steps – depending on your experience and skill level.*
  - *Practice – You practice the steps of cleaning your bedroom, and your caregiver observes and gives feedback and support as needed after each step. You can use your task analysis as a checklist to make sure that you did each step.*
  - *Do It Independently – You clean your bedroom on your own.*

- Ask and discuss the following:
  - *What steps of cleaning your bedroom do you feel you can do independently?*
  - *Are there steps to cleaning your bedroom that you do not yet know how to do or may need some help with?*
  - *It can be helpful to watch your caregiver do steps that you have not yet learned or mastered. Are there specific steps that it might be helpful to watch your caregiver do before you start practicing the steps?*
  - *How do you feel about getting feedback and support from your caregiver as you complete the steps when practicing?*

- *In session today, we discussed the steps for cleaning your bedroom using a task analysis. Now, and as part of your DLS contract, you may need to watch your caregiver complete the steps before you start to practice cleaning your room. Over time and with more practice and feedback, you will be able to clean your room completely independently.*
- Ask: *Any questions?*

Elements of an Effective System for Achieving DLS Goals (5–6 mins)

- The therapist should briefly ask the teen and caregiver about each of the elements and then incorporate their responses into the discussion on developing the DLS contract.
- *As we work to add the goal of cleaning your bedroom to your DLS contract, let's make sure we are thinking about all of the following elements to build an effective system for achieving DLS goals:*
  - *Teen – are we considering your strengths, challenges, preferred learning style, and commitment?*
  - *Caregiver – are we considering your parenting style, time and effort, and commitment?*

- *Some caregivers find it easy to have teens practice cleaning their room at the same time that they are cleaning another part of the house. It can also be helpful for caregivers to do a "big room clean" with teens to show them all of the steps.*
  - *Are we using evidence-based strategies?*
    - *We are using a task analysis to break the skill down into simple steps. This can be used as a checklist as you are practicing some of the steps or all of the steps of cleaning your bedroom.*
    - *We are using the DLS Teaching Method to help you learn and then become independent in cleaning your bedroom.*
  - *Are we making sure that the cleaning your bedroom goal is obvious, attractive, easy, and satisfying?*
    - *Obvious – some ideas might be to put hamper in a place in your room to remind you to put dirty clothes in, post the task analysis, or put all cleaning supplies in one area of the house.*

    - *Attractive – some ideas might be to listen to music while cleaning or think about doing something fun in your room after it is clean and organized. It can also be helpful to schedule a time to clean with your whole family so that everyone is working together to clean.*
    - *Easy – some ideas might be to set a reminder/alarm to clean your room every Sunday after dinner or make sure your room has designated places to put all of your belongings.*
    - *Satisfying – some ideas might include to identify a reward that you will earn or the natural reward of having a clean bedroom where your belongings can be easily found.*
  - Ask and Discuss: *Any questions or comments?*

- *Let's apply all of this information to creating your DLS contract!*

Developing Your DLS Contract (8 mins)

- Refer to the DLS Contract handout
- *Let's spend the remainder of our time in today's session modifying your DLS contract to continue working on your morning routine goal and add in the goal of cleaning your room. Use a blank copy of the DLS Contract and the task analysis we created for cleaning your room. We will also keep in mind the importance of making sure the goal is easy, obvious, attractive, and satisfying so that you are more likely to achieve your goal. The DLS contract will have you track your progress and set up rewards for you to earn, which makes working on the goals satisfying!*

- The therapist should support the caregiver/teen dyad in creating the DLS contract by doing the following:
  - Incorporate all of the information from the last several sessions (e.g., rewards that are motivating for the teen, use of strategies to build independence with certain steps) and the Real World Practice Check-In to create the DLS contract. The therapist should also consider the goals that the caregiver and teen collaboratively developed during the Preparing for STRW session.
  - Use the task analysis for cleaning the bedroom to outline the steps that the teen will complete when working on the goal of cleaning their bedroom.
  - Use the DLS Contract handout to specify the (1) Goal, (2) Expectations, and (3) Reward for Morning Routine and Cleaning the Bedroom.
  - Encourage the caregiver/teen dyad to work together and model appropriate and supportive coaching as they develop the DLS contract.

- Possible discussion questions that may be helpful to ask and discuss when creating the contract for the Morning Routine and Cleaning the Bedroom goals include:
  - *How often are you going to need to do the goal – every day, every weekday, every other day, or once per week?*
  - *What steps of your goal do you need help with?*
  - *What steps do you not know how to do?*
  - *What steps are you doing independently?*

- *How easy/hard do you think it will be to meet your goal?*
- *What reward would you like to earn?*
- *Does the reward fit the goal? For example, earning 1 hour of screen time for doing your morning routine goal each day is a lot, but maybe earning 15–20 extra minutes of screen time would be a better fit.*
- *How will you check in about your goals daily to discuss if the goal was met?*
- *Where can you post your DLS contract so that you can track goals daily and remember to get your reward if it was earned?*

♦ The caregiver and teen should write each goal, expectation, and reward on the DLS Contract handout. It may be helpful for the therapist to share their screen and add/modify the goals, expectations, and rewards on a fillable PDF of the DLS Contract handout. The therapist can then email it to the caregiver and teen after the session.

♦ When the DLS contract has been completed, encourage the dyad to sign it and post it somewhere where they can easily see it so that the goals may be tracked.

Real World Practice (2 mins)

♦ Refer to the Real World Practice handout.

♦ Discuss the details of the Real World Practice assignment.
- *Work on your morning routine and cleaning the bedroom goals for the remainder of the week using your DLS contract.*
    - *Set aside a specific time such as on the way to school or after dinner to discuss how the morning routine went and how to problem-solve for the next day.*
    - *Schedule a day/time to work on watching and/or practicing how to clean your bedroom.*
    - *Make sure that if the teen earns the reward, they receive it immediately! This makes it more likely that they will continue to be motivated to meet their goal!*
- *While at the store or online, find and then compare the prices of different types of cleaning supplies you may use to clean your room. If any cleaning supplies are needed, purchase them using cash or a debit/credit card with the help of your caregiver.*

♦ Ask: *Any questions about your Real World Practice assignment?*

Guess the Price (3 mins) – OPTIONAL

♦ *Let's play a quick round of Guess the Price, which is just meant to be a fun way to build up your understanding of how much things cost.*

♦ *Let's see if you know the prices of some common cleaning items even if they are not necessarily items that you use!*

♦ The therapist can have the teen guess the price or have the caregiver and teen compete against each other.

♦ The therapist should click through the next four slides that contain examples of common cleaning items. Prior to the session, the therapist will need to look up the prices to ensure that they are accurate.

- Therapists can change the cleaning items for the Guess the Price game.
- This activity is meant to be fun and engaging! If the teen is averse to playing the game, it can be skipped. However, it would be helpful for the caregiver and teen to find other ways to build up an understanding of what things cost (e.g., compare the cost of products at the grocery store, involve the teen when purchasing cleaning items).

Preparing for the Next Dyad Session (2 mins)

- ***We will have our next caregiver/teen dyad session on DAY and TIME. At this session, we will discuss how to do your laundry and will add that as the third goal on your DLS contract. We will need you to prepare for the session by gathering a clean basket of laundry, and we will plan on being in your laundry area and the teen's room.***
  - NOTE: If the teen does not have access to a washing machine and dryer in their home, they can hold this session at another location (e.g., relative's house, laundromat), or they can rehearse the steps of using a washing machine and dryer with the pictures on next session's PowerPoint presentation slides.
- ***It will be important to complete your Real World Practice assignment before our next dyad session and come prepared to discuss it. We will spend a lot of time next session talking about how the DLS contract went!***
- Ask: *Are there any questions before we end the session?*

Wrap-Up

- The therapist should send a calendar invite with the next caregiver/teen dyad session's day/time to the caregiver and teen. The therapist may also want to send the caregiver/teen a copy of the DLS contract if they completed it using a fillable PDF.

Task Analysis

Skill: ______________________________

Steps:

Evidence-Based Strategy: **Daily Life Skills Teaching Method**

Cleaning Your Bedroom

LEARN

Create a task analysis for cleaning your bedroom.
Read through and discuss the task analysis steps.

WATCH

Your parent/caregiver will demonstrate how to clean your bedroom by going through all of the steps and using all of the cleaning products and supplies.

PRACTICE

You will practice the steps of cleaning your bedroom.
Your parent/caregiver will observe and give feedback and support after you complete each step.

DO IT INDEPENDENTLY

You will clean your bedroom on your own using the task analysis steps.

Daily Living Skills Contract

Date ____________________

Goal	Expectations	Reward	MONDAY	TUESDAY	WEDNESDAY	THURSDAY	FRIDAY	SATURDAY	SUNDAY

____________________ Teen

____________________ Parent / Caregiver

Surviving and Thriving in the Real World Session 4 – Real World Practice

- Work on your (1) morning routine and (2) cleaning the bedroom goals for the remainder of the week using your DLS contract.
  - Set aside a specific time (e.g., on the way to school, after dinner) to discuss how the morning routine went and how to problem-solve for the next day.
  - Schedule a day/time to work on watching and/or practicing how to clean the bedroom.
  - Make sure that if a reward is earned, it is provided immediately!

- At the store (or online), find and then compare the prices of different types of cleaning supplies you may use to clean your room. If any cleaning supplies are needed, purchase them using cash or a debit/credit card with the help of your caregiver.
  - Schedule a day/time to complete the money assignment.

Surviving & Thriving in the Real World

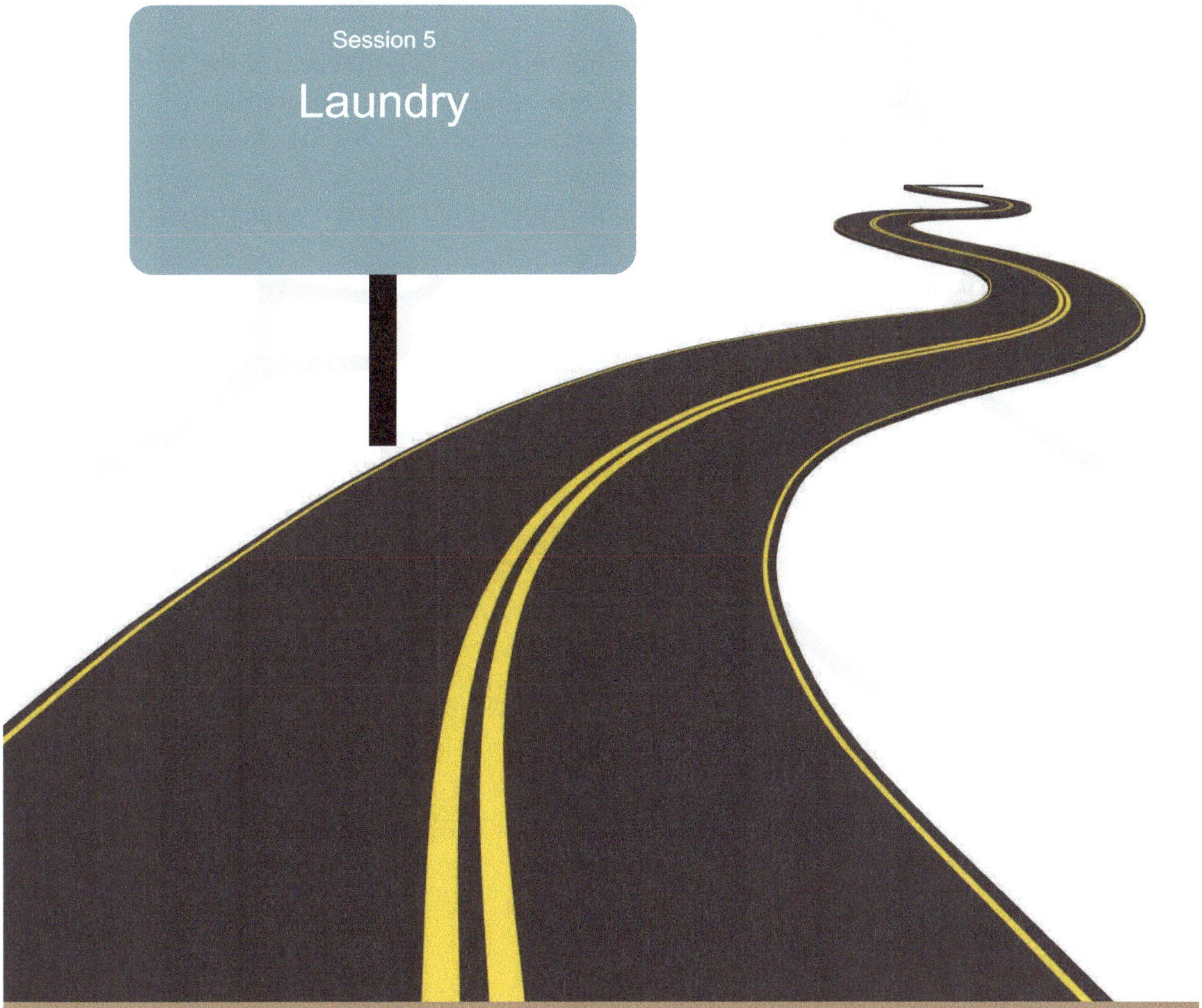

Session 5

Laundry

Aims

- Continue to build rapport between caregiver group members and the therapist
- Continue to build rapport between the teen, caregiver, and therapist
- Further develop ability to use a DLS contract to set a DLS goal, define expectations, and identify a reward for meeting the goal
- Review the four elements for developing an effective system to achieve the teen's DLS goals
- Identify the steps for doing laundry from start to finish (i.e., sorting, using the washing machine and dryer, and folding and putting clothes away)
- Understand how to use the DLS Teaching Method to learn the steps for doing laundry
- Create and implement a DLS contract to target the goals of morning routine, cleaning the bedroom, and doing laundry

Structure

- Caregiver group session via telehealth
- Caregiver/teen dyad session via telehealth

Session Supplies

- Caregiver Group Handouts
  - DLS Contract
  - STRW Resources (from Session 1)

- Caregiver/Teen Dyad Handouts
  - Laundry Task Analysis
  - Task Analysis Steps
  - DLS Teaching Method for Doing Your Laundry
  - Washing Machine and Dryer Settings
  - DLS Contract

DOI: 10.4324/9781003458838-8

- ❍ Session 5 – Real World Practice
- ❍ STRW Resources (from Session 1)

- Videos (optional links available on the STRW website and the STRW Resources handout)

Caregiver/Teen Preparation for Session

- For the dyad session, the caregiver and teen should gather a basket of clean clothing to practice doing laundry (i.e., sort, use washing machine and dryer, and fold and put clothing away). The caregiver and teen should also gather any laundry products that would be used when doing the laundry (e.g., detergent, fabric softener, dryer sheets).
- The session will be held in the laundry area of the home and also the teen's bedroom.
- If the teen does not have access to a washing machine and dryer in their home, they can hold this session at another location (e.g., relative's house, laundromat), or they can rehearse the steps of using a washing machine and dryer with the pictures in the PowerPoint presentation slides.

Therapist Preparation for Session

- The therapist may want to review the Example Task Analyses handout (see appendix), which includes examples of how STRW teen participants broke down the steps for the tasks of morning routine, nighttime routine, cleaning the bedroom, and laundry. These may be helpful to get an understanding of how detailed to get when creating task analyses with caregiver and teen participants.
- The therapist may want to review the Strategies Commonly Used to Target Goals on the DLS Contract handout (see appendix), which includes the evidence-based strategies, supports, and tools that teens utilize as they work on their DLS goals of morning routine, cleaning the bedroom, laundry, cooking, grocery shopping, and money management. It may be beneficial for therapists to review these prior to facilitating these sessions and developing the DLS contract with the caregiver/teen dyads.
- The therapist should use the Real World Practice Tracking Sheet for each caregiver/teen dyad in all subsequent STRW sessions to track progress on their DLS contract goals.
- The therapist will need to be mindful about individualizing the session for each dyad based on whether they have access to a washing machine and dryer and also based on how their family prefers to do laundry (e.g., washes all laundry on the cold cycle, uses a specific sorting method, etc.).
- The therapist should consider reviewing the Tips for STRW Therapists: How to Facilitate Achievement of DLS Goals handout prior to each caregiver group session or dyad session for tips and strategies on how to help teens achieve the goals on their DLS contract. Tips that may be beneficial for Session 5 include:
  - *Emphasize that any progress is good progress.* As the caregiver and teen work towards the goals on their DLS contract, the therapist should emphasize that any progress towards a DLS goal (e.g., becoming more independent, practicing a new skill, effectively implementing a strategy) is a step in the right direction.

- *Provide instruction and guidance in a focused and manageable way.* Therapists should let caregivers and teens know when they plan on providing instruction, giving feedback, and/or engaging in problem solving, especially as they work towards increasing independence. It will also be critical for the therapist to ensure that any guidance they provide fits with what the caregiver/teen needs. At times, therapists may find it beneficial to discuss what has worked (or not worked) for other teens as they targeted a DLS goal.
- *Be a good listener.* The therapist should take the time to listen to the caregiver and teen as they discuss their progress with the goals on the DLS contract. It can sometimes be easy to rush through parts of the session (e.g., asking the questions in the Real World Practice Check-In), but by really listening and reflecting on the dyad's responses, the therapist will be able to effectively address any obstacles or challenges.

Session 5 Notes

- The therapist can choose to go over Group Rules whenever it is beneficial for the caregivers or teens. However, it will no longer be included in the PowerPoint slides.
- Fillable PDFs of handouts from this session (i.e., Task Analysis Steps) are available on the STRW website.
- Teens may also struggle to acquire DLS due to challenges with executive functioning (e.g., cannot remember when to start the laundry), anxiety (e.g., are nervous about cooking on the stovetop, worry about the responsibility of carrying a debit card), fine or gross motor issues (e.g., struggle to fold clothing neatly, struggle to chop vegetables with a sharp knife), or sensory issues (e.g., become overwhelmed by the smells of food when cooking, do not like how water feels on their face when showering). It will be important to make individual adaptations as needed to set adolescents up for success as they are working on DLS. For example, it may be important to consult with an occupational therapist about how fine motor, gross motor, or sensory issues impact the acquisition of DLS and what adaptations may be available (e.g., using a handheld showerhead to control the flow of water when showering).
- For this session and all future sessions, it may be helpful to use a fillable PDF of the DLS Contract handout (available on the STRW website) when reviewing progress during the Real World Practice Review. This may also streamline the discussion when developing the new DLS Contract at the end of the session (e.g., modifying goals, changing rewards, etc.). Further, the DLS Contract handout can then document the progress the teen is making on their goals over the course of the STRW intervention (e.g., how the morning routine goal changed from Session 3 to Session 14). The DLS Contract handout can then be emailed to the caregiver and teen after the dyad session.

- Caregiver Group Session
  - The therapist should plan on devoting the majority of the caregiver group session to reviewing how the DLS contract is progressing for each caregiver. This is an opportunity to identify any issues and brainstorm solutions prior to the dyad session.
  - The therapist should utilize the caregiver group session to get an understanding of how it may be necessary to personalize the dyad session content (e.g., discuss

options if the teen does not have access to washing machine or dryer; identify any issues with putting clothing away in the teen's bedroom).
- During the caregiver group session, the therapist should make an active effort to foster collaboration between the group members by encouraging active discussion and problem solving of challenges or questions about the DLS contract.
- The therapist should refer to the Tips for Creating a Successful DLS Contract handout as needed in this session and in future sessions. This handout reviews some of the important points to keep in mind when working towards a goal on the DLS contract (e.g., clearly defining expectations, re-evaluating rewards regularly to ensure they are motivating, etc.).

♦ Dyad Session
  - The dyad session has a lot of content because it covers all of the steps of doing laundry. Thus, therapists will need to prepare so that they can manage time efficiently. Optional session components are clearly indicated in the manual and the PowerPoint slides (i.e., Laundry Basics video, Guess the Price activity, pictures of washing machine and dryers for those who do not have these in their home).
  - The therapist should strive to spend about 10 minutes on each of the following six main sections of the dyad session: (1) Real World Practice Check-In, (2) Sorting Laundry, (3) Using the Washing Machine, (4) Using the Dryer, (5) Folding and Putting Clothing Away, and (6) Real World Practice Assignment.
  - While the caregiver and teen are encouraged to write down the steps for doing laundry on the Task Analysis Steps handout in their workbook, the therapist can also use a fillable PDF of the Task Analysis Steps handout to write down the steps for doing laundry. This may increase the likelihood of getting through all of the material quickly and efficiently, while also allowing for effective modeling and practicing.
  - Therapists should observe the caregivers as they instruct, practice, and provide feedback and support to their teen. It will be important to model how to give constructive feedback to teens about a DLS they are learning and practicing. Therapists may also need to give caregivers feedback on how they deliver feedback or provide verbal praise and support as they are working to build DLS with their teen. This can often be addressed in the caregiver group session by reviewing the importance of constructive feedback and initiating a group discussion about how to do this with teens. It may also need to be directly addressed in the dyad session if a caregiver is being overly critical or unsupportive as their teen works on their DLS.
  - When developing the DLS contract at the end of the caregiver/teen dyad session, the therapist should continue to incorporate all of the information and knowledge gained from the past several sessions (e.g., issues that were brought up during the caregiver group session, task analysis steps, discussing how to incorporate the essential elements of an effective system for achieving DLS goals, identifying appropriate rewards, etc.). The therapist should also consider the goals that the caregiver and teen collaboratively developed during the Preparing for STRW session.

Caregiver Group Session 5 Content (90 mins)

Review – Real World Practice Assignment (50 mins)

- The therapist should greet the caregivers and welcome them to the session.
- Discuss the Real World Practice assignment in detail by having all caregivers share how the second week of using the DLS contract to target the morning routine and cleaning the bedroom goals went with their teen. Encourage caregivers to jot down notes or questions on a blank copy of the DLS Contract handout that they may want to discuss or incorporate into their teen's DLS contract at the next dyad session.
- ***We will have everyone share how the second week of using the DLS contract to target their teen's morning routine and cleaning the bedroom goals went. This is an opportunity to celebrate successes and also problem-solve any challenges or obstacles that occurred. We will spend the majority of our session discussing each teen's progress with the DLS contract. It may be helpful to jot down notes or questions on a copy of the DLS Contract handout, and feel free to ask questions or add to the discussion.***
- It may be helpful to refer caregivers to the Tips for Creating a Successful DLS Contract handout (from Session 4) when discussing the goals on the DLS contract (e.g., clearly defining expectations, re-evaluating rewards regularly to ensure they are motivating, etc.).
- Points of discussion or questions to ask each caregiver include the following:
  - DLS contract
    - ***Did the teen make progress at becoming more independent with each of their goals – morning routine and cleaning the bedroom?***
    - ***What went well?***
    - ***What was difficult?***
    - ***Did they receive a reward?***
    - ***Did they use any strategies to help them to learn the skill or become more independent?***
    - ***Any obstacles or barriers?***
    - ***Do you plan on modifying any goals on the current DLS contract?***
  - Purchasing an item
    - ***Was your teen able to compare the prices of any items?***
    - ***Was your teen able to purchase an item at the store?***
    - ***What went well?***
    - ***What skills still need to be practiced?***

- Ask: ***Any questions about the Real World Practice assignment?***

STRW Session 5 Goals (1 min)

- *The goal of today's session is to discuss how we will be targeting the third DLS goal of doing laundry from start to finish using a DLS contract and other evidence-based strategies. We will also review how to build an effective system to help you and your teen achieve their DLS goals now and in the future.*
- *At this point, we are really starting to build your teen's DLS, and it may seem overwhelming to add in another goal. With laundry, it will be helpful to keep in mind if there are ways that the teen can incorporate this into their daily or weekly schedule. For example, it may be easiest for you if the teen begins assisting you at the times that you do laundry. The goal is to still encourage independence, but depending on their skill level with laundry, this may be a great place to start instructing, modeling, and having the teen practice.*
- Ask and Discuss: *Any questions?*

Review Dyad Session 5 Content (37 mins)

- *Now we will briefly review the material that will be covered in the upcoming dyad session with your teen. This will allow you to have some time to prepare for the upcoming session. Please feel free to ask any questions as we go over the content of the dyad session.*
- *For this session, we will plan on teaching skills in the laundry area of your home. We will also plan on going into the teen's bedroom to practice folding and putting clothing away. It is a session that has a lot of content because we review all of the steps of doing laundry. It will be important to be prepared for this session by having a basket of clean clothes to practice sorting and putting clothing away. It will also be important to have your washing machine, dryer, and laundry products available so that we can review how to use these with your teen.*
- *If you do not have a washing machine and dryer at home, we can still practice this skill at home and/or we can practice it wherever you typically do laundry – such as a laundromat or a relative's home.*
- Ask: *Any questions about practicing the skill of doing laundry in your home with your teen at the upcoming dyad session?*
- *Before we review the dyad session content, let's have each caregiver briefly share their teen's experience with sorting laundry, using the washing machine and dryer, and folding and putting clothing away.*
- After each caregiver has shared their teen's experience with doing laundry, the therapist should refer to the PowerPoint presentation slides for Dyad Session 5 while reviewing the content for the session.
- The therapist should have also prepared for the session by reviewing the Dyad Session 5 content discussed in the manual, which has detailed information about the content that will be covered.
- The important points to make while reviewing the Dyad Session 5 Content are:
  - We will do a Real World Practice Check-In, which will ask you and your teen specific questions about the goals on the DLS contract. This will be an opportunity to problem-solve any challenges and celebrate successes.
  - The elements of an effective system for achieving DLS goals will be reviewed with the teens as it relates to the goals on the DLS contract. This will be our main

opportunity each session to revise the goals that are currently being targeted on the DLS contract before we add in a new goal at the end of the session.
- There are four main steps to doing laundry – sorting clothing, using the washing machine, using the dryer, and folding and putting clean clothing away.
- A task analysis is a great way to learn the steps for doing laundry – and it will be personalized for the way that your family does the laundry.
- The DLS Teaching Method is another evidence-based strategy that we have learned that is particularly useful for learning, watching, practicing, and doing the steps of laundry independently.
- Video modeling is an evidence-based strategy that may also be helpful for learning the steps of doing laundry by watching someone else discuss and demonstrate how to do laundry from start to finish.
- It is important for teens to become familiar with how to operate the washing machine and dryer that they will use and also what products, such as laundry detergent or fabric softener, they should be using.
- Teens may benefit from learning different and fun ways to fold their clothing. There are many videos that demonstrate how to quickly fold clothing. A folding board may also be a useful tool to help make folding easy and quick!

♦ Ask: ***Any questions about the content for the upcoming dyad session?***

Prep for the Next Caregiver Session (2 mins)

♦ ***We will have our next caregiver group session on DAY and TIME. At this session, we will discuss how setting up and implementing the DLS contract went. We will also discuss how to add the goal of cooking in the microwave to your teen's DLS contract.***

♦ ***To prepare for the upcoming dyad session with your teen, please gather a clean basket of clothing to practice doing laundry from start to finish. Also make sure that the washing machine, dryer, and laundry products are available at the time of the session.***

♦ ***After your dyad session with your teen, it will be important to prioritize working on the goals on the DLS contract and the Real World Practice assignment so that we can celebrate successes and also discuss any challenges or questions that arose in the caregiver group session.***

♦ Ask: ***Are there any questions before we end the session?***

Wrap-Up

♦ The therapist should send a calendar invite with the next caregiver group session's day/time to the caregiver.

♦ The therapist may also want to email caregivers a blank copy of the DLS contract or refer them to the STRW website.

♦ The therapist should email the caregiver a copy of the STRW Resources handout (see "Therapist Resources") that contains resources and links related to doing laundry (e.g., videos, visual supports). This handout is available on the STRW website (www.strw.org).

Daily Living Skills Contract

Date ______________________

Goal	Expectations	Reward	MONDAY	TUESDAY	WEDNESDAY	THURSDAY	FRIDAY	SATURDAY	SUNDAY

______________________ Teen

______________________ Parent / Caregiver

Caregiver/Teen Dyad Session 5 Content (60 mins)

STRW Session 5 Schedule (1 min)

- The therapist should greet the caregiver and teen.
- *Let's get started! As a reminder, it will be helpful to sit together at a table so that we can all see each other and work together. Please pull out your STRW workbook that contains the handouts for all STRW sessions. This session is called Session 5 – Laundry. Please turn to that section in your workbook.*
- *Let's go over the session schedule so that you know what we will be doing. Please feel free to ask any questions about our schedule!*
- Briefly go over each item on the Session Schedule.
- Check to make sure that the caregiver and teen have a basket of clean clothing that can be used to practice sorting, using the washing machine and dryer, and folding and putting clothing away. If not, they should get a basket of clothing now.

Real World Practice Check-In: Contract and Morning Routine (3 mins)

- Refer to the Session 4 Real World Practice handout and the DLS Contract handout.
- *Let's check in on how you are doing with each goal on your DLS contract. Please be honest, as this is an opportunity to talk about what is working and what is not and do some brainstorming to address any challenges.*
- The following questions should be asked (if applicable), and the responses and any relevant notes should be entered into the Real World Practice Tracking Sheet:
  - *Did you use your DLS contract this week?*
  - *Did you work on your morning routine goal during the week?*
    - *What went well?*
    - *What was challenging?*
    - *How many days did you work on your morning routine goal?*
    - *Did you earn a reward for your morning routine goal?*
    - *How many days did you earn a reward?*

- The therapist may need to spend more time this session on modifying the DLS contract and problem-solving how to make a more effective system to target the DLS goal (e.g., make expectations more specific, change reward, increase/decrease number of prompts, modify the strategies being used to help with goals).
- If the therapist used a fillable PDF of the DLS Contract handout in the previous session, it may be helpful to share this on the screen so that the goal, expectations, and reward can be easily discussed.

Real World Practice Check-In: Cleaning the Bedroom and Money (5 mins)

- The following questions should be asked (if applicable), and the responses and any relevant notes should be entered into the Real World Practice Tracking Sheet:
  - *Did you work on your cleaning the bedroom goal during the week?*
    - *What went well?*
    - *What was challenging?*
    - *How many days did you work on your cleaning the bedroom goal?*
    - *Did you earn a reward for your cleaning the bedroom goal?*
  - *For your Real World Practice, you were also given a money assignment.*
    - *Did you work on or complete a money assignment?*
    - *What did you do?*
    - *What went well?*
    - *What was challenging?*

- Ask: *Any questions or comments about your Real World Practice assignments?*
- If the caregiver/teen dyad struggled to complete the Real World Practice assignments, the therapist should spend some time discussing how to identify days/times that they could designate to commit to working on the assignments.
- If the therapist used a fillable PDF of the DLS Contract handout in the previous session, it may be helpful to share this on the screen so that the goal, expectations, and reward can be easily discussed.

Elements of an Effective System for Achieving DLS Goals (2 mins)

- Ask: *Are there any issues you want to discuss or troubleshoot related to the DLS contract?*
- Ask and Discuss: *Are we considering all of the important elements to increase the likelihood of you achieving your DLS goals by developing the most effective system?*
- If applicable, discuss how to modify any DLS goals to address (1) qualities of the teen and their caregiver; (2) use of evidence-based strategies to teach and master DLS; and (3) ensuring that goals are obvious, attractive, easy, and satisfying.

Laundry Basics (3 mins)

- *Today we are going to talk about how to break down the steps for doing your laundry. Doing your laundry will be the third goal that you will work on using your DLS contract. We will first break down and discuss the basics of doing each step of laundry using a task analysis. The task analysis that we create can be used as a checklist to help you with learning the steps, practicing the steps, and then checking to make sure that you completed each step.*
- *We also use the DLS teaching method of Learn, Watch, Practice, and Do Independently as we work on the skill of laundry. For example, if you have never done laundry, it may be helpful to watch your caregiver as they teach you the steps for loading the washing machine, measuring the detergent, and choosing the correct*

cycle. If you have some experience using the washing machine, you may have your caregiver watch you load laundry and have them give you feedback if needed.

- *There are four main steps of laundry that we will be discussing today, which are illustrated by the picture showing the journey of a shirt.*
  - *The first step is sorting and separating dirty clothes into categories such as whites, darks, and delicates.*
  - *The second step is loading and using the washing machine.*
  - *The third step is loading and operating the dryer.*
  - *The final step is folding and putting clean clothing away.*

- Ask the teen the following questions to get an understanding of their current process, challenges, and use of strategies when doing laundry:
  - *Do you currently do your own laundry?*
  - *What steps do you do independently?*
  - *What steps do you need help with?*
  - *What strategies work well for doing laundry and putting it away?*

- If a teen has mastered the skill of laundry, discuss if there are ways to refine their skills (e.g., helping out with the entire family's laundry, washing bedding or towels, putting clothing away more neatly, etc.).

Laundry Basics Video (1 min)

- *Watching videos to learn new skills is another evidence-based strategy that can be used to learn DLS. On the* STRW Resources *handout that you were given in Session 1, we included a video of a college student doing his laundry at home that includes all four steps of sorting/separating clothing, using the washing machine, using the dryer, and folding clothing before putting it away. The student describes how he does laundry while also demonstrating the steps. It may be helpful to watch this video and some of the other videos on the* STRW Resources *handout to learn more about doing your laundry and other DLS.*

Task Analysis: Sorting (2–3 mins)

- Refer to the Laundry Task Analysis handout and the Task Analysis Steps handout. The steps on the Laundry Task Analysis handout should be used as a guide, and the dyad should write down the steps for sorting on the Task Analysis Steps handout that is specific to how they sort dirty laundry in their family. It may also be helpful for the therapist to write down the steps for doing laundry on a fillable PDF of the Task Analysis Steps handout.
- Have the dyad move the session to the laundry area (i.e., where the washing machine and dryer are located) and bring a laundry basket of clean clothes that can be used to practice doing laundry.
- If the family does not have a washing machine/dryer, the pictures of the washing machine and dryer in the PowerPoint slides should be used to illustrate how to go through the steps of using the washing machine and dryer. Dyads can also practice doing their laundry at the laundromat or another location if they feel comfortable doing this.

- If time allows, the therapist and the dyad could also watch a video on how to do laundry (see STRW Resources handout for possible videos to watch).

- ***We will go through the steps for each of the four parts of doing laundry, and we want you to write down the steps on the Task Analysis Steps handout that apply to how you and your family do the laundry. This task analysis will be longer than the ones for your morning routine and cleaning your room, but it can still be used as a checklist as you work towards doing all of the steps of laundry independently.***
- Have the teen read the steps for sorting laundry. The goal of this activity is to get the teens thinking about the steps that need to be completed each and every time that they do their laundry.
- Ask and Discuss:
  - ***Is this the same way that your family sorts laundry?***
  - ***Are there steps of sorting laundry that are hard or easy for you?***

Evidence-Based Strategy: DLS Teaching Method-Doing Your Laundry (1 min)

- Refer to DLS Teaching Method for Doing Your Laundry handout.
- ***Just like for cleaning your bedroom, we will use a task analysis and the DLS Teaching Method to increase the likelihood that you will be able meet your goal of doing your own laundry. In session today, you will learn the steps for doing laundry, watch your caregiver demonstrate the steps, and get some practice doing the steps of laundry. As part of your DLS contract in the coming weeks, you will continue to practice and then do the steps of laundry independently.***
- Ask: *Any questions?*

Sorting Activity (3 mins)

- ***We are now going to use the DLS Teaching Method to work on our laundry skills. The first skill we will work on is the skill of sorting. We will have your caregiver do the steps of Learn and Watch, and then we will have you Practice sorting.***
- The therapist should do the following for the first three steps of the DLS Teaching Method as it relates to sorting:
  - LEARN – First, instruct the caregiver to use the task analysis to review how they sort laundry.
  - WATCH – Then, instruct the caregiver to demonstrate how to sort three to four pieces of laundry while explaining how and why they sorted it the way that they did.
  - PRACTICE – Finally, instruct the teen to practice the skill and instruct the caregiver to provide feedback or support as needed.

- The therapist should provide feedback and support to the caregiver as needed, including giving clear directions about what to sort, giving their teen an opportunity to sort the clothing before providing any feedback, and modeling how to give feedback (e.g., explanation of how to tell if a load is too large and needs to be broken into two loads, verbal reminder to check pockets, and explanation of why a sweater may be considered delicate).

Task Analysis: Using the Washing Machine (2 mins)

- Refer to the Laundry Task Analysis handout and the Task Analysis Steps handout.
- Dyad should write down the steps for using the washing machine on the Task Analysis Steps handout that is specific to how they use the washing machine. It may also be helpful for the therapist to write down the steps for using the washing machine on a fillable PDF of the Task Analysis Steps handout.
- *Let's read through the steps of Using the Washing Machine, and then we want you to write down the steps on the Task Analysis Steps handout that apply to how you and your family will be using the washing machine to do laundry.*
- Ask and Discuss:
  - *Is this the same way that your family uses the washing machine?*
  - *Are there steps of using the washing machine that are hard or easy for you?*

Washing Machine Products (2 mins)

- *These products are commonly used when washing clothing in the washing machine.*
- *The top row of products are all various types of detergent. Detergent is basically soap that gets your clothes clean. Detergent can come in the form of a pod, liquid, or powder. Depending on your washing machine, you may put the detergent directly in the washing machine with your clothing or in a slot located on your washing machine.*
- *Bleach is used to clean white clothing. Most washing machines have a specific slot for you to pour bleach into. You do not want to pour bleach directly on clothing because it could ruin the clothing. The product labeled Clorox on the slide is bleach.*
- *Fabric softener is used to make clothes feel softer, smell better, and may keep clothes from fading or accumulating fuzz. You will either put the fabric softener directly into the washing machine with your clothing or in a slot located on your washing machine. The product labeled Downy on the slide is fabric softener.*
- Ask: *What kind of products does your family use to wash clothing?*
- Instruct the caregiver to identify the actual washing machine product(s) that are used.

Washing Machine Settings (2 mins)

- Refer to the Washing Machine and Dryer Settings handout.
- *In this Washing Machine Settings table, you can see the different options for both water temperature and the washing machine cycle or setting for various types of clothing. Each washing machine is different, and you will need to work with your caregiver to identify the correct settings on your own washing machine. You will also want to talk with your caregiver about how they do laundry. For example, some families wash everything on the Permanent Press cycle, while some families wash different clothes on different settings.*
- Instruct the caregiver to discuss and demonstrate the washing machine cycles that they typically use and refer to the Washing Machine and Dryer Settings handout as needed:
  - Normal/Regular setting – select this when washing items such as socks, underwear, light-colored cotton clothing, towels, and bedding.

- Permanent Press setting – select this for brightly colored clothes. This cycle washes with warm water and ends with cooler water, which keeps clothing looking brighter. Darker cotton shirts and sweatpants, jeans, khakis, polo shirts, hoodies, and sweatshirts should be washed on this cycle.
- Delicates/Gentle setting – select this when washing delicate clothing such as cotton sweaters, dress shirts, dress pants, bras, some types of activewear, and dresses.
- Whites setting – select this when washing white clothing because this cycle uses hot water to keep clothing bright white instead of fading.

Example Washing Machine – OPTIONAL

- If the caregiver and teen do not have access to a washing machine, this slide can be used to discuss the different settings and what settings the caregiver typically uses to do laundry throughout the session (i.e., Washing Machine Settings, Washing Machine Activity).

Washing Machine Activity (3 mins)

- ***We are now going to use the DLS Teaching Method to practice using the washing machine. We will have your caregiver do the steps of Learn and Watch, and then we will have you Practice using the washing machine.***
- The therapist should do the following for the first three steps of the DLS Teaching Method as it relates to using the washing machine:
  - LEARN – First, instruct the caregiver to use the task analysis to review how they use the washing machine to do a load of laundry.
  - WATCH – Then, instruct the caregiver to demonstrate how to choose the wash cycle, put the detergent in, and start the washing machine.
  - PRACTICE – Finally, instruct the teen to practice the skill of choosing the cycle, putting the detergent in, and starting the washing machine, and instruct the caregiver to provide feedback or support as needed.

- The therapist should provide feedback and support to the caregiver as needed, including giving clear directions (e.g., which cycle to choose) and modeling various steps (e.g., how much liquid detergent to put in).

Task Analysis: Using the Dryer (2 mins)

- Refer to the Laundry Task Analysis handout and the Task Analysis Steps handout.
- The dyad should write down the steps for using the dryer on the Task Analysis Steps handout that is specific to how they use the dryer. It may also be helpful for the therapist to write down the steps for using the dryer on a fillable PDF of the Task Analysis Steps handout.
- ***Read through the steps of Using the Dryer and then write down the steps on the Task Analysis Steps handout that apply to how you and your family will be using the dryer.***
- Ask and Discuss:
  - ***Is this the same way that your family uses the dryer?***
  - ***Are there steps to using the dryer that are hard or easy for you?***

Dryer Products (1 min)

- ***These products are commonly used when drying clothes. Both dryer sheets and dryer balls are meant to reduce the time it takes for your clothes to dry, decrease static cling, and soften your clothes.***
- Ask and Discuss:
  - ***Does your family use dryer sheets or dryer balls?***
  - ***Does your family use any other products when drying their clothes?***

- Instruct the caregiver to identify the actual product(s) they use for the dryer.

Dryer Settings (3 mins)

- Refer to the Washing Machine and Dryer Settings handout.
- ***In this Dryer Settings table, you can see the different options for dryer cycles or settings for various types of clothing. Each dryer is different, and you will need to work with your caregiver to identify the correct settings on your own dryer and how to use the dryer to do laundry.***
- Instruct the caregiver to discuss and demonstrate the dryer cycles/settings that they typically use and refer to the following information on dryer settings as needed:
  - Permanent Press setting – dark and light cottons, jeans, socks and underwear, bedding, and towels should be dried on this setting because it uses medium heat that makes it less likely that fabrics will fade.
  - Regular/Normal setting – white clothing should be dried on this setting because it can handle more intense heat
  - Delicates/Gentle setting – any clothing that was washed on the delicate cycle should be dried on the delicate cycle. This setting uses close to room temperature air and a slow drying cycle to decrease the likelihood of damage to clothing.

Example Dryer – OPTIONAL

- If the caregiver and teen do not have access to a dryer, this slide can be used to discuss the different settings and what settings the caregiver typically uses to do laundry throughout the session (i.e., Dryer Settings, Dryer Activity).

Dryer Activity (2 mins)

- ***We are now going to use the DLS Teaching Method to practice using the dryer. We will have your caregiver do the steps of Learn and Watch, and then we will have you Practice using the dryer.***
- The therapist should do the following for the first three steps of the DLS Teaching Method as it relates to using the dryer:
  - LEARN – First, instruct the caregiver to use the task analysis to review how they use the dryer.
  - WATCH – Then, instruct the caregiver to demonstrate how to choose the dryer cycle, put the clothing in, put any products in, and start the dryer.

- PRACTICE – Finally, instruct the teen to practice the skill of choosing the cycle, putting the clothing in, putting the products in, and starting the dryer. Instruct the caregiver to provide feedback or support as needed.

♦ The therapist should provide feedback and support to the caregiver as needed, including giving clear directions (e.g., choosing the correct dryer setting) and modeling various steps (e.g., using fabric softener).

Task Analysis: Folding and Putting Clothing Away (2–3 mins)

♦ Have the dyad move the session to an area where they can either fold laundry easily (e.g., kitchen table) or to the teen's bedroom so that the caregiver and teen can practice how to fold and put clothing away in the teen's bedroom. A basket of clean clothing will be needed to practice folding.

♦ *The last step in doing laundry is folding clothing and putting it away in your bedroom. This may mean folding clothing and putting it in a dresser drawer or on a closet shelf or hanging clothing in a closet. The exact way that you do this depends on your own preferences and how you organize the clothing in your room.*

♦ *Ideally, you want to immediately fold and put your clothes away after they have finished drying so that they are less likely to become wrinkled. Some people may also fold their clothes into a laundry basket before putting them away. Some people may also use a "wrinkle release" setting on their dryer if time has passed and the clothes have remained in the dryer for a long time.*

♦ *Read through the steps of Folding and Putting Clothing Away on the Task Analysis Steps handout, and then write down the steps that apply to you and your family.*
  - It may also be helpful for the therapist to write down the steps for folding and putting clothing away on a fillable PDF of the Task Analysis Steps handout.

♦ Ask and Discuss:
  - *How does your family typically get ready to fold clothing and put it away?*
  - *Do either of you have any tips or ideas to increase the likelihood of being successful with folding and putting clothing away?*

Videos on Folding Clothing (1 min)

♦ *There are several videos that you may find useful on the STRW Resources handout that illustrate how to quickly fold shirts, hoodies, pants, and other clothing. You can watch these after the session if you are interested in in learning how to fold quickly!*

Using a Flipboard to Fold (1 min)

♦ *A flipboard is another tool that can be used to easily fold pants, shirts, sweaters, and even towels and sheets. These can be made out of stiff cardboard boxes or bought at a store. There are several videos on the STRW Resources handout that demonstrate how to use a flipboard to fold clothing.*

Folding Activity (4 mins)

- *We are now going to use the DLS Teaching Method to practice folding clothing. We will have your caregiver do the steps of Learn and Watch, and then we will have you Practice folding.*
- The therapist should do the following for the first three steps of the DLS Teaching Method as it relates to folding clothing:
  - LEARN – First, instruct the caregiver to use the task analysis to review how they fold and put clothing away. The caregiver should discuss where the teen should put away clothing items such as shirts, pants, socks, shorts, underwear, socks, and dress clothes.
  - WATCH – Then, instruct the caregiver to demonstrate how to fold and put clothing away. It would be helpful for them to demonstrate folding a shirt, pair of pants, pair of socks, and long-sleeved shirt/dress shirt.
  - PRACTICE – Finally, instruct the teen to practice the skill of folding and putting clothing away. They should practice using the same items of clothing that their caregiver demonstrated with.

- The therapist should provide feedback and support to the caregiver as needed, including giving clear directions (e.g., how to fold a pair of pants) and modeling how to fold and put clothing away.
- The therapist should also problem-solve or brainstorm any potential issues (e.g., difficulties with hanging items up, putting all short-sleeve t-shirts in one drawer and all long-sleeve shirts in a different drawer).

Elements of an Effective System for Achieving DLS Goals (3 mins)

- The therapist should briefly ask the teen and caregiver about each of the elements and then incorporate their responses into the discussion on developing the DLS contract.
- *As we work to add the goal of doing your laundry to the DLS contract, let's make sure we are thinking about all of the following elements to build an effective system for achieving DLS goals:*
  - *Teen – are we considering your strengths, challenges, preferred learning style, and commitment?*
    - *If you are a visual learner, it can be helpful to put a sticker or Post-It note on the washing machine cycle that you will likely be using. You could also use number stickers to indicate the order that buttons are pushed on the washer or dryer.*
  - *Caregiver – are we considering your parenting style, time and effort, and commitment?*
    - *Some caregivers find it easy to have teens practice doing laundry alongside them or on a particular day or time that they typically do the laundry.*
  - *Are we using evidence-based strategies?*
    - *We are using a task analysis to break the skill down into simple steps that can be used as a checklist as you learn, practice, and master laundry.*

    - *We are also using the DLS Teaching Method to help you learn and become independent in doing the skill of laundry.*
    - *There are several videos you can use to help with folding and putting clothing away on the* **STRW Resources** *handout.*
  - *Is the goal of doing your laundry obvious, attractive, easy, and satisfying?*
    - *Obvious – some ideas might be that the task analysis is posted, all laundry supplies are in one area, or the washing machine and dryer settings are posted.*
    - *Attractive – some ideas might be to do something fun while waiting to switch laundry from the washer to the dryer.*
    - *Easy – some ideas might be to set a reminder or alarm to do laundry every Wednesday after school or to use a folding board to fold laundry.*
    - *Satisfying – some ideas include earning a reward for completing this goal on the DLS contract or the natural reward of having clean clothing and an empty hamper!*

- Ask and Discuss: *Any questions or comments?*
- *Let's apply all of this information to creating your DLS contract!*

Developing Your DLS Contract (6 mins)

- Refer to the DLS Contract handout.
- *Let's spend the remainder of our time in today's session modifying your DLS contract to continue working on your morning routine and cleaning your bedroom goals and add in the goal of doing laundry. Use a blank copy of the DLS Contract and the task analysis we created for doing laundry. We will also keep in mind the importance of making sure the goal is easy, obvious, attractive, and satisfying so that you are more likely to achieve your goal. The DLS contract will have you track your progress and identify rewards for you to earn, which makes working on the goals satisfying!*
- The therapist should support the caregiver/teen dyad in creating the DLS contract by doing the following:
  - Incorporate all of the information from the last several sessions (e.g., rewards that are motivating for the teen, use of strategies and supports to build independence with certain steps) and the Real World Practice Check-In to create the DLS contract. The therapist should also consider the goals that the caregiver and teen collaboratively developed during the Preparing for STRW session.
  - Use the task analysis for doing laundry to outline the steps that the teen will complete when working on the goal of doing laundry.
  - Incorporate information from the teen practicing the steps of doing laundry over the course of the dyad session (e.g., if folding was difficult, this step could be added later, or the caregiver may need to provide some assistance).
  - Use the DLS Contract handout to specify the (1) Goal, (2) Expectations, and (3) Reward for Morning Routine, Cleaning the Bedroom, and Doing Laundry.
  - Encourage the caregiver/teen dyad to work together and model appropriate and supportive coaching as they develop the DLS contract.

- Possible discussion questions that may be helpful to ask and discuss when creating the DLS contract for the Morning Routine, Cleaning the Bedroom, and Laundry goals include:
  - *How often are you going to need to do the goal – every day, every weekday, every other day, or once per week?*
  - *What steps of your goal do you need help with?*
  - *What steps do you not know how to do?*
  - *What steps are you doing independently?*
  - *How easy or hard do you think it will be to meet your goal?*
  - *What reward would you like to earn?*
  - *Does the reward fit the goal? For example, earning 1 hour of screen time for doing your morning routine goal each day is a lot, but maybe earning 15–20 extra minutes of screen time would be a better fit.*
  - *How will you check in about your goals daily to discuss if goal was met?*
  - *Where can you post your DLS contract so that you can track goals daily and remember to get your reward if it was earned?*

- The caregiver and teen should write each goal, expectation, and reward on the DLS Contract handout. It may be helpful for the therapist to share their screen and add/modify the goals, expectations, and rewards on a fillable PDF of the DLS Contract handout. The therapist can then email it to the caregiver and teen after the session.
- When the DLS contract has been completed, encourage the dyad to sign it and post it somewhere where they can easily see it so that the goals may be tracked.

Real World Practice (1 min)

- Refer to the Real World Practice handout.
- Discuss the details of the Real World Practice assignment.
  - *Work on your morning routine, cleaning the bedroom, and laundry goals for the remainder of the week using your DLS contract.*
    - *Set aside a specific time such as on the way to school or after dinner to discuss how the morning routine went and how to problem-solve for the next day.*
    - *Schedule a day/time to work on watching and/or practicing how to clean your bedroom or do laundry.*
    - *Make sure that if a reward is earned, it is received immediately! This makes it more likely that you will continue to be motivated to meet your goal!*
  - *Practice making a small purchase at the store using cash. Make sure to get the correct change.*

- Ask: *Any questions about your Real World Practice assignment?*

Guess the Price (3 mins) – OPTIONAL

- NOTE: This activity can be skipped if there is not enough time to complete it.
- *Let's play a quick round of Guess the Price, which is just meant to be a fun way to build up your understanding of how much things cost.*
- *Let's see if you know the prices of some common laundry items even if they are not necessarily items that you use!*

- The therapist can have the teen guess the price or have the caregiver and teen compete against each other.
- The therapist should click through the next four slides that contain examples of common laundry items. Prior to the session, the therapist will need to look up the prices to ensure that they are accurate.
  - Therapists can change the laundry items for the Guess the Price game.
  - This activity is meant to be fun and engaging! If the teen is averse to playing the game, it can be skipped. However, it would be helpful for the caregiver and teen to find other ways to build up an understanding of what things cost (e.g., compare the cost of products at the store, involve the teen when purchasing cleaning items).

Preparing for the Next Dyad Session (2 mins)

- ***We will have our next caregiver/teen dyad session on DAY and TIME. At this session, we will discuss how to use a knife, make no-cook recipes, and use the microwave to cook. You will add a cooking goal as the fourth goal on your DLS contract. We will need you to prepare for the session by doing the following:***
  - ***Make sure that you have a knife, cutting board, and fruits or vegetables to practice cutting.***
  - ***Gather ingredients for no-cook recipes. Examples are a hummus wrap, bagel and cream cheese, or a peanut butter and jelly sandwich. Think about what you might like to learn how to cook!***
  - ***Gather ingredients for a microwave recipe. Examples include mug desserts, quesadilla, soup, or mac and cheese. Think about a recipe you would like to master or one that you have been wanting to learn!***
  - ***We will also be spending the majority of the session in your kitchen.***

- ***I will check in with you by email in a few days to remind you to get the items you need to make the no-cook and microwave recipes. It is sometimes easiest to just use ingredients you already have at home!***
- ***It will be important to complete your Real World Practice assignment before our next dyad session and come prepared to discuss it. We will spend a lot of time next session talking about how the DLS contract went!***
- Ask: ***Are there any questions before we end the session?***

Wrap-Up

- The therapist should send a calendar invite with the next caregiver/teen dyad session's day/time to the caregiver and teen. The therapist may also want to send the caregiver/teen a copy of the DLS contract if they completed it using a fillable PDF.
- The therapist can email the caregiver and teen some ideas for no-cook recipes or microwave recipes if needed or refer them to the STRW Resources handout.

Laundry Task Analysis

Sorting:

1. Remove clothes from hamper or basket
2. Check pockets and remove items from pockets
3. Make pile of light everyday clothes
4. Make pile of dark everyday clothes
5. Make pile of delicate clothes
6. Make pile for towels and/or bedding
7. If too large, separate piles into two loads

Washing:

1. Choose pile of clothes to wash
2. Set correct temperature and cycle on washing machine
3. Open lid or door to washing machine
4. Measure cup of laundry detergent
5. Pour cup of detergent into washer
6. Put clothes into washer without over-filling
7. Close lid or door
8. Push/pull button or knob to start the machine
9. Set timer on phone for reminder to check load

Drying:

1. Remove lint from dryer filter if dirty
2. Check tags of clothing if needed (to make sure they can go in the dryer)
3. Place appropriate clothing items into dryer one at a time (not a huge pile all at once)
4. For items that air dry, hang on hanger or lay flat on table to dry
5. Put dryer sheet in dryer
6. Close dryer door
7. Set appropriate cycle for dryer
8. Push/pull knob or button to start
9. Set timer on phone for reminder to check load

Folding:

1. Check dryer when timer goes off
2. Clean lint out of dryer filter
3. Immediately remove and fold clothes to prevent wrinkling
4. Put appropriate clothes on hangers
5. Hang up clothes on hangers in closet
6. Fold t-shirts, shorts, pants, underwear appropriately
7. Put away appropriate clothes in dresser and in correct drawer
8. Match pairs of socks and put away

Task Analysis

Skill: ______________________________

Steps:

____

____

____

____

____

____

____

____

____

____

____

____

____

____

____

____

____

____

____

Evidence-Based Strategy: **Daily Life Skills Teaching Method**

Laundry

LEARN

Create a task analysis for doing your laundry.
Read through and discuss the task analysis steps.

WATCH

Your parent/caregiver will demonstrate how to sort clothing, use the washing machine and dryer, and fold and put clothing away.

PRACTICE

You will practice the steps of doing your laundry.
Your parent/caregiver will observe and give feedback and support after you complete each step.

DO IT INDEPENDENTLY

You will do laundry on your own using the task analysis steps.

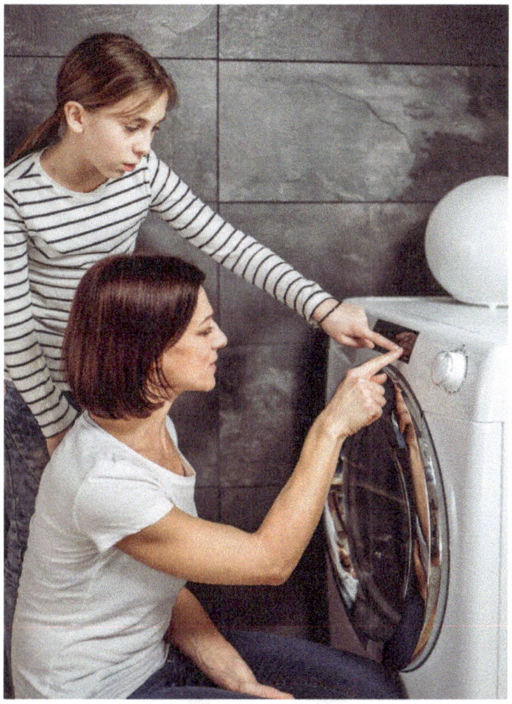

Washing Machine Settings

Clothing Type	Temp	Wash Cycle/ Setting
• Light everyday cottons • Socks and underwear • Bedding • Towels	Warm/Cold	Normal/ Regular
• Dark everyday cottons • Denim jeans	Cold	Permanent Press
• Dress clothes • Sweaters	Cold	Delicate/ Gentle
• Whites	Hot	Whites

Dryer Settings

Clothing Type	Dryer Cycle/ Setting
• Dark everyday cottons • Light everyday cottons • Denim Jeans • Socks and underwear • Bedding • Towels	Permanent Press
• Whites	Regular/Normal
• Dress clothes • Sweaters	Delicate/Gentle

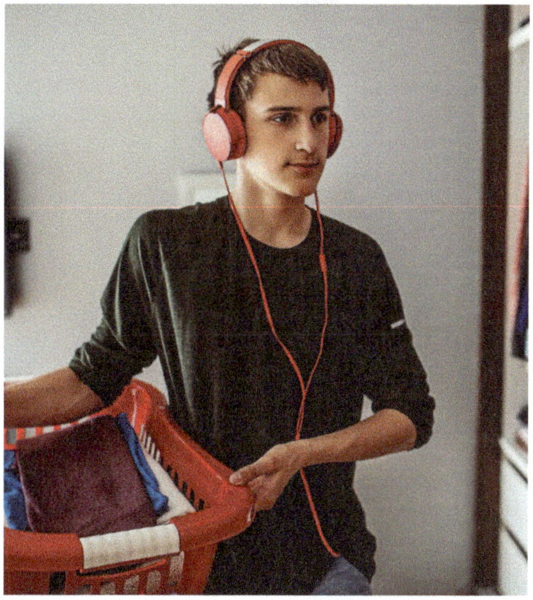

Daily Living Skills Contract

Date ______________________

Goal	Expectations	Reward	MONDAY	TUESDAY	WEDNESDAY	THURSDAY	FRIDAY	SATURDAY	SUNDAY

____
Teen

____
Parent / Caregiver

Surviving and Thriving in the Real World Session 5 – Real World Practice

- Work on your (1) morning routine, (2) cleaning the bedroom, and (3) doing laundry goals for the remainder of the week using your DLS contract.
  - Set aside a specific time (e.g., on the way to school, after dinner) to discuss how the morning routine went and how to problem-solve for the next day.
  - Schedule a day/time to work on watching and/or practicing how to clean the bedroom and do laundry.
  - Make sure that if a reward is earned, it is provided immediately!

- Practice making a small purchase at the store using cash. Make sure to get the correct change!
  - Schedule a day/time to complete the money assignment.

Surviving & Thriving in the Real World

Session 6

Kitchen Safety and Microwave Cooking

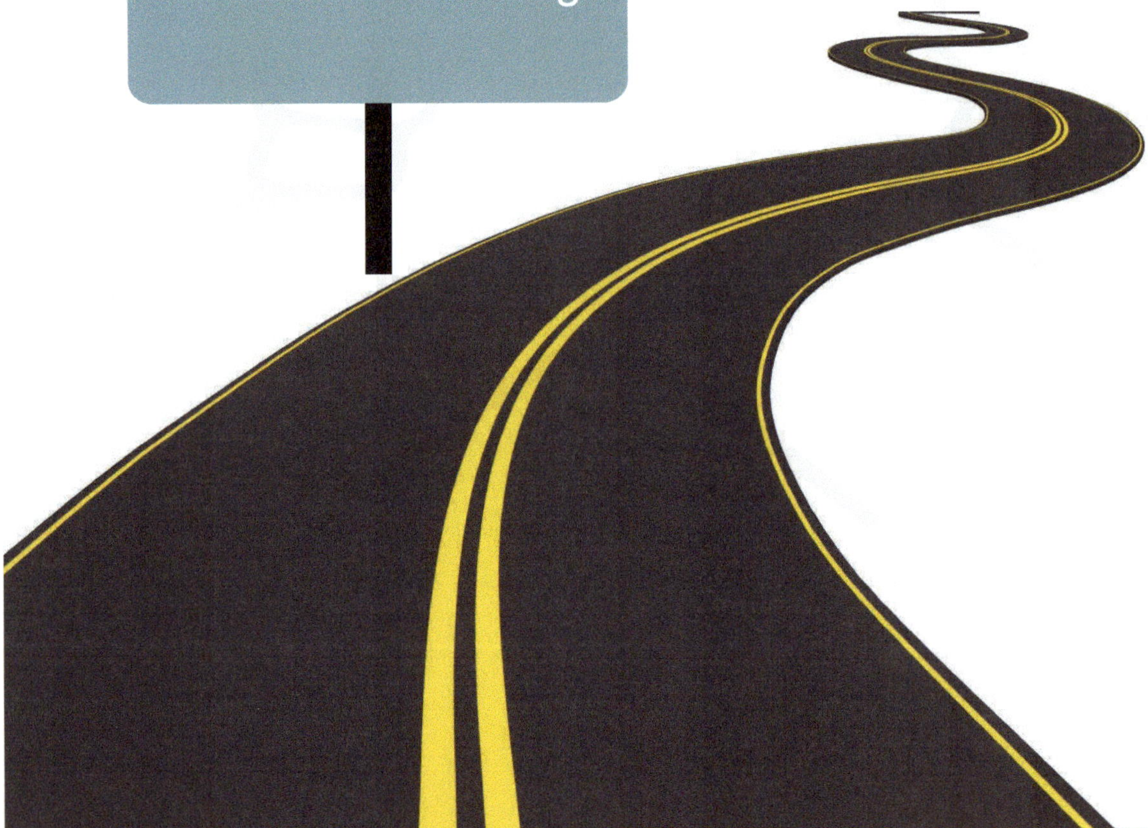

Session 6

Kitchen Safety and Microwave Cooking

Aims

- Continue to build rapport between caregiver group members and the therapist
- Continue to build rapport between the teen, caregiver, and therapist
- Further develop ability to use a daily living skills (DLS) contract to set a DLS goal, define expectations, and identify a reward for meeting the goal
- Review the four elements for developing an effective system to achieve the teen's DLS goals
- Understand basic kitchen safety concepts
- Understand how to use the DLS Teaching Method to learn the steps for using a knife to cut up fruits/vegetables, cooking a no-cook recipe, and cooking a microwave recipe
- Create and implement a DLS contract to target the goals of morning routine, cleaning the bedroom, doing laundry, and cooking

Structure

- Caregiver group session via telehealth
- Caregiver/teen dyad session via telehealth

Session Supplies

- Caregiver Group Handouts
  - DLS Contract

- Caregiver/Teen Dyad Handouts
  - DLS Teaching Method for Cooking in the Microwave
  - Task Analysis Steps
  - Microwave Cheese Quesadilla Recipe
  - Kitchen Safety Rules
  - DLS Teaching Method for Cutting with a Knife
  - DLS Teaching Method for No-Cook Recipes

DOI: 10.4324/9781003458838-9

- DLS Contract
- Session 6 – Real World Practice

- Videos (optional links available on the STRW website and the STRW Resources handout)

Caregiver/Teen Preparation for Session

- For the dyad session, the caregiver and teen should have identified a no-cook recipe and a microwave recipe that they want to cook during this session. They should also have the ingredients needed to make both of these recipes.
- For the dyad session, the caregiver and teen should also have access to a cutting board, knife, and fruit/vegetable so that they can practice cutting with a knife.
- It would be highly beneficial for the caregiver and teen to practice these skills in the kitchen area that is free from as many distractions as possible (e.g., siblings, noise from the television, etc.).

Therapist Preparation for Session

- The therapist may want to review the Strategies Commonly Used to Target Goals on the DLS Contract handout (see appendix), which includes the evidence-based strategies, supports, and tools that teens utilize as they work on their DLS goals of morning routine, cleaning the bedroom, laundry, cooking, grocery shopping, and money management. It may be beneficial for therapists to review these prior to facilitating these sessions and developing the DLS contract with the caregiver/teen dyads.
- The therapist may want to review the Recipe Ideas for the STRW Cooking Sessions handout (see appendix), which includes ideas of recipes to cook if the caregiver/teen are having trouble identifying what to cook in Sessions 6–8.
- The therapist should use the Real World Practice Tracking Sheet for each caregiver/teen dyad in all subsequent STRW sessions to track progress on their DLS contract goals.
- The therapist will need to be mindful about individualizing the session for each dyad based on whether they have access to a microwave and also based on the foods that their family cooks and eats on a regular basis (e.g., have the dyad work together to identify recipes to cook and recipes that include ingredients that they often have readily available in their kitchen).
- The STRW Resources handout has resources for adaptive kitchen equipment that may be helpful for some teens (e.g., cutting gloves, adaptive cutting boards).
- The therapist should consider reviewing the Tips for STRW Therapists: How to Facilitate Achievement of DLS Goals handout prior to each caregiver group session or dyad session for tips and strategies on how to help teens achieve the goals on their DLS contract. Tips that may be beneficial for Session 6 include:
  - *Be a good observer.* The therapist has the unique opportunity to "be" in the teen's home while they receive instruction and practice new DLS with the support of their caregiver. It can often be beneficial to observe whether there are any environmental modifications that can easily be made (e.g., how to organize

the teen's closet to make putting clothing away easier, where to post visual reminders, how to streamline morning routine steps).

- *Label the teen's progress to instill a sense of pride.* Therapists should identify and describe the teen's progress with a goal to stimulate internal feelings of pride, accomplishment, and independence. Many teens may prefer this to the therapist or caregiver praising them ("Great work!"), labeling emotions ("It must be exciting to make this much progress!"), or stating their own emotions ("I am so proud of you.").
- *Establish an open and collaborative relationship with the teen and caregiver.* STRW therapists have expertise in how to target the development of age-appropriate daily living skills in adolescents using evidence-based strategies and supports. However, caregivers and teens are truly experts in themselves (e.g., strengths, challenges, what strategies work for them, what motivates them), which is equally critical when creating, targeting, and modifying DLS goals. Some things to keep in mind:
- Teens should be encouraged to think about what strategies will work best for them when developing or modifying goals and expectations!
- Caregivers should be given an opportunity to provide their feedback and thoughts about what is working or not working. It can be helpful to discuss this in the caregiver group session so that the caregiver can openly share and then make a plan for how to discuss it with the teen. For example, the therapist may provide ideas on how the caregiver can balance providing honest feedback with praise when discussing the DLS contract.

Session 6 Notes

- Fillable PDFs of handouts from this session (i.e., Task Analysis Steps, DLS Contract) are available on the STRW website.
- The use of notifications, alarms, and reminders is particularly helpful for reminding a teen to get started on or complete a task. These can be set on phones, laptops/tablets, smart speakers (e.g., Amazon Echo), smart watches, or alarm clocks. It can be helpful to set recurring notifications or alarms (e.g., alarm to wake up at 6:30 am on Monday–Friday, calendar reminder to cook dinner on Tuesdays at 5 pm, alarm to remember to switch the laundry to the dryer).
- If a teen has too many notifications and reminders on their phone, they may not pay attention to reminders or alarms for their DLS goals. It can be helpful to adjust their notification settings to make it more likely that the technology strategies will be effective for building DLS.

- Caregiver Group Session
  - The therapist should plan on devoting the majority of the caregiver group session to reviewing how the DLS contract is progressing for each caregiver. This is an opportunity to identify any issues and brainstorm solutions prior to the dyad session.
  - The therapist should utilize the caregiver group session to get an understanding of how it may be necessary to personalize the dyad session content (e.g., discuss options if the teen does not have a microwave, brainstorm possible recipes for the teen to cook with the caregiver).

- The therapist should make an active effort to foster collaboration between the group members by encouraging active discussion and problem solving of challenges or questions about the DLS contract.
- The therapist should have caregivers discuss how they can encourage cooking on a regular basis and get ideas from other caregivers. It can often feel overwhelming to add in another goal to the DLS contract, but cooking is a goal that can typically be done alongside a caregiver because there are likely several times during the week that they are preparing food or cooking a meal.

♦ Dyad Session
- The therapist should encourage the caregiver, in collaboration with their teen, to choose a recipe that they are motivated to learn how to cook (and eat) but should also encourage them to identify recipes for ingredients that they consistently have in their kitchen and/or may be beneficial for the teen to learn how to cook (e.g., to help with dinner prep, to become more independent with making their own breakfast, etc.).
- It may be helpful to have the caregiver/teen dyad complete a <u>Task Analysis Steps</u> handout for both the no-cook recipe and the microwave recipe. This would help them get into the habit of following the steps of a recipe when cooking.
- If the teen does not have access to a microwave, they can choose another appliance to practice cooking (e.g., blender, air fryer, grill, toaster, etc.) or prepare another no-cook recipe.
- The therapist will need to manage time effectively so that teens get an opportunity to cut with a knife and make both a no-cook and microwave recipe. Some suggestions include:
    - Incorporate the cutting activity into the actual recipe that the teen is cooking in the microwave (if applicable).
    - The session can end prior to the item being completely cooked or ready to eat.
    - Have a copy of the recipe available to share on the therapist's computer screen so that the steps are displayed while the caregiver and teen are cooking.
- It is highly recommended that the therapist use video modeling to demonstrate how to use a knife safely (video link is available on the <u>STRW Resources</u> handout and the STRW website). While the caregiver can also demonstrate, it can be highly beneficial for the teen to see the appropriate technique demonstrated via video.
- The therapist can encourage caregivers to point out where various items can be found in the kitchen (e.g., fire extinguisher, knife, cutting board) if the teen is not aware of where to find these items.
- When developing the DLS contract at the end of the dyad session, the therapist should continue to incorporate all of the information and knowledge gained from the past several sessions (e.g., issues that were brought up during the caregiver group session, task analysis steps, discussing how to incorporate the essential elements of an effective system for achieving DLS goals, identifying appropriate rewards, etc.).

Caregiver Group Session 6 Content (90 mins)

Review – Real World Practice Assignment (50 mins)

- The therapist should greet the caregivers and welcome them to the session.
- Discuss the Real World Practice assignment in detail by having all caregivers share how using the DLS contract to target the morning routine, cleaning the bedroom, and laundry goals went with their teen. Encourage caregivers to jot down notes or questions on a blank copy of the DLS Contract handout that they may want to discuss or incorporate into their teen's contract at the next dyad session.
- ***We will have everyone share how using the DLS contract to target the morning routine, cleaning the bedroom, and laundry goals went for their teen. This is an opportunity to celebrate successes and also problem-solve any challenges or obstacles that occurred. We will spend the majority of our session discussing each teen's progress with the DLS contract. It may be helpful to jot down notes or questions on a copy of the DLS Contract handout, and feel free to ask questions or add to the discussion.***
- It may be helpful to refer caregivers to the Tips for Creating a Successful DLS Contract handout (from Session 4) when discussing the goals on the DLS contract (e.g., clearly defining expectations, re-evaluating rewards regularly to ensure they are motivating, etc.).
- Points of discussion or questions to ask each caregiver include the following:
  - DLS contract
    - ***Did the teen make progress at becoming more independent with each of their goals – morning routine, cleaning the bedroom, laundry?***
    - ***What went well?***
    - ***What was difficult?***
    - ***Did they receive a reward?***
    - ***Did they use any strategies to help them to learn the skill or become more independent?***
    - ***Any obstacles or barriers?***
    - ***Do you plan on modifying any goals on the current DLS contract?***
  - Purchasing an item
    - ***Was your teen able to purchase an item at the store?***
    - ***What went well?***
    - ***What skills still need to be practiced?***

- Ask: ***Any questions about the Real World Practice assignment?***

STRW Session 6 Goals (1 min)

- *The goal of today's session is to discuss how we will be targeting the next DLS goals of understanding kitchen safety concepts, cutting with a knife, making a no-cook recipe, and cooking in the microwave. We will also review how to build an effective system to help you and your teen achieve their DLS goals now and in the future.*
- *At this point, we are really starting to build your teen's DLS, and it may seem overwhelming to add in another goal. With cooking, it will be helpful to keep in mind if there are ways that the teen can incorporate this into their daily or weekly schedule. For example:*
    - *Could the teen make their own breakfast – such as a waffle or oatmeal?*
    - *Could the teen make their own lunch – such as a sandwich or cheese quesadilla?*
    - *Could the teen make a snack for themselves after school?*
    - *Could the teen help you prepare a meal during the week? For example, they could chop up vegetables or get all of the ingredients for a recipe.*

- Ask and Discuss: *Any questions?*

Review Dyad Session 6 Content (36 mins)

- *Now we will briefly review the material that will be covered in the upcoming dyad session with your teen. This will allow you to have some time to prepare for the upcoming session. Please feel free to ask any questions as we go over the content of the dyad session.*
- *For this session, we will plan on teaching skills in the kitchen area of your home. It is a session that has a lot of hands-on practice as the teen practices cutting with a knife, making a no-cook recipe, and making a microwave recipe. It will be important to be prepared for this session by having a no-cook recipe, a microwave recipe, a knife, a cutting board, a fruit or vegetable to cut up, and any ingredients needed for the recipes. We also want you to think about possible recipes that your teen can cook to further build their skills and are not just recipes that they already have experience cooking.*
- *It will also be important to have your microwave available. If you do not have a microwave, we can still practice the skill of cutting and no-cook recipes and can possibly identify another appliance that your teen could use to practice cooking such as an air fryer, toaster, or blender.*
- Ask: *Any questions about practicing these cooking skills in your home with your teen at the upcoming dyad session?*
- *Before we review the dyad session content, let's all briefly share our teen's abilities to do the following:*
    - *Use a knife to cut up fruits or vegetables*
    - *Make no-cook recipes such as a sandwich, cereal, waffles in the toaster, or a smoothie in the blender*
    - *Use the microwave to cook soup, popcorn, macaroni and cheese, or oatmeal*

- The therapist should refer to the PowerPoint presentation slides for Dyad Session 6 while reviewing the content for the session. The therapist should have also prepared for the session by reviewing the Dyad Session 6 content discussed in the manual, which has detailed information about the content that will be covered.

- The important points to make while reviewing the Dyad Session 6 Content are:
  - We will do a Real World Practice Check-In, which will ask you and your teen specific questions about the goals on the DLS contract. This will be an opportunity to problem-solve any challenges and celebrate successes.
  - The elements of an effective system for achieving DLS goals will be reviewed with the teens as it relates to the goals on the DLS contract. This will be our main opportunity each session to revise the goals that are currently being targeted on the DLS contract before we add in a new goal at the end of the session.
  - The DLS Teaching Method will be used to teach cooking skills for the next several sessions, and teens will become familiar with the steps of learning, watching, practicing, and doing it independently.
  - A recipe is basically a task analysis that not only breaks down what ingredients are needed but also specifies each step that needs to be completed when cooking. Many recipes also have corresponding videos that can be particularly helpful if a teen benefits from learning new skills from video modeling.
  - Basic safety rules related to wiping up spills, fire safety, and hygiene will be discussed briefly so that teens have a basic understanding that can be discussed in more detail as they develop their cooking skills.
  - Knife skills will be taught using video modeling and the DLS Teaching Method as caregivers demonstrate and then teens practice cutting a fruit or vegetable with a knife.
  - Teens will use the DLS Teaching Method and a recipe to make a no-cook recipe and a microwave recipe.
  - Teens will learn about the features of their microwave and how to operate it before cooking a recipe.

- Ask: ***Any questions about the content for the upcoming dyad session?***

Prep for the Next Caregiver Session (2 mins)

- ***We will have our next caregiver group session on DAY and TIME. At this session, we will discuss how setting up and implementing the DLS contract went. We will also discuss how to add the goal of cooking in the oven to your teen's DLS contract.***
- ***To prepare for the upcoming dyad session with your teen, please choose a no-cook recipe and a microwave recipe and have the ingredients available. These can be items that you have in your home already. You should try to involve your teen in choosing the recipes so that they are more motivated to build their cooking skills.***
- ***Also make sure to have a knife, cutting board, and a fruit or vegetable to cut.***
- ***Last, make sure that the kitchen is available at the time of your session.***
- ***After your dyad session with your teen, it will be important to prioritize working on the goals on the DLS contract and the Real World Practice assignment so that we can celebrate successes and also discuss any challenges or questions that arose in the caregiver group session.***
- Ask: ***Are there any questions before we end the session?***

Wrap-Up

- The therapist should send a calendar invite with the next caregiver group session's day/time to the caregiver.
- The therapist may also want to email caregivers a blank copy of the DLS contract or refer them to the STRW website.
- Prior to the dyad session, the therapist may want to check in with caregivers about the recipes they are planning on cooking. It is particularly helpful to have a copy of the recipe so that it can be displayed on the therapist's screen while the teen practices cooking.

Daily Living Skills Contract

Date ______________________

Goal	Expectations	Reward	MONDAY	TUESDAY	WEDNESDAY	THURSDAY	FRIDAY	SATURDAY	SUNDAY

______________________ Teen

______________________ Parent / Caregiver

Caregiver/Teen Dyad Session 6 Content (60 mins)

STRW Session 6 Schedule (1 min)

- The therapist should greet the caregiver and teen.
- *Let's get started! As a reminder, it will be helpful to sit together at a table so that we can all see each other and work together. Please pull out your STRW workbook that contains the handouts for all STRW sessions. This session is called Session 6 – Kitchen Safety and Microwave Cooking. Please turn to that section in your workbook.*
- *Let's go over the session schedule so that you know what we will be doing. Please feel free to ask any questions about our schedule!*
- Briefly go over each item on the Session Schedule.
- Check to make sure that the caregiver and teen have the following materials: knife, cutting board, fruit/vegetable to practice cutting, and ingredients for the no-cook and microwave recipes. The teen and caregiver can gather these materials now if needed.

Real World Practice Check-In: Contract and Morning Routine (3 mins)

- Refer to the Session 5 Real World Practice handout and DLS Contract handout.
- *Let's check in on how you are doing with each goal on your DLS contract. Please be honest, as this is an opportunity to talk about what is working and what is not working and do some brainstorming to address any challenges.*
- As needed, the therapist should spend time modifying the DLS contract and problem solving how to make a more effective system to target the DLS goal (e.g., make expectations more specific, change reward, increase/decrease number of prompts, modify the strategies being used to help with goals).
- If the therapist used a fillable PDF of the DLS Contract handout in the previous session, it may be helpful to share this on the screen so that the goal, expectations, and reward can be easily discussed.
- The following questions should be asked (if applicable), and the responses and any relevant notes should be entered into the Real World Practice Tracking Sheet:
  - *Did you use your DLS contract this week?*
  - *Did you work on your morning routine goal during the week?*
    - *What went well?*
    - *What was challenging?*
    - *How many days did you work on your morning routine goal?*
    - *Did you earn a reward for your morning routine goal?*
    - *How many days did you earn a reward?*

Real World Practice Check-In: Cleaning the Bedroom and Laundry (5 mins)

- The following questions should be asked (if applicable), and the responses and any relevant notes should be entered into the Real World Practice Tracking Sheet:
  - *Did you work on your cleaning the bedroom goal during the week?*
    - *What went well?*
    - *What was challenging?*
    - *How many days did you work on your cleaning the bedroom goal?*
    - *Did you earn a reward for your cleaning the bedroom goal?*
  - *Did you work on your laundry goal during the week?*
    - *What went well?*
    - *What was challenging?*
    - *How many days did you work on your laundry goal?*
    - *Did you earn a reward for your laundry goal?*

Real World Practice Check-In: Money (2 mins)

- The following questions should be asked (if applicable), and the responses and any relevant notes should be entered into the Real World Practice Tracking Sheet:
  - **For your Real World Practice, you were also given a money assignment.**
    - *Did you work on or complete a money assignment?*
    - *What did you do?*
    - *What went well?*
    - *What was challenging?*

- Ask: *Any questions or comments about your Real World Practice assignments?*
- If the caregiver/teen dyad struggled to complete the Real World Practice assignments, the therapist should spend some time discussing how to identify days/times that they could designate to commit to working on the assignments.
- If the therapist used a fillable PDF of the DLS Contract handout in the previous session, it may be helpful to share this on the screen so that the goal, expectations, and reward can be easily discussed.

Elements of an Effective System for Achieving DLS Goals (2 mins)

- Ask: *Are there any issues you want to discuss or troubleshoot related to the DLS contract?*
- Ask and Discuss: *Are we considering all of the important elements to increase the likelihood of you achieving your DLS goals by developing the most effective system?*
- If applicable, discuss how to modify any DLS goals to address (1) qualities of the teen and their caregiver; (2) use of evidence-based strategies to teach and master DLS; and (3) ensuring that goals are obvious, attractive, easy, and satisfying.

Evidence-Based Strategy: DLS Teaching Method – Cooking in the Microwave (2 mins)

- Refer to the DLS Teaching Method for Cooking in the Microwave handout.
- *Just like for cleaning your bedroom and doing laundry, we will be using the DLS Teaching Method to build up your skills in the kitchen, including cutting up fruits or vegetables and cooking recipes in the microwave, oven, and stovetop. Depending on your skill level, you may need to learn, watch, and practice with your caregiver so that you can meet your goal of cooking on your own.*
- *In session today, you will learn how to be safe in the kitchen, cut with a knife, make no-cook recipes, and cook a recipe in the microwave. As part of your DLS contract in the coming weeks, you will have a cooking goal. It can be helpful to make your cooking goal related to the other goals on your DLS contract. For example, you could practice making your own breakfast in the morning or make a no-cook recipe when packing your lunch.*

Evidence-Based Strategy: Task Analysis (1 min)

- Refer to the Microwave Cheese Quesadilla Recipe handout and Task Analysis Steps handout.
- *In the last several sessions we have used a task analysis to break down the steps of cleaning your bedroom and doing your laundry. A recipe already breaks down the steps needed to cook and also includes all of the ingredients that you will need to cook. Just like a task analysis, a recipe can be used to make sure you are doing the steps in the correct order. For the next several sessions, we will use recipes that you and your caregiver choose to cook in the microwave, oven, and stovetop.*

Kitchen Safety Rules: The Basics (2 mins)

- Have the dyad move the session to the kitchen for the remainder of the session.
- Refer to Kitchen Safety Rules handout.
- *We will be discussing basic safety concepts in the kitchen before working on the skill of cooking in the next few sessions. These safety rules are on your handout. Let's take turns reading through each safety rule and then discussing if you have questions or concerns. We will also have you identify the location of items in your kitchen such as a fire extinguisher and potholders.*
- For this slide, have the caregiver and teen take turns reading each safety rule and discuss as needed. Instruct the caregiver to point out where items are if the teen does not know (e.g., location of fire extinguisher, where potholders are stored). The safety rules to discuss include:
  - Wash your hands before and after handling food.
  - Use potholders and oven mitts.
  - Wipe up spills immediately.
  - Turn pot handles away from the front of the stove to prevent them from being knocked over.
  - Store knives safely in an area that is out of reach (e.g., wooden block, drawer).

- Be mindful of what you are wearing when you cook.
  - Do not wear loose clothing.
  - Keep hair tied back.
  - Do not wear dangling jewelry.
- Stay in the kitchen when you are cooking on the stovetop.

Kitchen Safety Rules: The Basics (2 mins)

- Refer to Kitchen Safety Rules handout.
- For this slide, have the caregiver and teen take turns reading each safety rule and discuss as needed. Instruct the caregiver to point out where items are if the teen does not know (e.g., location of fire extinguisher, where potholders are stored). The safety rules to discuss include:
  - Make sure your kitchen has a fire extinguisher that is easily accessible.
  - Make sure you know how to use the fire extinguisher.
  - Do not place any items near an open flame.
  - Dish rags, potholders, etc. can easily catch fire if left near an open flame.
  - Do not let temperature sensitive foods – such as raw meat, fish, dairy products – sit out in the kitchen.
    - Put items back in the refrigerator after you use them.
    - If you are defrosting frozen meat products, make sure you monitor how long they have been left out.
  - Keep raw meat separate from other food items whenever you use it.
    - Wash your hands after touching raw meat.
    - Thoroughly wash any utensils or cooking equipment after you have used it to prepare raw meat.

Kitchen Safety Rules: How to Put Out Kitchen Fires (2 mins)

- Refer to the Kitchen Safety Rules handout.
- ***When a fire starts in the kitchen, you need to act fast to keep the fire from getting out of control. But how you act depends on what kind of fire you have and where it is. Let's take turns reading these instructions for putting out kitchen fires.***
- Have caregiver and teen take turns reading each safety rule on the handout and discuss as needed. The safety rules to discuss include:
  - If you have a fire in the oven or the microwave, close the door or keep it closed and turn off the appliance.
  - If you have a fire in a pan, use an oven mitt to put the lid on, then move the pan off the burner, and turn off the stove.
  - If you can't safely put the lid on a pan that is on fire, use a fire extinguisher to aim at the base of the fire.
  - Use baking soda or salt (NOT WATER OR FLOUR!) to put out a grease fire.
  - Don't attempt to put out a fire with a towel, apron, or clothing.
  - If the fire is spreading and you can't control it, evacuate the house and call 911!

- Ask: *Any questions before we move on to discussing how to use knives in the kitchen?*

Evidence-Based Strategy: DLS Teaching Method – Cutting with a Knife (1 min)

- Refer to the DLS Teaching Method for Cutting with a Knife handout.
- ***We are going to use the DLS Teaching Method to learn how to safely use a knife to cut up food. We will first learn how to use a knife to cut and then you will get an opportunity to watch your caregiver cut with a knife before you practice.***
- The therapist should do the following for the first three steps of the DLS Teaching Method as it relates to using a knife (see detailed instructions on the next two slides):
  - LEARN – First, have the caregiver and teen review basic knife safety rules on the Kitchen Safety Rules handout.
  - WATCH – Then, watch a video on how to cut safely and instruct the caregiver to demonstrate how to cut up a fruit/vegetable with a knife.
  - PRACTICE – Finally, instruct the teen to practice the skill of cutting up a fruit/vegetable with a knife.

- The therapist should provide feedback and support to the caregiver as needed with an emphasis on safety.

Kitchen Safety Rules: How to Use Kitchen Knives Safely (2 mins)

- Refer to the Kitchen Safety Rules handout.
- ***Let's do the first step of the DLS Teaching Method – which is to learn how to use kitchen knives safely. As we do this, please get a knife, cutting board, and the fruit or vegetable that you will use to practice cutting.***
- ***Let's take turns reading each safety rule about kitchen knives and please feel free to bring up any questions or concerns you have!***
- Have caregiver and teen take turns reading each safety rule on the handout and discuss as needed. The safety rules to discuss include:
  - Always use a cutting board.
    - Do not use the palm of your hand as a cutting board!
  - Make sure the cutting board and knife is clean.
  - Keep your knives sharp.
    - Dull knives can slip while you're cutting and cause injury.
  - Curl your fingers under and hold the food with your fingertips when cutting.
  - Slice away from your hand and keep your fingers clear of the blade.

Practice Knife Skills (6 mins)

- ***Let's first watch a video demonstrating how to cut up fruits and vegetables with a knife.***

- It is strongly recommended that therapist show a video demonstrating how to use kitchen knives safely that is available on the STRW Resources handout and the STRW website.
- ***Let's watch your caregiver demonstrate how to cut up the fruit or vegetable before you practice.***
- Instruct the caregiver to use the cutting board and fruit/vegetable to demonstrate how to safely cut with a knife.
- Ask: ***Any questions on how to use a knife safely?***
- Instruct the teen to practice cutting and provide feedback as needed.
- The therapist should provide feedback and support to the caregiver as needed, including giving clear directions and demonstrations on cutting with a knife.

No-Cook Recipes (2 mins)

- ***No-cook recipes do not require any cooking and are typically easy and quick to make. Examples of no-cook recipes include a bagel with cream cheese, pretzels and hummus, a peanut butter and jelly sandwich, tortilla chips and guacamole, yogurt and granola, and smoothies.***
- Ask and Discuss: ***What are no-cook recipes that you could make and eat at home?***

DLS Teaching Method – No-Cook Recipes (5 mins)

- Refer to the DLS Teaching Method for No-Cook Recipes handout.
- ***We are now going to use the DLS Teaching Method of Learn, Watch, Practice, and then Do It Independently to practice making a no-cook recipe.***
- ***What is the no-cook recipe you will be making today?***
  - If a recipe has not been identified, assist the teen/caregiver by finding a recipe in a cookbook or on the internet.

- After a recipe is identified, review the steps of the recipe. If possible, the therapist should display the recipe on their computer screen. The Task Analysis Steps handout could be used to write down the steps of the no-cook recipe if needed.
- The therapist should do the following for the first three steps of the DLS Teaching Method as it relates to making a no-cook recipe:
  - LEARN – First, instruct the caregiver to review the no-cook recipe steps and the ingredients and supplies (e.g., plate, knife, etc.) that are needed.
  - WATCH – Then, instruct the caregiver to demonstrate (as needed) how to prepare the recipe. This can be done by demonstrating the steps or talking through the steps.
  - PRACTICE – Finally, instruct the teen to practice making the no-cook recipe and instruct the caregiver to provide feedback or support as needed.

- The therapist should provide feedback and support to the caregiver as needed, including giving clear directions and demonstrations on making the no-cook recipe.

Microwave Cooking (3 mins)

- ***Next, we are going to learn about cooking recipes in the microwave.***

- Ask and discuss the following questions:
  - ***What have you cooked in the microwave?***
  - ***What would you like to learn to cook in the microwave?***

- ***Let's review the features of your microwave.***
- Depending on the teen's experience, instruct the caregiver to show the teen the following buttons/functions and discuss as needed:
  - Power button
  - Cook time
  - Start
  - Clear
  - Defrost
  - Automatic buttons (e.g., popcorn)
  - Timer

DLS Teaching Method – Cooking in the Microwave (5 mins)

- Refer to the <u>DLS Teaching Method for Cooking in the Microwave</u> handout.
- ***We are now going to use the DLS Teaching Method of Learn, Watch, Practice, and then Do It Independently to practice cooking in the microwave.***
- ***What is the microwave recipe you will be making today?***
  - If a recipe has not been identified, assist the teen/caregiver by finding a recipe in a cookbook or on the internet.

- After a recipe is identified, review the steps of the recipe. If possible, the therapist should display the recipe on their computer screen. The <u>Task Analysis Steps</u> handout could be used to write down the steps of the microwave recipe if needed.
- The therapist should do the following for the first three steps of the DLS Teaching Method as it relates to making a microwave recipe:
  - LEARN – First, instruct the caregiver to review the recipe and the ingredients and supplies (e.g., bowl, measuring cup, etc.) that are needed.
  - WATCH – Then, instruct the caregiver to demonstrate (as needed) how to cook the recipe. This should involve the caregiver demonstrating (e.g., showing how to measure 1 cup of water) or talking through each step (e.g., fill the measuring cup to the top) and providing the support that the teen may need.
  - PRACTICE – Finally, instruct the teen to practice making the recipe and instruct the caregiver to provide feedback or support (including kitchen safety) as needed.

- The therapist should provide feedback and support to the caregiver as needed, including giving clear directions and demonstrations on making the recipe in the microwave.

Elements of an Effective System for Achieving DLS Goals (3 mins)

- The therapist should briefly ask the teen and caregiver about each of the elements and then incorporate their responses into the discussion on developing the DLS contract.
- *As we work to add the goal of cooking to the DLS contract, let's make sure we are thinking about all of the following elements to build an effective system for achieving DLS goals:*
  - *Teen – are we considering your strengths, challenges, preferred learning style, and commitment?*
  - *Caregiver – are we considering your parenting style, time and effort, and commitment?*
    - *Some caregivers find it easy to have teens practice cooking alongside them – while they are making breakfast, packing lunches, making after-school snacks, or making dinner.*
  - *Are we using evidence-based strategies?*
    - *We are using a recipe, which is very similar to a task analysis, to break the skill down into simple steps.*
    - *We are also using the DLS Teaching Method to help you learn and become independent in cooking.*
    - *You could also look up videos that go along with recipes to teach you and demonstrate the steps of how to cook the recipe.*
  - *Is the goal of cooking obvious, attractive, easy, and satisfying?*
    - *Obvious – some ideas might be to print out the recipe so that the steps can be crossed off as they are completed.*
    - *Attractive – some ideas might be to listen to music while cooking or cook with your caregiver.*
    - *Easy – some ideas might be to have all of the ingredients available and on the counter, to set a reminder to cook at a specific day/time, or to choose a recipe that you regularly cook during the week such as pizza on Friday.*
    - *Satisfying – some ideas include getting to eat whatever it is that you cook!*

- Ask and Discuss: *Any questions or comments?*
- *Let's apply all of this information to creating your DLS contract!*

Developing Your DLS Contract (5 mins)

- Refer to the DLS Contract handout
- *Let's spend the remainder of our time in today's session modifying your DLS contract to continue working on your morning routine, cleaning your bedroom, and laundry goals and add in the goal of cooking. Use a blank copy of the DLS Contract. We will also keep in mind the importance of making sure the goal is easy, obvious, attractive, and satisfying so that you are more likely to achieve your goal.*

The DLS contract will have you track your progress and set up rewards for you to earn, which makes working on the goals satisfying!

- The therapist should support the caregiver/teen dyad in creating the DLS contract by doing the following:
  - Incorporate all of the information from the last several sessions (e.g., rewards that are motivating for the teen, use of strategies and supports to build independence with certain steps) and the Real World Practice Check-In to create the DLS contract. The therapist should also consider the goals that the caregiver and teen collaboratively developed during the Preparing for STRW session.
  - While the teen worked on many cooking skills today, they only need to identify one cooking goal. Examples include making a no-cook recipe for breakfast or lunch during the week, cutting up vegetables for dinner one day, or making an after-school snack in the microwave. The therapist should encourage the dyad to make sure the teen is prepared by having a recipe available and any materials or ingredients to make it more likely they will achieve their cooking goal.
  - Incorporate information from the teen practicing cooking and cutting with a knife over the course of the dyad session (e.g., if cutting with a knife was difficult, it may be best to have the caregiver present to support and give feedback as the teen practices this skill).
  - Use the <u>DLS Contract</u> handout to specify the (1) Goal, (2) Expectations, and (3) Reward for Morning Routine, Cleaning the Bedroom, Doing Laundry, and Cooking.
  - Encourage the caregiver/teen dyad to work together and model appropriate and supportive coaching as they develop the DLS contract.

- Possible discussion questions that may be helpful to ask and discuss when creating the contract for the Morning Routine, Cleaning the Bedroom, Laundry, and Cooking goals include:
  - ***How often are you going to need to do the goal – every day, every weekday, every other day, or once per week?***
  - ***What steps of your goal do you need help with?***
  - ***What steps do you not know how to do?***
  - ***What steps are you doing independently?***
  - ***How easy/hard do you think it will be to meet your goal?***
  - ***What reward would you like to earn?***
  - ***Does the reward fit the goal? For example, earning 1 hour of screen time for doing your morning routine goal each day is a lot, but maybe earning 15–20 extra minutes of screen time would be a better fit.***
  - ***How will you check in about your goals daily to discuss if the goal was met?***
  - ***Where can you post your DLS contract so that you can track goals daily and remember to get your reward if it was earned?***

- The caregiver and teen should write each goal, expectation, and reward on the <u>DLS Contract</u> handout. It may be helpful for the therapist to share their screen and add/modify the goals, expectations, and rewards on a fillable PDF of the <u>DLS Contract</u> handout. The therapist can then email it to the caregiver and teen after the session.
- When the DLS contract has been completed, encourage the dyad to sign it and post it somewhere where they can easily see it so that the goals may be tracked.

Real World Practice (1 min)

- Refer to the Real World Practice handout.
- Discuss the details of the Real World Practice assignment.
  - *Work on your morning routine, cleaning the bedroom, laundry, and cooking goals for the remainder of the week using your DLS contract.*
    - *Set aside a specific time such as on the way to school or after dinner to discuss how the morning routine went and how to problem-solve the next day.*
    - *Schedule a day/time to work on watching and/or practicing how to clean your bedroom, do laundry, and cook.*
    - *Make sure that if the teen earns the reward, they receive it immediately! This makes it more likely that they will continue to be motivated to meet their goal!*
  - *Make a list of ingredients for a recipe you want to cook. Find and purchase the ingredients at the grocery store and pay for the items with either cash or credit/ debit card.*

- Ask: *Any questions about your Real World Practice assignment?*

Guess the Price (3 mins) – OPTIONAL

- NOTE: This activity can be skipped if there is not enough time to complete it.
- *Let's play a quick round of Guess the Price, which is just meant to be a fun way to build up your understanding of how much things cost.*
- *Let's see if you know the prices of some common grocery items even if they are not necessarily items that you use!*
- The therapist can have the teen guess the price or have the caregiver and teen compete against each other.
- The therapist should click through the next four slides that contain examples of common grocery items. Prior to the session, the therapist will need to look up the prices to ensure that they are accurate.
  - Therapists can change the grocery items for the Guess the Price game.
  - This activity is meant to be fun and engaging! If the teen is averse to playing the game, it can be skipped. However, it would be helpful for the caregiver and teen to find other ways to build up an understanding of what things cost (e.g., compare the cost of products at the store, involve the teen when purchasing cleaning items).

Preparing for the Next Dyad Session (2 mins)

- *We will have our next caregiver/teen dyad session on DAY and TIME. At this session, we will discuss how to measure and mix ingredients and cook in the oven. We will need you to prepare for the session by doing the following:*
  - *Make sure that you have measuring cups and spoons to practice measuring ingredients.*

- *Gather ingredients for an oven recipe. Examples include cookies, brownies, homemade pizza, or Chex mix. Think about a recipe you would like to master or one that you have been wanting to learn!*
- *We will also be spending the majority of the session in your kitchen.*

- *I will check in with you by email in a few days to remind you to get the items you need to make the oven recipe. It is sometimes easiest to just use ingredients you already have at home!*
- *It will be important to complete your Real World Practice assignment before our next dyad session and come prepared to discuss it. We will spend a lot of time next session talking about how the DLS contract went!*
- Ask: *Are there any questions before we end the session?*

Wrap-Up

- The therapist should send a calendar invite with the next caregiver/teen dyad session's day/time to the caregiver and teen. The therapist may also want to send the caregiver/teen a copy of the DLS contract if they completed it using a fillable PDF.

Evidence-Based Strategy: **Daily Life Skills Teaching Method**

Cooking in the Microwave

LEARN

Review the steps of the microwave recipe.
Gather the ingredients and cooking supplies that are needed.

WATCH

Your parent/caregiver will demonstrate (as needed) how to make the microwave recipe by going through each step of the recipe.

PRACTICE

You will practice following the steps of the microwave recipe
Your parent/caregiver will observe and give feedback and support after you complete each step.

DO IT INDEPENDENTLY

You will make the microwave recipe on your own.

Task Analysis

Skill: ____

Steps:

Microwave Cheese Quesadilla Recipe

Preparation Time: 2 mins
Cook Time: 1 min

Ingredients:

- Two 10-inch flour tortillas
- ½ cup shredded cheddar cheese (or your choice of cheese)

Directions:

- Place one flour tortilla onto a large microwave-safe plate.
- Sprinkle the cheese onto the tortilla.
- Put the other flour tortilla on top.
- Microwave on high for 1 minute until the cheese is melted.
- Wait 2–3 mins for the quesadilla to cool.
- Use a pizza cutter to cut the tortilla.

Kitchen Safety Rules

- **The Basics**
  - Wash your hands before and after handling food.
  - Use potholders and oven mitts.
  - Wipe up spills immediately.
  - Turn pot handles away from the front of the stove to prevent them from being knocked over.
  - Store knives safely in an area that is out of reach (e.g., wooden block, drawer).
  - Be mindful of what you are wearing when you cook.
    - Do not wear loose clothing.
    - Keep hair tied back.
    - Do not wear dangling jewelry.
  - Stay in the kitchen when you are cooking on the stovetop.
  - Make sure your kitchen has a fire extinguisher that is easily accessible.
    - Make sure you know how to use the fire extinguisher.
  - Do not place any items near an open flame.
    - Dish rags, potholders, and so on can easily catch fire if left near an open flame.
  - Do not let temperature-sensitive foods – such as raw meat, fish, and dairy products – sit out in the kitchen.
    - Put items back in the refrigerator after you use them.
    - If you are defrosting frozen meat products, make sure you monitor how long they have been left out.
  - Keep raw meat separate from other food items whenever you use or store it.
    - Wash your hands after touching raw meat.
    - Thoroughly wash any utensils or cooking equipment after you have used it to prepare raw meat.

Kitchen Safety Rules

- **How to Put Out Kitchen Fires**
  - If you have a fire in the oven or the microwave, close the door or keep it closed and turn off the appliance.
  - If you have a fire in a pan, use an oven mitt to put the lid on, then move the pan off the burner, and turn off the stove.
  - If you can't safely put the lid on a pan that is on fire, use a fire extinguisher to aim at the base of the fire.
  - Use baking soda or salt (NOT WATER OR FLOUR!) to put out a grease fire.
  - Don't attempt to put out a fire with a towel, apron, or clothing.
  - If the fire is spreading and you can't control it, evacuate the house and call 911!

- **How to Use Kitchen Knives Safely**
  - Always use a cutting board.
    - Do not use the palm of your hand as a cutting board!
  - Make sure the cutting board and knife is clean.
  - Keep your knives sharp.
    - Dull knives can slip while you're cutting and cause injury.
  - Curl your fingers under and hold the food with your fingertips when cutting.
  - Slice away from your hand and keep your fingers clear of the blade.

Evidence-Based Strategy: **Daily Life Skills Teaching Method**

Cutting with a Knife

LEARN

Read the safety guidelines on how to cut with a knife.
Identify where your knives and cutting boards are stored in your kitchen.

WATCH

Your parent/caregiver will demonstrate (as needed) how to cut with a knife.
You can watch a video on how to safety use a knife to cut and chop up food.

PRACTICE

You will practice cutting up food with a knife.
Your parent/caregiver will observe and give feedback and support as you practice.

DO IT INDEPENDENTLY

You will cut up food with a knife on your own.

Evidence-Based Strategy: **Daily Life Skills Teaching Method**

No-Cook Recipes

LEARN

Review the steps of the no-cook recipe.
Gather the ingredients and cooking supplies (e.g., plate, knife) that are needed.

WATCH

Your parent/caregiver will demonstrate (as needed) how to make the no-cook recipe by going through each step of the recipe.

PRACTICE

You will practice following the steps of the no-cook recipe
Your parent/caregiver will observe and give feedback and support after you complete each step.

DO IT INDEPENDENTLY

You will make the no-cook recipe on your own.

Daily Living Skills Contract

Date ______________________

Goal	Expectations	Reward	MONDAY	TUESDAY	WEDNESDAY	THURSDAY	FRIDAY	SATURDAY	SUNDAY

____
Teen

____
Parent / Caregiver

Surviving and Thriving in the Real World Session 6 – Real World Practice

- Work on your (1) morning routine, (2) cleaning the bedroom, (3) doing laundry, and (4) cooking goals for the remainder of the week using your DLS contract.
  - Set aside a specific time (e.g., on the way to school, after dinner) to discuss how the morning routine went and how to problem-solve for the next day.
  - Schedule a day/time to work on watching and/or practicing how to clean the bedroom, do laundry, and cook.
  - Make sure that if a reward is earned, it is provided immediately!

- Make a list of ingredients for a recipe you want to cook. Find and purchase the ingredients at the grocery store and pay for the items with either cash or credit/debit card.

Surviving & Thriving in the Real World

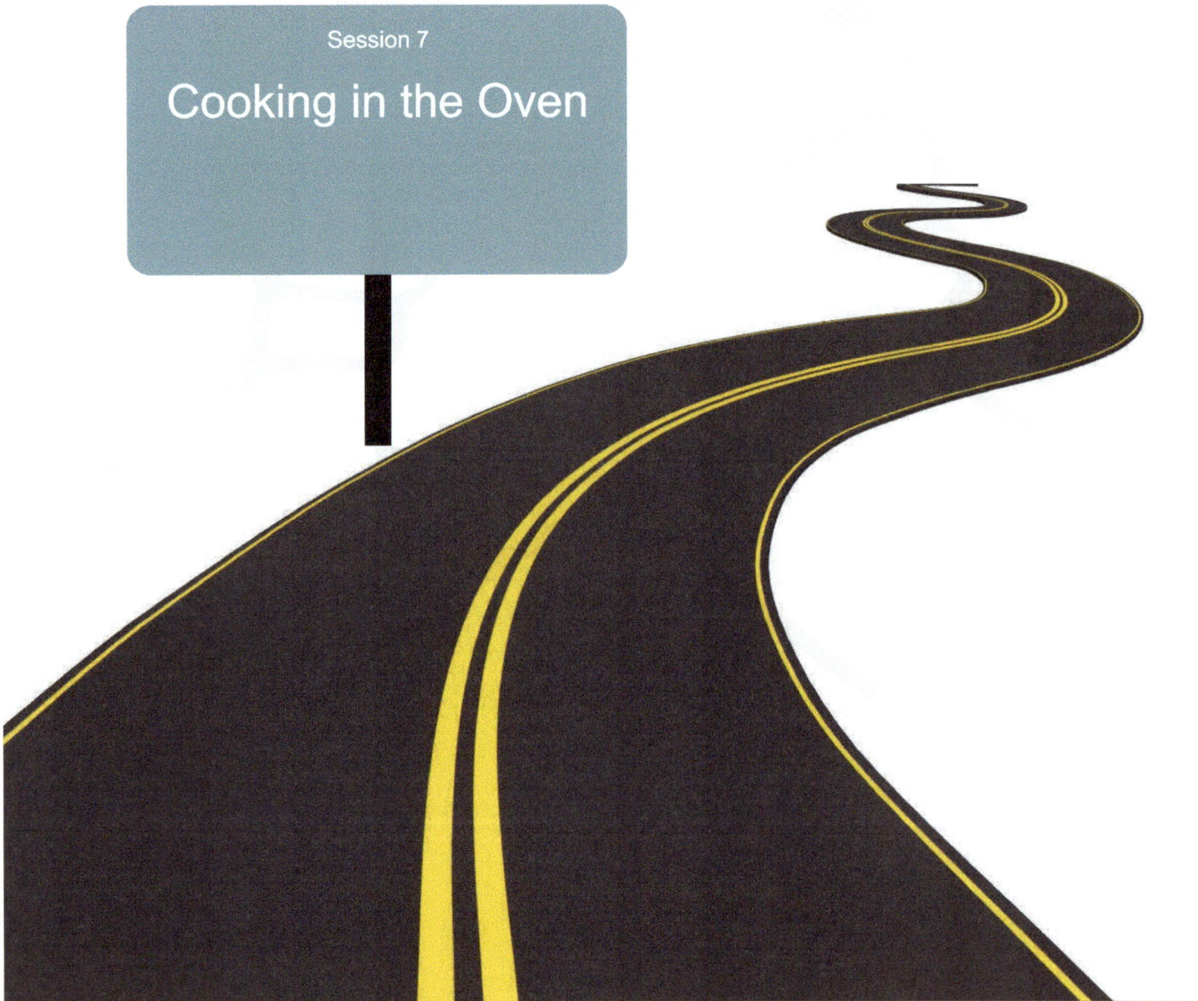

Session 7

Cooking in the Oven

Aims

- Continue to build rapport between caregiver group members and the therapist
- Continue to build rapport between the teen, caregiver, and therapist
- Further develop ability to use a DLS contract to set a DLS goal, define expectations, and identify a reward for meeting the goal
- Review the four elements for developing an effective system to achieve the teen's DLS goals
- Understand how to measure and mix wet and dry ingredients
- Understand how to use the DLS Teaching Method to learn the steps for cooking a recipe in the oven
- Create and implement a DLS contract to target the goals of morning routine, cleaning the bedroom, doing laundry, and cooking

Structure

- Caregiver group session via telehealth
- Caregiver/teen dyad session via telehealth

Session Supplies

- Caregiver Group Handouts
  - DLS Contract

- Caregiver/Teen Dyad Handouts
  - DLS Teaching Method for Cooking in the Oven
  - Chocolate Chip Cookies Recipe
  - Task Analysis Steps
  - Measuring Cups
  - Measuring Spoons
  - Oven Settings

DOI: 10.4324/9781003458838-10

- DLS Contract
- Session 7 – Real World Practice

- Videos (optional links available on the STRW website and the STRW Resources handout)

Caregiver/Teen Preparation for Session

- For the dyad session, the caregiver and teen should have identified a recipe that they want to cook in the oven during this session. They should also have the ingredients needed to make the recipe.
- The caregiver and teen should also get measuring cups and spoons so that they can practice measuring wet and dry ingredients. They will be measuring water for the wet ingredient and will also need to make sure they have access to a dry ingredient such as flour, sugar, or salt.
- It would be highly beneficial for the caregiver and teen to practice these skills in the kitchen area that is free from as many distractions as possible (e.g., other siblings, noise from the television, etc.).

Therapist Preparation for Session

- The therapist may want to review the Recipe Ideas for the STRW Cooking Sessions handout (see appendix), which includes ideas of recipes to cook if the caregiver/teen are having trouble identifying what to cook in Sessions 6–8.
- The therapist may want to review the Possible Solutions to Common Challenges that Arise for STRW Therapists handout (see appendix), which includes ideas for how STRW therapists can address common challenges that arise when facilitating the caregiver group and dyad sessions, including commitment; engagement; inattention; too much prompting; and family factors such as time, use of rewards, and caregiver/teen relationship.
- The therapist should use the Real World Practice Tracking Sheet for each caregiver/teen dyad in all subsequent STRW sessions to track progress on their DLS contract goals.
- The therapist will need to be mindful about individualizing the session for each dyad based on whether they have access to an oven to cook and also based on the foods that their family cooks and eats on a regular basis (e.g., have caregiver and teen work together to identify recipes that they want to cook and identify recipes that include ingredients that they often have readily available in their kitchen).
- The therapist should consider reviewing the Tips for STRW Therapists: How to Facilitate Achievement of DLS Goals handout prior to each caregiver group session or dyad session for tips and strategies on how to help teens achieve the goals on their DLS contract. Tips that may be beneficial for Session 7 include:
    - *Acknowledge differences between teens.* The therapist should be mindful of the different goals, expectations, and rewards of the teens in the group. It may be helpful to directly acknowledge that each teen comes in with different experiences, strengths, and challenges, but the end goal of achieving independence by building age-appropriate DLS is the same for everyone.

- *Review past successes to build confidence.* It can be effective for therapists to take time to remind caregivers and/or teens of their past successes in building DLS or other skills as a way to instill confidence and increase motivation. This can be particularly beneficial when the teen/caregiver are feeling frustrated or impatient about their progress towards DLS goals (e.g., slow progress, plateau in gaining of skills, taking more time to learn and master a new skill than was originally anticipated).
- *Be a guide.* While the therapist may have to be more directive at times by providing instructions and feedback, particularly at the beginning of the STRW intervention, they should be mindful of fading back their support so that the caregiver and teen feel confident to continue to build their DLS and overall independence after completing the STRW intervention.

Session 7 Notes

- Fillable PDFs of handouts from this session (i.e., Task Analysis Steps, DLS Contract) are available on the STRW website.

- Caregiver Group Session
  - The therapist should continue to devote the majority of the caregiver group session to reviewing how the DLS contract is progressing for each caregiver. This is an opportunity to identify any issues and brainstorm solutions prior to the dyad session.
  - The therapist should utilize the caregiver group session to get an understanding of how it may be necessary to personalize the dyad session content (e.g., discuss options if the teen does not have an oven, brainstorm possible recipes for the teen to cook).
  - The therapist should make an active effort to foster collaboration between the group members by encouraging active discussion and problem-solving of challenges or questions about the DLS contract.
  - The therapist should have caregivers discuss how they can encourage cooking on a regular basis and get ideas from other caregivers (e.g., take items out of the oven, helping to prepare a dinner so that the teen can eventually cook dinner on their own).

- Dyad Session
  - The therapist should encourage the caregiver, in collaboration with their teen, to choose a recipe that they are motivated to learn how to cook and eat but should also encourage them to identify recipes for items that they consistently have in their kitchen and/or may be beneficial for the teen to learn how to cook (e.g., learn how to bake cookies that they can bring to family get-togethers, learn how to make a favorite family dinner in the oven).
  - The therapist should work with the caregiver/teen dyad to determine if they want to add in another cooking goal (e.g., make a homemade pizza in the oven) or continue working on the cooking goal from Session 6 (e.g., make a microwave quesadilla). While it can often feel overwhelming to add another goal to the DLS contract, cooking is a goal that can typically be done alongside the caregiver during the course of the week or as part of the teen's daily routine

(e.g., make an after school snack in the oven or microwave). It will be important to encourage the teen to find ways to practice the cooking skills that they are learning the session or make a plan for practicing these skills in the future.

- If the teen does not have access to an oven, they can choose another appliance to practice cooking (e.g., grill, griddle, toaster oven, air fryer, crock pot, etc.).
- The therapist can choose to use video modeling to demonstrate how to cook a recipe such as chocolate chip cookies. Many websites or cooking blogs have pictures and videos that break down how to prepare and cook a recipe, which may be particularly helpful for some teens. There are several cooking websites that may be useful on the STRW Resources handout on the STRW website.
- The therapist will need to manage time effectively so that teens get an opportunity to make a recipe in the oven. Some suggestions include:
  - Incorporate the measuring and mixing activity into the actual recipe the teen is cooking in the oven (if applicable).
  - The session can end prior to the item being completely cooked or ready to eat.
  - Have a copy of the recipe available to share on the therapist's computer screen so that the steps are displayed while the caregiver and teen are cooking.
  - It can be helpful to preheat the oven at the start of the session.
- The therapist can encourage caregivers to point out where various items can be found in the kitchen (e.g., mixing spoons, large bowls, cookie sheet) if the teen is not aware of where to find these items.
- When developing the DLS contract at the end of the caregiver/teen dyad session, the therapist should continue to incorporate all of the information and knowledge gained from the past several sessions (e.g., issues that were brought up during the caregiver group session, task analysis steps, discussing how to incorporate the essential elements of an effective system for achieving DLS goals, identifying appropriate rewards, etc.).

Caregiver Group Session 7 Content (90 mins)

Review – Real World Practice Assignment (50 mins)

- The therapist should greet the caregivers and welcome them to the session.
- Discuss the Real World Practice assignment in detail by having all caregivers share how using the DLS contract to target the morning routine, cleaning the bedroom, laundry, and cooking goals went with their teen. Encourage caregivers to jot down questions and notes on a blank copy of the DLS Contract handout that they may want to discuss or incorporate into their teen's DLS contract at the next dyad session.
- ***We will have everyone share how using the DLS contract to target the morning routine, cleaning the bedroom, laundry, and cooking goals went for their teen. This is an opportunity to celebrate successes and also problem-solve any challenges or obstacles that occurred. We will spend the majority of our session discussing each teen's progress with the DLS contract. It may be helpful to jot down questions and notes on a copy of the*** **DLS Contract** ***handout, and feel free to ask questions or add to the discussion.***
- It may be helpful to refer caregivers to the Tips for Creating a Successful DLS Contract handout (from Session 4) when discussing the goals on the DLS contract (e.g., clearly defining expectations, re-evaluating rewards regularly to ensure they are motivating, etc.).
- Points of discussion or questions to ask each caregiver include the following:
  - DLS contract
    - ***Did the teen make progress at becoming more independent with each of their goals – morning routine, cleaning the bedroom, laundry, and cooking?***
    - ***What went well?***
    - ***What was difficult?***
    - ***Did they receive a reward?***
    - ***Did they use any strategies to help them to learn the skill or become more independent?***
    - ***Any obstacles or barriers?***
    - ***Do you plan on modifying any goals on the current DLS contract?***
  - Making a list and purchasing items
    - ***Was your teen able to make a list of ingredients for a recipe that they want to cook?***
    - ***Was your teen able to find and purchase the items at the store?***
    - ***What went well?***
    - ***What skills still need to be practiced?***
- Ask: ***Any questions about the Real World Practice assignment?***

STRW Session 7 Goals (1 min)

- *The goals of today's session are to continue discussing how to target the DLS goals of understanding basic kitchen concepts such as measuring and mixing ingredients and cooking in the oven. We will also review how to build an effective system to help you and your teen achieve their DLS goals now and in the future.*
- *At this point, we are really starting to build your teen's DLS, and it may seem overwhelming to add in another goal. With cooking, it will be helpful to keep in mind if there are ways that the teen can incorporate this into their daily or weekly schedule. For example:*
    - *Could the teen make their own snack after school?*
    - *Could the teen help you prepare a meal during the week? For example, could they help make a casserole in the oven or a homemade pizza?*
    - *Could the teen help you prepare a dessert such as brownies or cookies?*

- Ask and Discuss: *Any questions?*

Review Dyad Session 7 Content (36 mins)

- *Now we will briefly review the material that will be covered in the upcoming dyad session with your teen. This will allow you to have some time to prepare for the upcoming session. Please feel free to ask any questions as we go over the content of the dyad session.*
- *For this session, we will plan on teaching skills in the kitchen area of your home. It is a session that has a lot of hands-on practice as the teen practices measuring and mixing ingredients and cooking a recipe in the oven. It will be important to be prepared for this session by having an oven recipe and any ingredients needed. You will also need kitchen supplies such as measuring cups and spoons and will need to have your oven available.*
- *If you do not have an oven, we can still practice the skill of cooking a recipe and can possibly identify another appliance that your teen could use to practice cooking such as a crock pot or microwave oven.*
- Ask: *Any questions about practicing these cooking skills in your home with your teen at the upcoming dyad session?*
- *Before we review the dyad session content, let's all briefly share your teen's abilities to do the following:*
    - *Measure and mix dry and wet ingredients*
    - *Use the oven to cook food such as cookies, brownies, frozen pizza, and casserole*

- The therapist should refer to the PowerPoint presentation slides for Dyad Session 7 while reviewing the content for the session.
- The therapist should have also prepared for the session by reviewing the Dyad Session 7 content discussed in the manual, which has detailed information about the content that will be covered.
- The important points to make while reviewing the Dyad Session 7 Content are:
    - We will do a Real World Practice Check-In, which will ask you and your teen specific questions about the goals on the DLS contract. This will be an opportunity to problem-solve any challenges and celebrate successes.
    - The elements of an effective system for achieving DLS goals will be reviewed with the teens as it relates to the goals on the DLS contract. This will be our main

opportunity each session to revise the goals that are currently being targeted on the DLS contract before we add in a new goal at the end of the session.
- The DLS Teaching Method will be used to teach the skill of cooking in the oven by using the steps of learning, watching, practicing, and doing it independently.
- Recipes and videos that demonstrate how to cook recipes may be useful strategies as teens are learning to cook in the oven.
- The teens will learn how to measure dry and wet ingredients using measuring cups and spoons.
- Teens will learn about the features of their oven and how to operate it before cooking a recipe. They will also learn about the types of containers that can be used to cook in the oven.
- Teens will use the DLS Teaching Method to cook a recipe in the oven.

♦ Ask: ***Any questions about the content for the upcoming dyad session?***

Prep for the Next Caregiver Session (3 mins)

♦ ***We will have our next caregiver group session on DAY and TIME. At this session, we will discuss how setting up and implementing the DLS contract went. We will also discuss how to add the goal of cooking on the stovetop to your teen's DLS contract.***
♦ ***To prepare for the upcoming dyad session with your teen, please choose an oven recipe and have the ingredients available. These can be items that you have in your home already. You should try to involve your teen in choosing the recipe so that they are more motivated to cook the items and build their cooking skills.***
♦ ***Also, make sure to have measuring cups and spoons available to practice measuring dry and wet ingredients. You will also need to have a dry ingredient that the teen can use to practice measuring such as salt, sugar, or flour. We will use water to practice measuring wet ingredients.***
♦ ***Last, make sure that the kitchen is available at the time of your session.***
♦ ***After your dyad session with your teen, it will be important to prioritize working on the goals on the DLS contract and the Real World Practice assignment so that we can celebrate successes and also discuss any challenges or questions that arose in the caregiver group session.***
♦ Ask: ***Are there any questions before we end the session?***

Wrap-Up

♦ The therapist should send a calendar invite with the next caregiver group session's day/time to the caregiver.
♦ The therapist may also want to email caregivers a blank copy of the DLS contract or refer them to the STRW website.
♦ Prior to the dyad session, the therapist may want to check in with caregivers about the recipes they are planning on cooking. It is particularly helpful to have a copy of the recipe so that it can be displayed on the therapist's computer screen while the teen practices cooking.

Daily Living Skills Contract

Date ____________________

Goal	Expectations	Reward	MONDAY	TUESDAY	WEDNESDAY	THURSDAY	FRIDAY	SATURDAY	SUNDAY

____
Teen

____
Parent / Caregiver

Caregiver/Teen Dyad Session 7 Content (60 mins)

STRW Session 7 Schedule (1 min)

- The therapist should greet the caregiver and teen.
- ***Let's get started! As a reminder, it will be helpful to sit together at a table so that we can all see each other and work together. Please pull out your STRW workbook that contains the handouts for all STRW sessions. This session is called Session 7 – Cooking in the Oven. Please turn to that section in your workbook.***
- ***Let's go over the session schedule so that you know what we will be doing. Please feel free to ask any questions about our schedule!***
- Briefly go over each item on the Session Schedule.
- Check to make sure that the caregiver and teen have the following materials for the session: measuring cups and spoons, large mixing bowl, dry measuring ingredients (e.g., flour, salt, sugar), and ingredients and supplies (e.g., cookie sheet) for the oven recipe. The teen and caregiver can gather these materials now if needed.
- It may also be helpful to preheat the oven now and to have the caregiver demonstrate how to do this while referring to the recipe.

Real World Practice Check-In: Contract and Morning Routine (3 mins)

- Refer to the Session 6 Real World Practice handout and the DLS Contract handout.
- ***Let's check in on how you are doing with each goal on your DLS contract. Please be honest, as this is an opportunity to talk about what is working and what is not working and do some brainstorming to address any challenges.***
- As needed, the therapist should spend time modifying the DLS contract and problem-solving how to make a more effective system to target the DLS goal (e.g., make expectations more specific, change reward, increase/decrease number of prompts, modify the strategies being used to help with goals).
- If the therapist used a fillable PDF of the DLS Contract handout in the previous session, it may be helpful to share this on the screen so that the goal, expectations, and reward can be easily discussed.
- The following questions should be asked (if applicable), and the responses and any relevant notes should be entered into the Real World Practice Tracking Sheet:
  - ***Did you use your DLS contract this week?***
  - ***Did you work on your morning routine goal during the week?***
    - ***What went well?***
    - ***What was challenging?***
    - ***How many days did you work on your morning routine goal?***
    - ***Did you earn a reward for your morning routine goal?***
    - ***How many days did you earn a reward?***

Real World Practice Check-In: Cleaning the Bedroom and Laundry (3 mins)

- The following questions should be asked (if applicable), and the responses and any relevant notes should be entered into the Real World Practice Tracking Sheet:
  - *Did you work on your cleaning the bedroom goal during the week?*
    - *What went well?*
    - *What was challenging?*
    - *How many days did you work on your cleaning the bedroom goal?*
  - *Did you earn a reward for your cleaning the bedroom goal?*
    - *Did you work on your laundry goal during the week?*
    - *What went well?*
    - *What was challenging?*
    - *How many days did you work on your laundry goal?*
    - *Did you earn a reward for your laundry goal?*

Real World Practice Check-In: Cooking and Money (4 mins)

- The following questions should be asked (if applicable), and the responses and any relevant notes should be entered into the Real World Practice Tracking Sheet:
  - *Did you work on your cooking goal during the week?*
    - *What went well?*
    - *What was challenging?*
    - *How many days did you work on your cooking goal?*
    - *Did you earn a reward for your cooking goal?*
  - *For your Real World Practice, you were also given a money assignment.*
    - *Did you work on or complete a money assignment?*
    - *What did you do?*
    - *What went well?*
    - *What was challenging?*

- Ask: *Any questions or comments about your Real World Practice assignments?*
- If the caregiver/teen dyad struggled to complete the Real World Practice assignments, the therapist should spend some time discussing how to identify days/times that they could designate to commit to working on the assignments.
- If the therapist used a fillable PDF of the DLS Contract handout in the previous session, it may be helpful to share this on the screen so that the goal, expectations, and reward can be easily discussed.

Elements of an Effective System for Achieving DLS Goals (2 mins)

- Ask: *Are there any issues you want to discuss or troubleshoot related to the DLS contract?*
- Ask and Discuss: *Are we considering all of the important elements to increase the likelihood of you achieving your DLS goals by developing the most effective system?*

- If applicable, discuss how to modify any DLS goals to address (1) qualities of the teen and their caregiver; (2) use of evidence-based strategies to teach and master DLS; and (3) ensuring that goals are obvious, attractive, easy, and satisfying.

Evidence-Based Strategy: DLS Teaching Method-Cooking in the Oven (2 mins)

- Refer to the DLS Teaching Method for Cooking in the Oven handout.
- ***We will continue to use the DLS Teaching Method to build up your skills in the kitchen, including measuring and mixing ingredients and cooking recipes in the oven.***
- ***In session today, you will measure and mix ingredients and cook in the oven. As part of your DLS contract in the coming weeks, you will have a cooking goal. It can be helpful to make your cooking goal related to the other goals on your DLS contract. For example, you could practice baking cookies in the oven to reward yourself for doing your laundry.***

Evidence-Based Strategy: Task Analysis (3 mins)

- Refer to the Chocolate Chip Cookies Recipe handout and the Task Analysis Steps handout.
- ***As we discussed last week, a recipe already breaks down the steps needed to cook and also includes all of the ingredients that you will need to cook. Just like a task analysis, a recipe can be used to make sure you are doing the steps in the correct order.***
- ***Look at the*** Chocolate Chip Cookies Recipes ***handout that lists the ingredients and steps. Recipes in cookbooks and on websites and blogs will also list the ingredients and the steps for preparing and cooking the recipe.***
- OPTIONAL: The therapist can choose to use video modeling to demonstrate how to cook a recipe such as chocolate chip cookies. Many websites or cooking blogs have pictures and videos that break down how to prepare and cook a recipe, which may be particularly helpful for some teens. There are several cookbooks and cooking websites that may be useful resources to discuss with the caregiver and teen on the STRW Resources handout on the STRW website.

Measuring Ingredients (5 mins)

- ***We are going to learn how to measure and mix ingredients that are needed for making recipes. This is often really important for recipes that you cook in the oven such as chocolate chip cookies, muffins, or brownies.***
- OPTIONAL: The therapist can choose to use video modeling to demonstrate how to mix and measure ingredients. There are optional links to demonstrate this skill on the STRW Resources handout on the STRW website.

Liquid Measuring Cups (3 mins)

- Have the dyad move the session to the kitchen for the remainder of the session.
- Refer caregiver/teen to the Measuring Cups handout and the Measuring Spoons handout.

- ***These handouts list important information and guidelines for how to measure dry and wet ingredients using measuring cups and measuring spoons. Let's practice measuring liquid ingredients which may include water and oil.***
- Instruct the caregiver/teen to locate the measuring cups and spoons in their kitchen.
- Have the teen use a measuring cup to practice measuring wet ingredients and encourage the caregiver to provide feedback and coaching as needed:
  - ¼ cup of water
  - 1 cup of water

- The therapist should provide feedback and support to the caregiver as needed.
- NOTE: If applicable, it may be easier and a better use of time to have the teen measure the liquid ingredients needed in the oven recipe that they will be cooking.

Dry Measuring Cups (3 mins)

- Refer to the Measuring Cups handout
- ***Now we are going to practice measuring dry ingredients such as flour, salt, and sugar. You will need measuring cups and also a knife or spatula to measure dry ingredients.***
- Have the teen use a measuring cup and knife/spatula to practice measuring dry ingredients and encourage the caregiver to provide feedback and coaching as needed:
  - ½ cup of flour/sugar/salt
  - ¾ cup of flour/sugar/salt

- The therapist should provide feedback and support to the caregiver as needed.
- NOTE: If applicable, it may be easier and a better use of time to have the teen measure the dry ingredients needed in the oven recipe that they will be cooking.

Measuring Spoons (2 mins)

- Refer to the Measuring Spoons handout.
- ***Let's practice using measuring spoons to measure ingredients. You will need measuring spoons as we measure different amounts of water.***
- Have the teen use measuring spoons to measure the following with water and encourage the caregiver to provide feedback and coaching as needed:
  - ½ tsp of water
  - 1 tbsp of water
  - 1 tsp of water

- The therapist should provide feedback and support to the caregiver as needed.
- NOTE: If applicable, it may be easier and a better use of time to have the teen measure the ingredients needed in the oven recipe that they will be cooking.

Oven Settings (3 mins)

- Refer to the Oven Settings handout.
- ***Before we start cooking, let's go over some basics of using the oven.***
- Have the caregiver and teens take turns reading the bullet points on the Oven Settings handout. Encourage the caregiver to elaborate on or provide additional information on how they use their oven to cook.
- Have the caregiver demonstrate the basic settings on the oven including:
  - How to set the temperature on an oven
  - How to turn the oven off
  - How to safely put items in and out of the oven using potholders

- The therapist should provide feedback and support to the caregiver as needed.
- Ask: ***Any questions about how to use the oven?***

Common Oven Cooking Supplies (2 mins)

- ***Here are several examples of oven-safe cooking supplies. Items such as cookie sheets and glass casserole pans can be used to cook recipes in the oven. Cooking supplies will often have "oven safe" written on the bottom if they are safe to use in the oven. You can also ask your caregiver or search the internet if you are not sure if a container is safe to put in the oven.***
- Instruct the caregiver to go over where their oven safe containers are stored and what they typically use when cooking items in the oven.
- Ask: ***Any other questions before we practice cooking in the oven?***

DLS Teaching Method-Cooking in the Oven (10 mins)

- ***We are now going to use the DLS Teaching Method of Learn, Watch, Practice, and then Do It Independently to practice cooking in the oven.***
- ***What is the oven recipe that you will be making today?***
  - If a recipe has not been identified, assist the teen/caregiver by finding a recipe in a cookbook or on the internet.
  - The therapist may also need to add additional steps (e.g., preheat oven) or clarify steps that are vague or unclear

- After a recipe is identified, review the steps of the recipe. If possible, the therapist should display the recipe on their computer screen. The Task Analysis Steps handout could be used to write down the steps of the oven recipe if needed.
- The therapist should do the following for the first three steps of the DLS Teaching Method as it relates to making a recipe in the oven:
  - LEARN – First, instruct the caregiver to review the recipe steps and the ingredients and supplies (e.g., bowl, measuring cup, etc.) that are needed.
  - WATCH – Then, instruct the caregiver to demonstrate (as needed) how to cook the recipe. This should involve the caregiver demonstrating (e.g., pressing the buttons to preheat the oven) or talking through (e.g., verbally instructing the teen to preheat the oven) each step of the recipe and providing any support that

the teen may need. The caregiver may need to provide coaching on concepts such as preheating the oven, setting the correct temperature, measuring and mixing, setting a timer, and using a potholder.

- PRACTICE – Finally, instruct the teen to practice making the recipe and instruct the caregiver to provide feedback or support (including kitchen safety) as needed. Provide coaching on how to begin cleaning up (e.g., put ingredients away, wipe up spills) while waiting for the recipe to cook.

♦ The therapist should provide feedback and support to the caregiver as needed, including giving clear directions and demonstrations on making the oven recipe.
♦ The therapist can move on to additional content while waiting for the recipe to cook.

Elements of an Effective System for Achieving DLS Goals (3 mins)

♦ The therapist should briefly ask each teen about each of the elements and then incorporate the responses to the discussion on developing the DLS contract.
♦ *As we work to add or modify the goal of cooking to the DLS contract, let's make sure we are thinking about all of the following elements to build an effective system for achieving DLS goals:*
  - *Teen – are we considering your strengths, challenges, preferred learning style, and commitment?*
  - *Caregiver – are we considering your parenting style, time and effort, and commitment?*
    - *Some caregivers find it easy to have teens practice cooking alongside them while they are making breakfast, packing lunches, making after-school snacks, or making dinner.*
  - *Are we using evidence-based strategies?*
    - *We are using a recipe, which is very similar to a task analysis, to break the skill down into simple steps.*
    - *We are also using the DLS Teaching Method to help you learn and become independent in cooking.*
    - *You could look up videos that go along with recipes to teach you and demonstrate the steps of how to cook a recipe.*
  - *Is the goal of cooking obvious, attractive, easy, and satisfying?*
    - *Obvious – some ideas might be to print out the recipe so that the steps can be crossed off as they are completed.*
    - *Attractive – some ideas might be to listen to music while cooking or cook with your caregiver.*
    - *Easy – some ideas might be to have all of the ingredients available and on the counter, to set a reminder to cook at a specific day/time, or to choose a recipe that you typically cook during the week such as pizza on Friday.*
    - *Satisfying – some ideas include getting to eat whatever it is that you cook.*

♦ Ask and Discuss: *Any questions or comments?*
♦ *Let's apply all of this information to creating your DLS contract!*

Developing Your DLS Contract (5 mins)

- Refer to the DLS Contract handout
- ***Let's spend the remainder of our time in today's session modifying your DLS contract to continue working on your morning routine, cleaning your bedroom, and laundry goals and add in or modify the goal of cooking. You can work on the same goal as last week or we can add another cooking goal based on what you have learned this week. Use a blank copy of the* DLS Contract. *We will also keep in mind the importance of making sure the goal is easy, obvious, attractive, and satisfying so that you are more likely to achieve your goal. The DLS contract will have you track your progress and set up rewards for you to earn, which makes working on the goals satisfying!***
- The therapist should support the caregiver/teen dyad in creating the DLS contract by doing the following:
  - Incorporate all of the information from the last several sessions (e.g., rewards that are motivating for the teen, use of strategies and supports to build independence with certain steps) and the Real World Practice Check-In to create the DLS contract. The therapist should also consider the goals that the caregiver and teen collaboratively developed during the Preparing for STRW session.
  - While the teen worked on many cooking skills today and in the previous session, they need to determine if they want to have one cooking goal or multiple cooking goals. The therapist should help the dyad determine whether they should modify or change their cooking goals for the DLS contract.
  - Examples of cooking goals include mixing and measuring ingredients for cookies or brownies, making the same oven recipe they made in session, making a no-cook recipe for breakfast or lunch during the week, cutting up vegetables for dinner one day, and making an after-school snack in the microwave. The therapist should encourage the dyad to make sure the teen is prepared by having a recipe and any materials or ingredients available to make it more likely they will achieve their cooking goal.
  - Incorporate information from the teen practicing measuring and mixing ingredients and cooking in the oven over the course of the dyad session (e.g., if operating the oven or mixing dry ingredients was difficult, it may be beneficial to have the caregiver present to support and give feedback as the teen practices various skills).
  - Use the DLS Contract handout to specify the (1) Goal, (2) Expectations, and (3) Reward for Morning Routine, Cleaning the Bedroom, Doing Laundry, and Cooking.
  - Encourage the caregiver/teen dyad to work together and model appropriate and supportive coaching as they develop the DLS contract.

- Possible discussion questions that may be helpful to ask and discuss when creating the contract for the Morning Routine, Cleaning the Bedroom, Laundry, and Cooking goals include:
  - ***How often are you going to need to do the goal – every day, every weekday, every other day, or once per week?***
  - ***What steps of your goal do you need help with?***
  - ***What steps do you not know how to do?***

- *What steps are you doing independently?*
- *How easy/hard do you think it will be to meet your goal?*
- *What reward would you like to earn?*
- *Does the reward fit the goal? For example, earning 1 hour of screen time for doing your morning routine goal each day is a lot, but maybe earning 15–20 extra minutes of screen time would be a better fit.*
- *How will you check in about your goals daily to discuss if the goal was met?*
- *Where can you post your DLS contract so that you can track goals daily and remember to get your reward if it was earned?*

♦ The caregiver and teen should write each goal, expectation, and reward on the DLS Contract handout. It may be helpful for the therapist to share their screen and add/modify the goals, expectations, and rewards on a fillable PDF of the DLS Contract handout. The therapist can then email it to the caregiver and teen after the session.

♦ When the DLS contract has been completed, encourage the dyad to sign it and post it somewhere where they can easily see it so that the goals may be tracked.

Real World Practice (1 min)

♦ Refer to the Real World Practice handout.

♦ Discuss the details of the Real World Practice assignment.

- *Work on your morning routine, cleaning the bedroom, laundry, and cooking goals for the remainder of the week using your DLS contract.*
    - *Set aside a specific time such as on the way to school or after dinner to discuss how the morning routine went and how to problem-solve the next day.*
    - *Schedule a day/time to work on watching and/or practicing how to clean your bedroom, do laundry, and cook.*
    - *Make sure that if the teen earns the reward, they receive it immediately! This makes it more likely that they will continue to be motivated to meet their goal!*
- *Make a list of ingredients for a recipe you want to cook. Find and purchase the ingredients at the grocery store and pay for the items with either cash or credit/debit card.*

♦ Ask: *Any questions about your Real World Practice assignment?*

Guess the Price (3 mins) – OPTIONAL

♦ NOTE: This activity can be skipped if there is not enough time to complete it.

♦ *Let's play a quick round of Guess the Price, which is just meant to be a fun way to build up your understanding of how much things cost.*

♦ *Let's see if you know the prices of some common grocery items even if they are not necessarily items that you use!*

♦ The therapist can have the teen guess the price or have the caregiver and teen compete against each other.

♦ The therapist should click through the next four slides that contain examples of common grocery items. Prior to the session, the therapist will need to look up the prices to ensure that they are accurate.

- The therapist can change the grocery items for the Guess the Price game.
- This activity is meant to be fun and engaging! If the teen is averse to playing the game, it can be skipped. However, it would be helpful for the caregiver and teen to find other ways to build up an understanding of what things cost (e.g., compare the cost of products at the grocery store, involve the teen when purchasing cleaning items).

Preparing for the Next Dyad Session (2 mins)

- *We will have our next caregiver/teen dyad session on DAY and TIME. At this session, we will discuss how to cook on the stovetop. We will need you to prepare for the session by doing the following:*
    - *Gather ingredients for one or two stovetop recipes. Examples include grilled cheese sandwich, scrambled eggs, spaghetti, macaroni and cheese, quesadilla, stir fry vegetables, or French toast. Think about a recipe you would like to master or one that you have been wanting to learn!*
    - *We will also be spending the majority of the session in your kitchen.*
- *I will check in with you by email in a few days to remind you to get the items you need to make the stovetop recipes. It is sometimes easiest to just use ingredients you already have at home!*
- *It will be important to complete your Real World Practice assignment before our next dyad session and come prepared to discuss it. We will spend a lot of time next session talking about how the DLS contract went!*
- Ask: *Are there any questions before we end the session?*

Wrap-Up

- The therapist should send a calendar invite with the next caregiver/teen dyad session's day/time to the caregiver and teen. The therapist may also want to send the caregiver/teen a copy of the DLS contract if they completed it using a fillable PDF.

Evidence-Based Strategy: **Daily Life Skills Teaching Method**

Cooking in the Oven

LEARN

Review the steps of the oven recipe.
Gather the ingredients and cooking supplies that are needed.

WATCH

Your parent/caregiver will demonstrate (as needed) how to make the oven recipe by going through each step of the recipe.

PRACTICE

You will practice following the steps of the oven recipe
Your parent/caregiver will observe and give feedback and support after you complete each step.

DO IT INDEPENDENTLY

You will make the oven recipe on your own.

Chocolate Chip Cookies Recipe

Preparation Time: 20 mins
Cook Time: 10–12 mins

Ingredients:

- 1 cup softened butter (not melted)
- 1 cup white sugar
- 1 cup packed brown sugar
- 2 eggs
- 2 tsp vanilla extract
- 1 tsp baking soda
- 2 tsp hot water
- ½ tsp salt
- 3 cups flour
- 2 cups semisweet chocolate chips

Directions:

- Preheat oven to 350 degrees Fahrenheit.
- Combine the butter, white sugar, and brown sugar and stir or blend until smooth.
- Add the eggs slowly and beat into the batter.
- Stir in the vanilla.
- Dissolve the baking soda into the hot water and then add to the batter.
- Stir in the salt.
- Add the flour and chocolate chips.
- Stir until well mixed.
- Put a spoonful of batter onto ungreased cookie sheet.

Bake for 10–12 minutes or until the edges start to brown slightly.

Task Analysis

Skill: ______________________________

Steps:

____

____

____

____

____

____

____

____

____

____

____

____

____

____

____

____

____

____

____

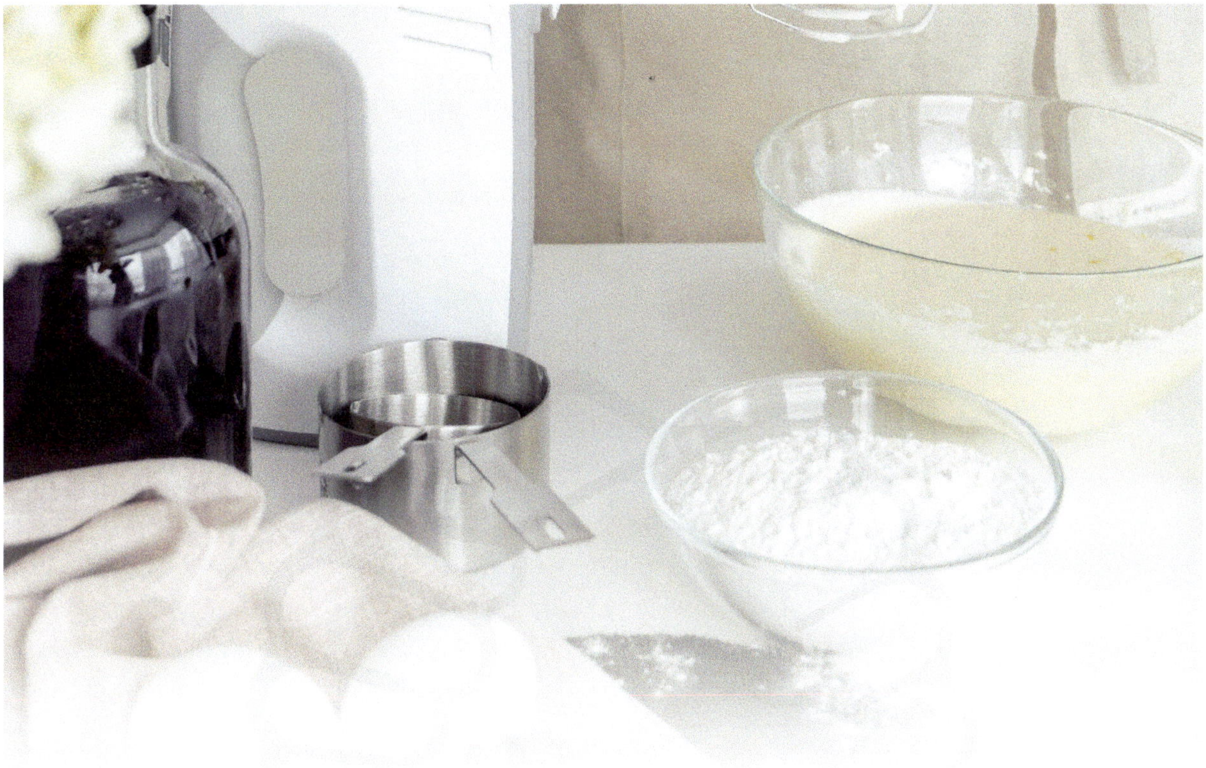

Dry Measuring Cups

Dry measuring cups measure dry ingredients such as flour, sugar, oats, butter, and peanut butter. They typically come in the sizes of 1 cup, 1/2 cup, 1/3 cup, and 1/4 cup.

Be sure not to measure your ingredients over the bowl or pan that you will be using.

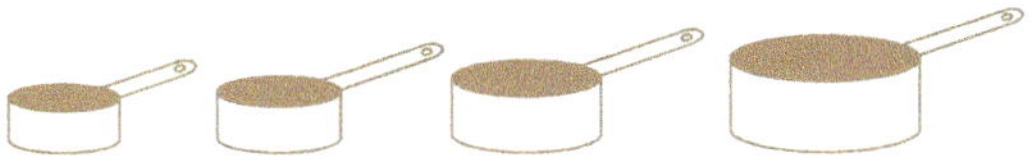

1/4 cup 1/3 cup 1/2 cup 1 cup

Liquid Measuring Cups

Liquid measuring cups measure liquids such as milk, water, and oil. They typically measure liquids in cups and/or ounces (or oz for short). Make sure that your liquid measuring cup is on a flat surface so that you measure accurately!

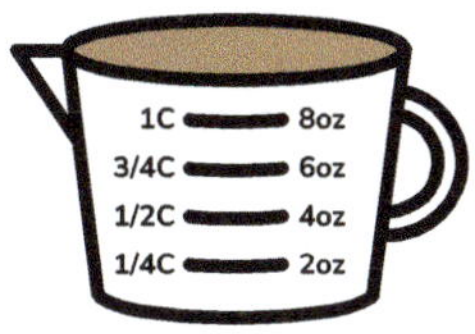

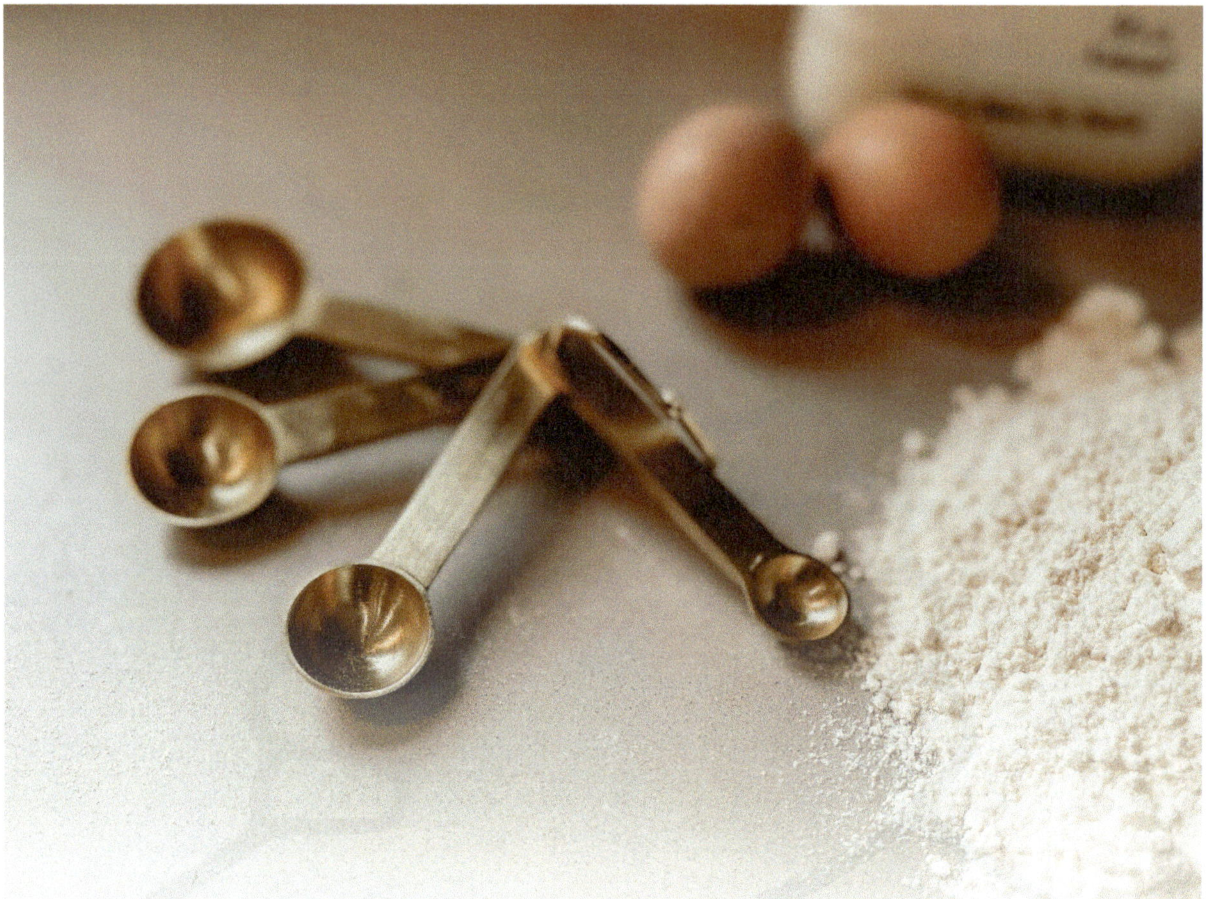

Measuring Spoons

Measuring spoons are used to measure small amounts. You can use them to measure liquids like milk or water and solids like salt and flour. They range in size from 1/8 teaspoon to 1 tablespoon.

A small 't' or 'tsp.' = **teaspoon**

A large 'T', 'Tbs.' or 'Tbsp.' = **tablespoon**

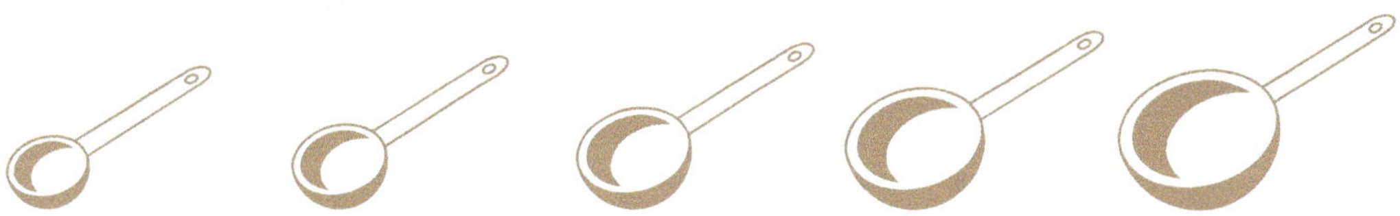

Oven Settings

1. **Preheat**
    - When you preheat an oven, you turn it on and set it to the correct temperature before cooking any food in it.
    - All cooking times in recipes are based on a preheated oven, so it is very important to preheat an oven before cooking!
    - When most ovens are preheated, they will beep or a light goes on or off, which means you can put the food in the oven.

2. **Bake**
    - The Bake setting is used to cook most things like pizza, French fries, chicken, fish, cookies, cakes, and brownies.
    - Food gets cooked from the outside in when it is baking in the oven.
        - For some foods, like pizza or French fries, you can use a timer to cook the food.
        - For foods like brownies or muffins, you can set a timer and check whether it is done by sticking a toothpick in and seeing if it comes out clean (i.e., without any batter on the toothpick).
        - For foods like meat, you can check whether it is done by measuring its internal temperatures by placing an oven thermometer into the meat. Different meats need to be cooked to specific temperatures.
    - While your food is baking, try not to open the door too often to check on it because this will cause a drop in the oven's temperature and extend the cooking time.

3. **Broil**
    - The Broil setting is used to cook foods such as steaks, hamburgers, and chicken under very direct heat.
    - With a gas oven, you actually see a flame. With an electric oven, you can see coils directly above the food.
    - Many recipes will tell you how to position your oven racks so that your food cooks evenly on the Broil setting.

Daily Living Skills Contract

Date ______________________

Goal	Expectations	Reward	MONDAY	TUESDAY	WEDNESDAY	THURSDAY	FRIDAY	SATURDAY	SUNDAY

______________________ Teen

______________________ Parent / Caregiver

Surviving and Thriving in the Real World
Session 7 – Real World Practice

- Work on your (1) morning routine, (2) cleaning the bedroom, (3) doing laundry, and (4) cooking goals for the remainder of the week using your DLS contract.
  - Set aside a specific time (e.g., on the way to school, after dinner) to discuss how the morning routine went and how to problem-solve for the next day.
  - Schedule a day/time to work on watching and/or practicing how to clean the bedroom, do laundry, and cook.
  - Make sure that if a reward is earned, it is provided immediately!

- Make a list of ingredients for a recipe you want to cook. Find and purchase the ingredients at the grocery store and pay for the items with either cash or credit/debit card.
  - Schedule a day/time to complete the money assignment.

Surviving & Thriving in the Real World

Session 8

Cooking on the Stove

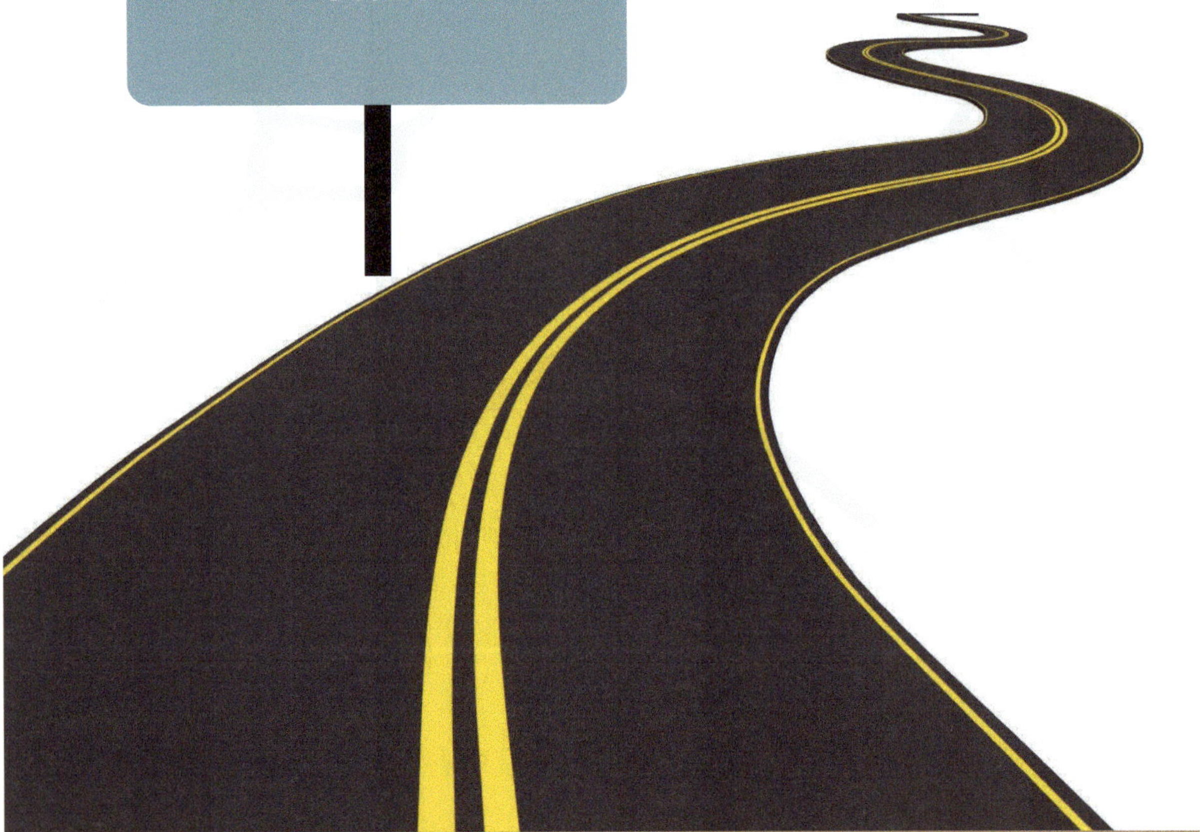

Session 8

Cooking on the Stove

Aims

- Continue to build rapport between caregiver group members and the therapist
- Continue to build rapport between the teen, caregiver, and therapist
- Further develop ability to use a DLS contract to set a DLS goal, define expectations, and identify a reward for meeting the goal
- Review the four elements for developing an effective system to achieve the teen's DLS goals
- Understand how to use the DLS Teaching Method to learn the steps for cooking a recipe on the stovetop
- Understand the steps for cleaning up the kitchen after cooking
- Create and implement a DLS contract to target the goals of morning routine, cleaning the bedroom, doing laundry, and cooking

Structure

- Caregiver group session via telehealth
- Caregiver/teen dyad session via telehealth

Session Supplies

- Caregiver Group Handouts
  - DLS Contract

- Caregiver/Teen Dyad Handouts
  - DLS Teaching Method for Cooking on the Stove
  - Grilled Cheese Sandwich Recipe
  - Task Analysis Steps (2 copies)
  - Kitchen Cleaning Checklist
  - DLS Contract
  - Session 8 – Real World Practice

- Videos (optional links available on the STRW website and the STRW Resources handout)

DOI: 10.4324/9781003458838-11

Caregiver/Teen Preparation for Session

- For the dyad session, the caregiver and teen should have identified a recipe that they want to cook on the stovetop during this session. They should also have the ingredients needed to make the recipe.
- The caregiver and teen should also get any cleaning supplies (e.g., sponge, broom, paper towels, etc.) that may be needed so that they can practice cleaning up the kitchen after cooking.
- It would be highly beneficial for the caregiver and teen to practice these skills in the kitchen area that is free from as many distractions as possible (e.g., other siblings, noise from the television, etc.).

Therapist Preparation for Session

- The therapist may want to review the Recipe Ideas for the STRW Cooking Sessions handout (see appendix), which includes ideas of recipes to cook if the caregiver/teen are having trouble identifying what to cook in Sessions 6–8.
- The therapist should use the Real World Practice Tracking Sheet for each caregiver/teen dyad in all subsequent STRW sessions to track progress on their DLS contract goals.
- The therapist will need to be mindful about individualizing the session for each dyad based on whether they have access to a stovetop to cook and also based on the foods that their family cooks and eats on a regular basis (e.g., have dyad work together to identify recipes to cook, identify recipes that include ingredients that they often have readily available in their kitchen).
- The therapist should consider reviewing the Tips for STRW Therapists: How to Facilitate Achievement of DLS Goals handout prior to each caregiver group session or dyad session for tips and strategies on how to help teens achieve the goals on their DLS contract. Tips that may be beneficial for Session 8 include:
  - *Identify the individual strategies that work best for a teen.* For many teens, there are likely four to five strategies that they can use over and over again to successfully meet their DLS goals. It is critical for therapists to assist with identifying successful strategies that can be used for current and future DLS goals. The therapist should regularly discuss what strategies work and do not work with the dyad.
  - *Encourage trying out a strategy before choosing another one.* Teens and caregivers may be resistant to trying out a strategy for a variety of reasons (e.g., it was not effective in the past, it seems too simple, it seems too hard). The therapist should encourage the teen and caregiver to try out a strategy before working to identify a new one. For example, a checklist can be a very effective tool for learning the steps of a task, starting a task, remembering the steps of a task, and completing a task – but the dyad may need to be strongly encouraged to incorporate it!

Session 8 Notes

- Fillable PDFs of handouts from this session (i.e., Task Analysis Steps, DLS Contract) are available on the STRW website.

- Caregiver Group Session
  - At approximately halfway through the STRW intervention, caregivers often benefit from a direct discussion and/or opportunity to reflect about how they are doing coaching their teen and supporting the goals on the DLS contract. Helpful points to address might include:
    - Caregivers are also putting a lot of time and effort into supporting their teen as they build their DLS.
    - It can feel overwhelming at times to be targeting many goals simultaneously, but the caregiver group can serve as a place for them to share their feelings and also engage in problem solving to decrease overwhelm.
    - Teens sometimes experience a sort of "honeymoon" period in the first few sessions after implementing the DLS contract, and then they may struggle to meet their goals. This is very normal and part of learning a new skill and making something a habit. Teens may need to incorporate additional strategies or may need to implement a previously used strategy to meet their goals.
    - Parenting neurodivergent teens can be challenging and takes a significant amount of time and effort, which can be exacerbated by working on new DLS goals, managing school and homework, balancing extracurricular activities, and managing relationships with family and friends. It can be beneficial to discuss these challenges and experiences in the caregiver group.
    - It may be helpful for the therapist to discuss the concept of self-efficacy and whether the teen's progress in learning new skills and becoming independent is increasing their confidence and sense of autonomy.
  - The therapist should continue to devote the majority of the caregiver group session to reviewing how the DLS contract is progressing for each caregiver. This is an opportunity to identify any issues and brainstorm solutions prior to the dyad session.
  - The therapist should utilize the caregiver group session to get an understanding of how it may be necessary to personalize the dyad session content (e.g., discuss options if the teen does not have a stovetop, develop an understanding of teen's ability and experience with cleaning up the kitchen, brainstorm possible recipes for the teen to cook with the caregiver).
  - The therapist should make an active effort to foster collaboration between the group members by encouraging active discussion and problem solving of challenges or questions about the DLS contract.
  - The therapist should have caregivers discuss how they can encourage cooking on a regular basis and get ideas from other caregivers (e.g., helping to prepare a specific family dinner so that the teen can eventually cook dinner on their own for their family).

- Dyad Session
  - The therapist should encourage the caregiver, in collaboration with their teen, to choose a recipe that they are motivated to learn how to cook and eat but should also encourage them to identify recipes for items that they consistently have in their kitchen and/or may be beneficial for the teen to learn how to cook (e.g., making scrambled eggs for themselves in the morning before they go to school).

- Teens may often feel nervous or anxious about cooking on the stovetop (e.g., turning burners on and off, transferring a pan from a burner, getting burned from boiling water or bubbling sauce). It may be helpful to implement any safety precautions (e.g., long cooking gloves, an apron, etc.). If the teen appears fearful of cooking on the stovetop, the therapist may need to coach caregivers and teens on how to gradually work up to cooking an item on the stovetop (e.g., learn about how to turn a burner on, watch the caregiver turn the burner on, have the caregiver watch the teen turn the burner on, turn the burner on while the caregiver gets ready to boil a pot of water, etc.). This type of gradual and systematic desensitization may be outside of the scope of the STRW session and may require additional support from a therapist.
- The therapist should work with the dyad to determine if they want to add in another cooking goal or continue working on the cooking goal from previous sessions. While it can often feel overwhelming to add in another goal to the DLS contract, cooking is a goal that can typically be done alongside the caregiver during the course of the week.
- It is often necessary to adjust the demands of a DLS contract goal to be more manageable so that the teen is more likely to acquire a skill. For example, if cooking an entire meal is overwhelming, the teen could start with just chopping up the vegetables needed to make the meal while the caregiver provides support as needed. If a teen is struggling to fold clothing as neatly as the caregiver would like, the expectation could be adjusted to increase success (e.g., clothes need to be folded so that the drawers can shut, teen can hang all shirts up in their closet if it is difficult to fold them).
- If the teen does not have access to a stovetop, they can choose another appliance to practice cooking (e.g., toaster oven, grill, griddle, air fryer, crock pot, etc.) and/or could practice making recipes that they would eat for breakfast or pack in their lunch.
- The therapist will need to manage time effectively so that teens get an opportunity to make one or two recipes on the stovetop. Some suggestions include:
    - Have a copy of the recipe available to share on the therapist's computer screen so that the steps are displayed while the caregiver and teen are cooking.
    - Review stovetop equipment in more detail as preparing to make recipe or while waiting for the recipe to cook.
    - The session can end prior to the item being completely cooked or ready to eat.
    - The caregiver and teen can finish cleaning the kitchen after the session ends.
- The therapists can encourage caregivers to point out where various items can be found in the kitchen (e.g., pots, spatula) if the teen is not aware of where to find these items.
- When developing the DLS contract at the end of the dyad session, the therapist should continue to incorporate all of the information and knowledge gained from the past several sessions (e.g., issues that were brought up during the caregiver group session, task analysis steps, discussing how to incorporate the essential elements of an effective system for achieving DLS goals, identifying appropriate rewards, etc.).

Caregiver Group Session 8 Content (90 mins)

Review – Real World Practice Assignment (50 mins)

- The therapist should greet the caregivers and welcome them to the session.
- Discuss the Real World Practice assignment in detail by having all caregivers share how using the DLS contract to target the morning routine, cleaning the bedroom, laundry, and cooking goals went with their teen. Encourage caregivers to jot down questions and notes on a blank copy of the DLS Contract handout that they may want to discuss or incorporate into their teen's contract at the next dyad session.
- ***We will have everyone share how using the DLS contract to target the morning routine, cleaning the bedroom, laundry, and cooking goals went for their teen. This is an opportunity to celebrate successes and also problem-solve any challenges or obstacles that occurred. We will spend the majority of our session discussing each teen's progress with the DLS contract. It may be helpful to jot down questions and notes on a copy of the*** **DLS Contract** ***handout, and feel free to ask questions or add to the discussion.***
- It may be helpful to refer caregivers to the Tips for Creating a Successful DLS Contract handout (from Session 4) when discussing the goals on the DLS contract (e.g., clearly defining expectations, re-evaluating rewards regularly to ensure they are motivating, etc.).
- Points of discussion or questions to ask each caregiver include the following:
  - DLS contract
    - ***Did the teen make progress at becoming more independent with each of their goals – morning routine, cleaning the bedroom, laundry, and cooking?***
    - ***What went well?***
    - ***What was difficult?***
    - ***Did they receive a reward?***
    - ***Did they use any strategies to help them to learn the skill or become more independent?***
    - ***Any obstacles or barriers?***
    - ***Do you plan on modifying any goals on the current DLS contract?***
  - Making a list and purchasing items
    - ***Was your teen able to make a list of ingredients for a recipe that they want to cook?***
    - ***Was your teen able to find and purchase the items at the store?***
    - ***What went well?***
    - ***What skills still need to be practiced?***
- Ask: ***Any questions about the Real World Practice assignment?***

STRW Session 8 Goals (1 min)

- *The goals of today's session is to discuss how we will be continuing to target the DLS goal of cooking on the stovetop and also cleaning up the kitchen after cooking. We will also review how to build an effective system to help you and your teen achieve their DLS goals now and in the future.*
- *We are more than halfway through STRW, and at this point, we are really starting to build your teen's DLS and it may seem overwhelming to add in another goal. With cooking, it will be helpful to keep in mind if there are ways that the teen can incorporate this into their daily or weekly schedule. For example:*
  - *Could the teen make their own breakfast during the week?*
  - *Could the teen make their own lunch on the weekends?*
  - *Could the teen help you prepare a meal during the week? For example, could they cook the meat for tacos?*

- Ask and Discuss: *Any questions?*

Review Dyad Session 8 Content (36 mins)

- *Now we will briefly review the material that will be covered in the upcoming dyad session with your teen. This will allow you to have some time to prepare for the upcoming session. Please feel free to ask any questions as we go over the content of the dyad session.*
- *For this session, we will plan on teaching skills in your kitchen. It is a session that is focused on cooking a recipe on the stovetop and going through the steps of cleaning up the kitchen. It will be important to be prepared for this session by having a stovetop recipe, pots or pans, supplies such as a spatula, and any ingredients that are needed. It will also be important to have your stove available.*
- *If you do not have a stovetop, we can still practice the skill of cooking a recipe and can possibly identify another appliance that your teen could use to practice cooking such as a crock pot or microwave oven.*
- Ask: *Any questions about practicing these cooking skills in your home with your teen at the upcoming dyad session?*
- *Before we review the dyad session content, let's all briefly share your teen's abilities to do the following:*
  - *Use the stovetop to cook foods such as grilled cheese, scrambled eggs, or spaghetti.*
  - *Clean up the kitchen after cooking, including wiping counters, mopping the floor, and putting ingredients away.*

- The therapist should refer to the PowerPoint presentation slides for Dyad Session 8 while reviewing the content for the session.
- The therapist should have also prepared for the session by reviewing the Dyad Session 8 content discussed in the manual, which has detailed information about the content that will be covered.
- The important points to make while reviewing the Dyad Session 8 Content are:
  - We will do a Real World Practice Check-In, which will ask you and your teen specific questions about the goals on the DLS contract. This will be an opportunity to problem-solve any challenges and celebrate successes.

- The elements of an effective system for achieving DLS goals will be reviewed with the teens as it relates to the goals on the DLS contract. This will be our main opportunity each session to revise the goals that are currently being targeted on the DLS contract before we add in a new goal at the end of the session.
- The DLS Teaching Method will be used to teach the skill of cooking on the stovetop by using the steps of learning, watching, practicing, and doing it independently.
- Recipes and videos that demonstrate how to cook recipes are useful evidence-based strategies for cooking on the stovetop.
- Teens will learn about the features of their stovetop and how to operate it before cooking a recipe. They will also learn about the types of cooking equipment that are used when cooking on the stovetop.
- Teens will use the DLS Teaching Method to cook a recipe on the stovetop.
- A task analysis for cleaning up the kitchen after cooking will be created that can be used as a checklist.

♦ Ask: *Any questions about the content for the upcoming dyad session?*

Prep for the Next Caregiver Session (3 mins)

♦ ***We will have our next caregiver group session on DAY and TIME. At this session, we will discuss how setting up and implementing the DLS contract went. We will also discuss how to add the goal of grocery shopping to your teen's DLS contract.***

♦ ***To prepare for the upcoming dyad session with your teen, please choose a stovetop recipe and have the ingredients available. These can be items that you have in your home already. You should try to involve your teen in choosing the recipe so that they are more motivated to cook the items and build their cooking skills.***

♦ ***After your dyad session with your teen, it will be important to prioritize working on the goals on the DLS contract and the Real World Practice assignment so that we can celebrate successes and also discuss any challenges or questions that arose in the caregiver group session.***

♦ Ask: ***Are there any questions before we end the session?***

Wrap-Up

♦ The therapist should send a calendar invite with the next caregiver group session's day/time to the caregiver.

♦ The therapist may also want to email caregivers a blank copy of the DLS contract or refer them to the STRW website.

♦ Prior to the dyad session, the therapist may want to check in with caregivers about the recipes they are planning on cooking. It is particularly helpful to have a copy of the recipe so that it can be displayed on the therapist's screen while the teen practices cooking.

Daily Living Skills Contract

Date ____________________

Goal	Expectations	Reward	MONDAY	TUESDAY	WEDNESDAY	THURSDAY	FRIDAY	SATURDAY	SUNDAY

____________________ Teen

____________________ Parent / Caregiver

Caregiver/Teen Dyad Session 8 Content (60 mins)

STRW Session 8 Schedule (1 min)

- The therapist should greet the caregiver and teen.
- *Let's get started! As a reminder, it will be helpful to sit together at a table so that we can all see each other and work together. Please pull out your STRW workbook that contains the handouts for all STRW sessions. This session is called Session 8 – Cooking on the Stove. Please turn to that section in your workbook.*
- *Let's go over the session schedule so that you know what we will be doing. Please feel free to ask any questions about our schedule!*
- Briefly go over each item on the Session Schedule.
- Check to make sure that the caregiver and teen have the following materials for the session: any pots or pans, cooking supplies such as a spatula or strainer, and ingredients for the stovetop recipe. The teen and caregiver can gather these materials now if needed.

Real World Practice Check-In: Contract and Morning Routine (3 mins)

- Refer to the Session 7 Real World Practice handout and the DLS Contract handout.
- *Let's check in on how you are doing with each goal on your DLS contract. Please be honest, as this is an opportunity to talk about what is working and what is not working and do some brainstorming to address any challenges.*
- As needed, the therapist should spend time modifying the DLS contract and problem solving how to make a more effective system to target the DLS goal (e.g., make expectations more specific, change reward, increase/decrease number of prompts, modify the strategies being used to help with goals).
- If the therapist used a fillable PDF of the DLS Contract handout in the previous session, it may be helpful to share this on the screen so that the goal, expectations, and reward can be easily discussed.
- The following questions should be asked (if applicable), and the responses and any relevant notes should be entered into the Real World Practice Tracking Sheet:
  - *Did you use your DLS contract this week?*
  - *Did you work on your morning routine goal during the week?*
    - *What went well?*
    - *What was challenging?*
    - *How many days did you work on your morning routine goal?*
    - *Did you earn a reward for your morning routine goal?*
    - *How many days did you earn a reward?*

Real World Practice Check-In: Cleaning the Bedroom and Laundry (3 mins)

- The following questions should be asked (if applicable), and the responses and any relevant notes should be entered into the Real World Practice Tracking Sheet:
  - *Did you work on your cleaning the bedroom goal during the week?*
    - *What went well?*
    - *What was challenging?*
    - *How many days did you work on your cleaning the bedroom goal?*
    - *Did you earn a reward for your cleaning the bedroom goal?*
  - *Did you work on your laundry goal during the week?*
    - *What went well?*
    - *What was challenging?*
    - *How many days did you work on your laundry goal?*
    - *Did you earn a reward for your laundry goal?*

Real World Practice Check-In: Cooking and Money (4 mins)

- The following questions should be asked (if applicable), and the responses and any relevant notes should be entered into the Real World Practice Tracking Sheet:
  - *Did you work on your cooking goal or goals during the week?*
    - *What went well?*
    - *What was challenging?*
    - *How many days did you work on your cooking goal or goals?*
    - *Did you earn a reward for your cooking goal or goals?*
  - *For your Real World Practice, you were also given a money assignment.*
    - *Did you work on or complete a money assignment?*
    - *What did you do?*
    - *What went well?*
    - *What was challenging?*

- Ask: *Any questions or comments about your Real World Practice assignments?*
- If the caregiver/teen dyad struggled to complete the Real World Practice assignments, the therapist should spend some time discussing how to identify days/times that they could designate to commit to working on the assignments.
- If the therapist used a fillable PDF of the DLS Contract handout in the previous session, it may be helpful to share this on the screen so that the goal, expectations, and reward can be easily discussed.

Elements of an Effective System for Achieving DLS Goals (2 mins)

- Ask: *Are there any issues you want to discuss or troubleshoot related to the DLS contract?*
- Ask and Discuss: *Are we considering all of the important elements to increase the likelihood of you achieving your DLS goals by developing the most effective system?*

- If applicable, discuss how to modify any DLS goals to address (1) qualities of the teen and their caregiver; (2) use of evidence-based strategies to teach and master DLS; and (3) ensuring that goals are obvious, attractive, easy, and satisfying.

Evidence-Based Strategy: DLS Teaching Method-Cooking on the Stove (2 mins)

- Refer to DLS Teaching Method for Cooking on the Stove handout.
- *We will continue to use the DLS Teaching Method to build up your skills of cooking recipes on the stovetop and making sure that you are cleaning up the kitchen after you finish cooking.*
- *In session today, you will cook a recipe on the stovetop and also clean up after you finish cooking. As part of your DLS contract in the coming weeks, you will have a cooking goal. It can be helpful to make your cooking goal related to the other goals on your DLS contract. For example, you could help cook tacos on the stovetop after earning your choice of dinner as a reward for cleaning your bedroom.*

Evidence-Based Strategy: Task Analysis (3 mins)

- Refer to Grilled Cheese Sandwich Recipe and Task Analysis Steps handout.
- *As we have previously discussed, a recipe already breaks down the steps needed to cook and also includes all of the ingredients that you will need to cook. Just like a task analysis, a recipe can be used to make sure you are doing the steps in the correct order.*
- *Look at the* **Grilled Cheese Sandwich Recipe** *handout that lists the ingredients and steps. It can be helpful to find a website or cookbook that includes pictures and/or videos to make it easier for you to learn and master the steps of a recipe.*
- The therapist can choose to use video modeling to demonstrate how to cook a recipe such as a grilled cheese sandwich.

Basic Stovetop Cooking Equipment-Pots and Pans (3 mins)

- Have the dyad move the session to the kitchen for the remainder of the session.
- *Today we will be talking about how to use the stovetop to cook. Let's start by going over some common cooking equipment you may use on the stove.*
- Have the teen read the description of each piece of stovetop cooking equipment on the slide and then have the teen find these items in their own kitchen.
- Have the caregiver discuss what they typically cook with each piece of cooking equipment that the teen identifies in the kitchen.

Basic Stovetop Cooking Equipment-Other Supplies (2 mins)

- *Here are other common supplies you may use when cooking on the stovetop.*
- Have the teen read the description of each piece of stovetop cooking equipment on the slide and then have the teen find these items in their own kitchen.

- Have the caregiver discuss what they typically cook with each piece of cooking equipment that teen identifies in the kitchen.
- Caregiver/teen can also identify any other stovetop cooking supplies/equipment that are not listed that their family often uses.
- Instruct the caregiver and teen to determine which equipment they are going to need to use for the recipes they are going to cook today (e.g., frying pan and spatula for scrambled eggs) and make sure it is placed to the side for later in the session.

Parts of the Stove (3 mins)

- ***Let's go over the basic parts and features of a stove that you will use when cooking.***
- Instruct the caregiver to go over the parts of the stovetop including burners, knobs, or other features (e.g., griddle) with an emphasis on the following:
  - How to turn the stove on and off.
  - The importance of turning burners off after cooking is complete.
  - The importance of leaving the stovetop surface free of items such as potholders and dish towels.
  - The difference between gas (e.g., have to use the knob to light the flame prior to cooking) and electric stoves (e.g., knob turns on the electric heat), and identification of which type the teen has in their kitchen.

- The therapist can also show a video demonstrating how to safely cook on a stovetop that is available on the STRW Resources handout and the STRW website.
- Ask: ***Any other questions or concerns before we practice cooking on the stovetop?***

DLS Teaching Method-Cooking on the Stove (15 mins)

- ***We are now going to use the DLS Teaching Method of Learn, Watch, Practice, and then Do It Independently to practice cooking on the stovetop.***
- ***What is the stovetop recipe you will be making today?***
  - If a recipe has not been identified, assist the teen/caregiver by finding a recipe in a cookbook or on the internet.

- After a recipe is identified, review the steps of the recipe. If possible, the therapist should display the recipe on their computer screen. The Task Analysis Steps handout could be used to write down the steps of the stovetop recipe if needed.
- The therapist should do the following for the first three steps of the DLS Teaching Method as it relates to making a recipe on the stovetop:
  - LEARN – First, instruct the caregiver to review the recipe steps and the ingredients and supplies (e.g., pan, pot, spatula, etc.) that are needed.
  - WATCH – Then, instruct the caregiver to demonstrate (as needed) how to cook the recipe. This should involve the caregiver demonstrating (e.g., turning on the burner) or talking through (e.g., verbally instructing the teen on how to turn the burner on) each step of the recipe. The caregiver may need to provide coaching on concepts such as turning the burner on, identifying the correct temperature, placement of the pot/pan on the burner, using a spatula, and so on.

  - PRACTICE – Finally, instruct the teen to practice making the recipe and instruct the caregiver to provide feedback or support (including kitchen safety) as needed. Provide coaching on how to begin cleaning up (e.g., put ingredients away, wipe up spills) while waiting for the recipe to cook or after it has been cooked.

- The therapist should provide feedback and support to the caregiver as needed, including giving clear directions and modeling how to make the stovetop recipe.
- The therapist can move on to additional content while waiting for the recipe to cook.

Kitchen Cleaning Checklist (5 mins)

- Refer to the Kitchen Cleaning Checklist.
- ***An important part of cooking is cleaning up the kitchen. This checklist has some of the steps that are common when cleaning up the kitchen area. Some may not be necessary to do each time you cook, and we will individualize this checklist so that it works for you by creating a task analysis for cleaning the kitchen.***
- It may be beneficial to have the caregiver and teen get any cleaning supplies (e.g., sponge, broom, paper towels, etc.) that may be needed so that they can practice cleaning up the kitchen after cooking.
- Refer to the Task Analysis Steps handout.
- ***Let's discuss the steps that should be included when cleaning the kitchen and write them down on the Task Analysis Steps handout.***
- Assist the caregiver and teen with creating a kitchen cleaning checklist of tasks specific to what they may need to do in their own home.
- If time allows, instruct the caregiver to demonstrate how to clean up the kitchen and allow the teen to practice the various steps.

Elements of an Effective System for Achieving DLS Goals (3 mins)

- The therapist should briefly ask each teen about each of the elements and then incorporate the responses to the discussion on developing the DLS contract.
- ***As we work to add or modify the goal of cooking to the DLS contract, let's make sure we are thinking about all of the following elements to build an effective system for achieving DLS goals:***
  - ***Teen – are we considering your strengths, challenges, preferred learning style, and commitment?***
    - ***If you are a visual learner, it can be helpful to mark the burners with a sticker or label. For example, you could mark low, medium, and high using a sticker if your stove does not have these labels.***
  - ***Caregiver – are we considering your parenting style, time and effort, and commitment?***
    - ***Some caregivers find it easy to have teens practice cooking alongside them – while they are making breakfast, packing lunches, making after-school snacks, or making dinner.***
  - ***Are we using evidence-based strategies?***
    - ***We are using a recipe, which is very similar to a task analysis, to break the skill down into simple steps.***

    - *We are also using the DLS Teaching Method to help you learn and become independent in cooking.*
    - *You could look up videos that go along with recipes to teach you and demonstrate the steps of how to cook.*
    - *We are using a task analysis to remember the steps for cleaning up the kitchen after cooking.*
  - *Is the goal of cooking obvious, attractive, easy, and satisfying?*
    - *Obvious – some ideas might be to print out the recipe so that the steps can be crossed off as they are completed.*
    - *Attractive – some ideas might be to listen to music while cooking or cook with your caregiver.*
    - *Easy – some ideas might be to have all of the ingredients available and on the counter, to set a reminder to cook at a specific day/time, or to choose a recipe that you typically cook during the week such as tacos on Tuesday.*
    - *Satisfying – some ideas include getting to eat whatever it is that you cook!*

- Ask and Discuss: *Any questions or comments?*
- *Let's apply all of this information to creating your DLS contract!*

Developing Your DLS Contract (5 mins)

- Refer to DLS Contract handout
- *Let's spend the remainder of our time in today's session modifying your DLS contract to continue working on your morning routine, cleaning your bedroom, and laundry goals and add in or modify the goal of cooking. You can work on the same goal as last week or you can add in a goal related to the skills that we worked on today – cooking on the stovetop or cleaning up the kitchen after cooking. This could even involve you helping your caregiver cook on the stovetop one day this week. Use a blank copy of the DLS Contract. We will also keep in mind the importance of making sure the goal is Obvious, Attractive, Easy, and Satisfying so that you are more likely to achieve your goal. The DLS contract will have you track your progress and set up rewards for you to earn, which makes working on the goals satisfying!*
- The therapist should support the caregiver/teen dyad in creating the DLS contract by doing the following:
    - Incorporate all of the information from the last several sessions (e.g., rewards that are motivating for the teen, use of strategies and supports to build independence with certain steps) and the Real World Practice Check-In to create the DLS contract. The therapist should also consider the goals that the caregiver and teen collaboratively developed during the Preparing for STRW session.
    - While the teen worked on many cooking skills today and in the previous sessions, they need to determine if they want to have one or multiple cooking goals. The therapist should help the dyad determine whether they should modify or change their cooking goals for the DLS contract.
    - Examples of cooking goals include chopping up and then cooking vegetables, making the same stovetop recipe they made in session, making a no-cook recipe for breakfast or lunch during the week, cleaning up the

kitchen after cooking, or making an after-school snack in the microwave. The therapist should encourage the dyad to make sure the teen is prepared by having a recipe available and any materials or ingredients to make it more likely they will achieve their cooking goal.
    - Incorporate information from the teen practicing cooking on the stovetop and cleaning up the kitchen over the course of the dyad session (e.g., if the teen forgot to turn off the burners, it may be beneficial to have the caregiver present to support and give feedback as the teen practices this skill).
    - Use the DLS Contract handout to specify the (1) Goal, (2) Expectations, and (3) Reward for Morning Routine, Cleaning the Bedroom, Doing Laundry, and Cooking.
    - Encourage the caregiver/teen dyad to work together and model appropriate and supportive coaching as they develop the DLS contract.

- Possible discussion questions that may be helpful to ask and discuss when creating the contract for the Morning Routine, Cleaning the Bedroom, Laundry, and Cooking goals include:
  - ***How often are you going to need to do the goal – every day, every weekday, every other day, or once per week?***
    - ***What steps of your goal do you need help with?***
    - ***What steps do you not know how to do?***
    - ***What steps are you doing independently?***
    - ***How easy/hard do you think it will be to meet your goal?***
    - ***What reward would you like to earn?***
    - ***Does the reward fit the goal? For example, earning 1 hour of screen time for doing your morning routine goal each day is a lot, but maybe earning 15–20 extra minutes of screen time would be a better fit.***
    - ***How will you check in about your goals daily to discuss if the goal was met?***
    - ***Where can you post your DLS contract so that you can track goals daily and remember to get your reward if it was earned?***

- The caregiver and teen should write each goal, expectation, and reward on the DLS Contract handout. It may be helpful for the therapist to share their screen and add/modify the goals, expectations, and rewards on a fillable PDF of the DLS Contract handout. The therapist can then email it to the caregiver and teen after the session.
- When the DLS contract has been completed, encourage the dyad to sign it and post it somewhere where they can easily see it so that the goals may be tracked.

Real World Practice (1 min)

- Refer to the Real World Practice handout.
- Discuss the details of the Real World Practice assignment.
  - ***Work on your morning routine, cleaning the bedroom, laundry, and cooking goals for the remainder of the week using your DLS contract.***
    - ***Set aside a specific time such as on the way to school or after dinner to discuss how the morning routine went and how to problem-solve the next day.***
    - ***Schedule a day/time to work on watching and/or practicing how to clean your bedroom, do laundry, and cook.***

    - *Make sure that if the teen earns the reward, they receive it immediately! This makes it more likely that they will continue to be motivated to meet their goal!*
  - *Make a list of ingredients for a recipe you want to cook. Find and purchase the ingredients at the grocery store and pay for the items with either cash or credit/debit card.*

- Ask: *Any questions about your Real World Practice assignment?*

Guess the Price (3 mins) – OPTIONAL

- NOTE: This activity can be skipped if there is not enough time to complete it.
- *Let's play a quick round of Guess the Price, which is just meant to be a fun way to build up your understanding of how much things cost.*
- *Let's see if you know the prices of some common grocery items even if they are not necessarily items that you use!*
- The therapist can have the teen guess the price or have the caregiver and teen compete against each other.
- The therapist should click through the next four slides that contain examples of common grocery items. Prior to the session, the therapist will need to look up the prices to ensure that they are accurate.
  - Therapists can change the grocery items for the Guess the Price game.
  - This activity is meant to be fun and engaging! If the teen is averse to playing the game, it can be skipped. However, it would be helpful for the caregiver and teen to find other ways to build up an understanding of what things cost (e.g., compare the cost of products at the grocery store, involve the teen when purchasing cleaning items).

Preparing for the Next Dyad Session (2 mins)

- *We will have our next caregiver/teen dyad session on DAY and TIME. At this session, we will discuss how to grocery shop. We will need you to prepare for the session by downloading any grocery shopping apps your family uses.*
- *It will be important to complete your Real World Practice assignment before our next dyad session and come prepared to discuss it. We will spend a lot of time next session talking about how the DLS contract went!*
- Ask: *Are there any questions before we end the session?*

Wrap-Up

- The therapist should send a calendar invite with the next caregiver/teen dyad session's day/time to the caregiver and teen. The therapist may also want to send the caregiver/teen a copy of the DLS contract if they completed it using a fillable PDF.

Evidence-Based Strategy: **Daily Life Skills Teaching Method**

Cooking on the Stovetop

LEARN

Review the steps of the stovetop recipe.
Gather the ingredients and cooking supplies that are needed.

WATCH

Your parent/caregiver will demonstrate (as needed) how to make the stovetop recipe by going through each step of the recipe.

PRACTICE

You will practice following the steps of the stovetop recipe
Your parent/caregiver will observe and give feedback and support after you complete each step.

DO IT INDEPENDENTLY

You will make the stovetop recipe on your own.

Grilled Cheese Sandwich

Preparation Time: 2 mins
Cook Time: 4–6 mins

Ingredients:

- 2 slices of your choice of bread
- 2 tbsp of butter, divided
- 1–2 slices of your choice of cheese

Directions:

- Preheat the pan over medium heat.
- Butter one side of the slice of bread.
- Place the bread slice butter-side-down onto the pan.
- Place 1 to 2 slices of cheese on top of the bread.
- Butter one side of the other bread slice.
- Place the bread butter-side-up on top of the cheese.
- Grill until lightly browned (2–3 minutes) and then flip the sandwich over using the spatula.
- Grill until lightly browned (2–3 minutes) and so that the cheese is melted.

Task Analysis

Skill: ____

Steps:

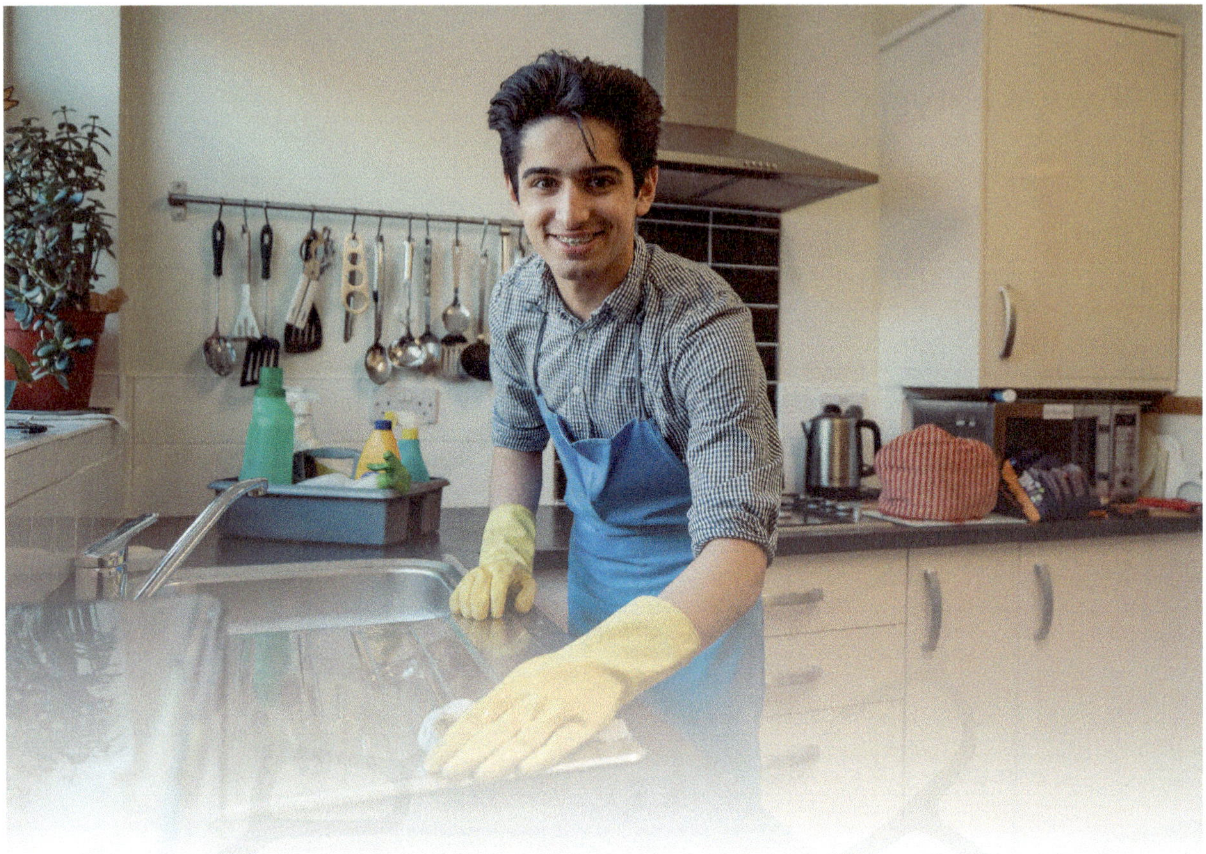

Kitchen Cleaning Checklist

☐ 1. Pick up and put everything on the counters and floor in its proper place.

☐ 2. Wipe down countertops and table.

☐ 3. Sweep/Vacuum the floor.

☐ 4. Empty/Load the dishwasher.

☐ 5. Clean out the sink.

☐ 6. If the garbage is full, take it out.

☐ 7. Double-check to make sure that everything was done correctly!

Task Analysis

Skill: ______________________________

Steps:

____

____

____

____

____

____

____

____

____

____

____

____

____

____

____

____

____

____

____

Daily Living Skills Contract

Date ______________________

Goal	Expectations	Reward	MONDAY	TUESDAY	WEDNESDAY	THURSDAY	FRIDAY	SATURDAY	SUNDAY

______________________ Teen

______________________ Parent / Caregiver

Surviving and Thriving in the Real World
Session 8 – Real World Practice

- Work on your (1) morning routine, (2) cleaning the bedroom, (3) doing laundry, and (4) cooking goals for the remainder of the week using your DLS contract.
    - Set aside a specific time (e.g., on the way to school, after dinner) to discuss how the morning routine went and how to problem-solve for the next day.
    - Schedule a day/time to work on watching and/or practicing how to clean the bedroom, do laundry, and cook.
    - Make sure that if a reward is earned, it is provided immediately!

- Make a list of ingredients for a recipe you want to cook. Find and purchase the ingredients at the grocery store and pay for the items with either cash or credit/debit card.
    - Schedule a day/time to complete the money assignment.

Surviving & Thriving in the Real World

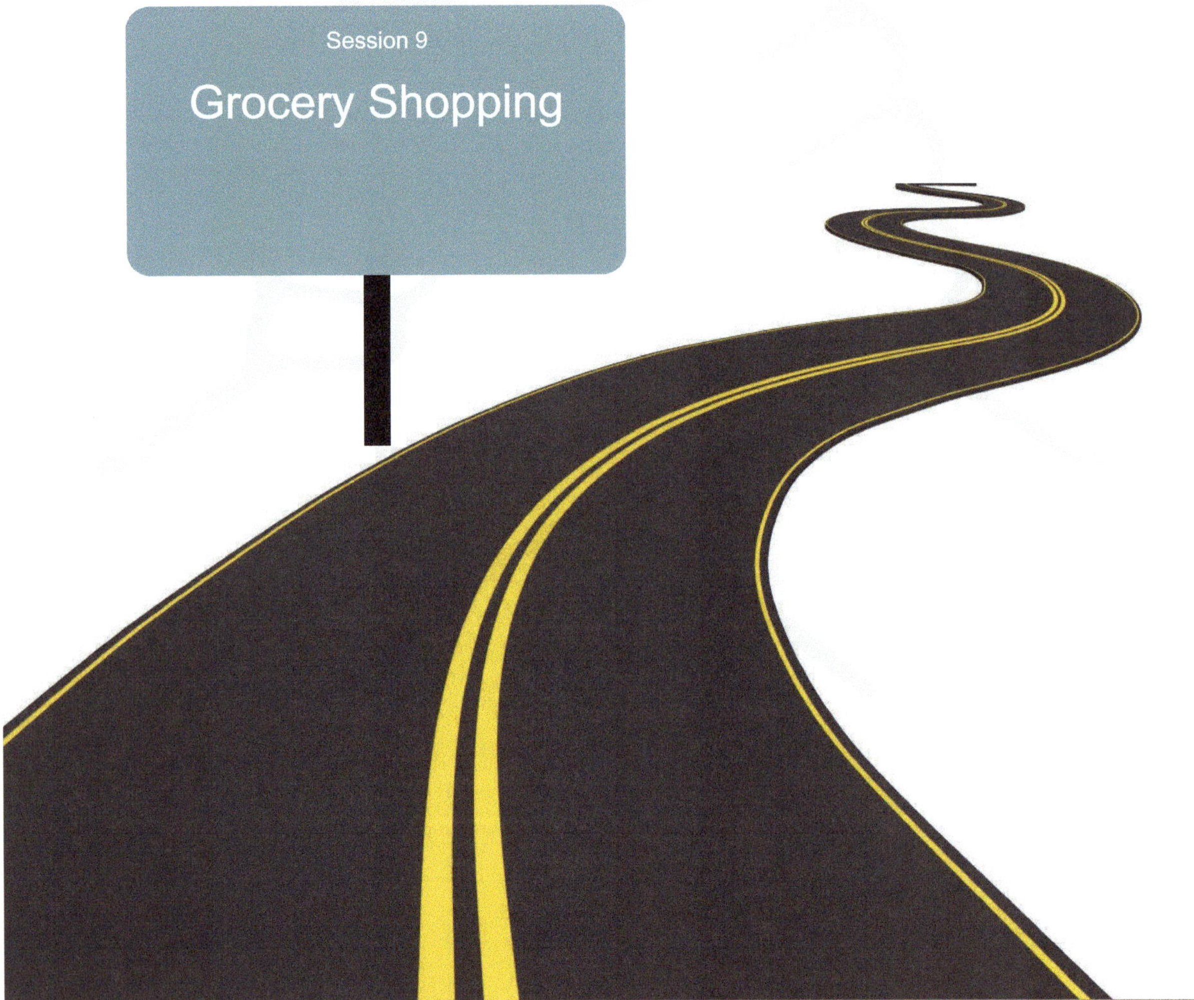

Session 9

Grocery Shopping

Aims

- Continue to build rapport between caregiver group members and the therapist
- Continue to build rapport between the teen, caregiver, and therapist
- Further develop ability to use a DLS contract to set a DLS goal, define expectations, and identify a reward for meeting the goal
- Review the four elements for developing an effective system to achieve the teen's DLS goals
- Understand how evidence-based strategies such as technology, visual supports, video modeling, and clear guidelines may be helpful when learning how to grocery shop
- Understand how to use the DLS Teaching Method to learn the steps for grocery shopping
- Create and implement a DLS contract to target the goals of morning routine, cleaning the bedroom, doing laundry, cooking, and grocery shopping

Structure

- Caregiver group session via telehealth
- Caregiver/teen dyad session via telehealth

Session Supplies

- Caregiver Group Handouts
  - DLS Contract
  - STRW Resources (from Session 1)

- Caregiver/Teen Dyad Handouts
  - DLS Teaching Method for Grocery Shopping
  - Grocery Store Map
  - Guidelines for Shopping at the Grocery Store
  - DLS Contract

DOI: 10.4324/9781003458838-12

- Session 9 – Real World Practice
- STRW Resources (from Session 1)

- Videos (optional links available on the STRW website and the STRW Resources handout)

Caregiver/Teen Preparation for Session

- For the dyad session, the caregiver should have the teen download any grocery shopping apps (e.g., specific grocery store app, grocery list app) that the caregiver uses.

Therapist Preparation for Session

- The therapist may want to review the Strategies Commonly Used to Target Goals on the DLS Contract handout (see appendix), which includes the evidence-based strategies, supports, and tools that teens utilize as they work on their DLS goals of morning routine, cleaning the bedroom, laundry, cooking, grocery shopping, and money management. It may be beneficial for therapists to review these prior to facilitating these sessions and developing the DLS contract with the caregiver/teen dyads.
- The therapist should use the Real World Practice Tracking Sheet for each caregiver/teen dyad in all subsequent STRW sessions to track progress on their DLS contract goals.
- The therapist will need to be mindful about individualizing the session for each dyad based on their experience with grocery shopping and how their family grocery shops (e.g., grocery shops at store, picks-up online grocery order, has grocery order delivered to their home, etc.).
- The therapist should individualize the session content on the use of a grocery store app to the specific grocery stores that the dyad uses. If an app is not used, this content can be omitted.
- For the Fridge, Freezer, or Pantry activity in the dyad session, the therapist can individualize this activity by modifying the food items to be specific to what the dyad often buy at the grocery store. The therapist can also look up the prices of some or all of the grocery items in this activity and have teens guess the price because there is no Guess the Price activity in this session.
- The therapist should consider reviewing the Tips for STRW Therapists: How to Facilitate Achievement of DLS Goals handout prior to each caregiver group session or dyad session for tips and strategies on how to help teens achieve the goals on their DLS contract. Tips that may be beneficial for Session 9 include:
  - *Be strategic about supporting the caregiver and teen in modifying the DLS contract.* At the beginning of the dyad session, the therapist should intentionally utilize the Real World Practice Check-In to identify how to possibly adapt the DLS contract by incorporating the characteristics of the caregiver and teen, successful evidence-based strategies, and the Four Laws of Behavior Change. These modifications can be discussed further and incorporated when developing the DLS contract at the end of the session in partnership

with the caregiver and the teen. The therapist should also utilize the relevant discussion questions (e.g., "What steps of the goal do you need help with?") when developing the new DLS contract to facilitate the likelihood of the teen achieving their goals.

- *Flexibility is critical when developing goals and expectations.* The therapist, teen, and caregiver will need to be flexible when identifying goals and defining expectations. Some teens may make progress very quickly such that their expectations may also increase quickly. Conversely, it may take some teens a lot of time to practice a skill such that expectations are changed more slowly. For example, some teens may have an expectation to complete most of their morning routine (e.g., eight out of ten steps) and other teens may only be working on one step at a time (e.g., waking up on their own).

Session 9 Notes

- ♦ Fillable PDFs of handouts from this session (i.e., Task Analysis Steps, DLS Contract) are available on the STRW website.

- ♦ Caregiver Group Session
  - At approximately halfway through the STRW intervention, caregivers often benefit from a direct discussion and/or opportunity to reflect about how they are doing coaching their teen and supporting the goals on the DLS contract. Helpful points to address might include:
    - Caregivers are also putting a lot of time and effort into supporting their teen as they build their DLS.
    - It can feel overwhelming at times to be targeting many goals simultaneously, but the caregiver group can serve as a place for them to share their feelings and also engage in problem solving to decrease overwhelm.
    - Teens sometimes experience a sort of "honeymoon" period in the first few sessions after implementing the DLS contract, and then they may struggle to meet their goals. This is very normal and part of learning a new skill and making something a habit. Teens may need to incorporate additional strategies or may need to implement a previously used strategy to meet their goals.
    - Parenting neurodivergent teens can be challenging and takes a significant amount of time and effort, which can be exacerbated by working on new DLS goals, managing school and homework, balancing extracurricular activities, and managing relationships with family and friends.
    - It may be beneficial to discuss whether caregivers are feeling like they are understanding their teen more (e.g., how they learn new skills, what strategies work for them) and if they notice their teen's self-understanding increasing.
  - The therapist may want to normalize that teens may have a "bad" week and that this is an opportunity to build understanding by examining what happened and brainstorming solutions.

- The therapist should continue to devote the majority of the caregiver group session to reviewing how the DLS contract is progressing for each caregiver. This is an opportunity to identify any issues and brainstorm solutions prior to the dyad session.
- The therapist should utilize the caregiver group session to get an understanding of how it may be necessary to personalize the dyad session content (e.g., how the family grocery shops, any apps that are used for grocery shopping).
- The therapist should make an active effort to foster collaboration between the group members by encouraging active discussion and problem solving of challenges or questions about the DLS contract.
- The therapist should have caregivers discuss how they can encourage participation in the grocery shopping process on a regular basis and get ideas from other caregivers (e.g., adding items that the teen needs to a grocery list, finding items at the grocery store, using an app to add items to the grocery cart, putting groceries away, etc.).

♦ Dyad Session

- Many caregivers and teens may be feeling overwhelmed by the goals on their DLS contract, so it may be beneficial to choose a grocery shopping goal that builds their skills but is also something that the family does on a regular basis (e.g., teen puts the groceries away with their caregiver, teen uses a list to find eight items at the grocery store with support from the caregiver, etc.).
- It is also critical to consider the work, school, and family schedules of the caregiver and teen so that DLS contract goals are doable. For example, it can be helpful for caregivers and teens to do DLS together (e.g., make dinner together, do the grocery shopping together, do several loads of laundry together) if the caregiver feels that they do not have the time to devote to providing instruction and feedback for the teen to do DLS independently. The therapist can provide support around how to fade back instruction and prompting as they work together to complete tasks so that the teen will eventually be doing the DLS independently.
- When developing the DLS contract at the end of the dyad session, the therapist should continue to incorporate all of the information and knowledge gained from the past several sessions (e.g., issues that were brought up during the caregiver group session, task analysis steps, discussing how to incorporate the essential elements of an effective system for achieving DLS goals, identifying appropriate rewards, etc.).

Caregiver Group Session 9 Content (90 mins)

Review – Real World Practice Assignment (50 mins)

- The therapist should greet the caregivers and welcome them to the session.
- Discuss the Real World Practice assignment in detail by having all caregivers share how using the DLS contract to target the morning routine, cleaning the bedroom, laundry, and cooking goals went with their teen. Encourage caregivers to jot down questions and notes on a blank copy of the DLS Contract handout that they may want to discuss or incorporate into their teen's contract at the next dyad session.
- ***We will have everyone share how using the DLS contract to target the morning routine, cleaning the bedroom, laundry, and cooking goals went for their teen. This is an opportunity to celebrate successes and also problem-solve any challenges or obstacles that occurred. We will spend the majority of our session discussing each teen's progress with the DLS Contract. It may be helpful to jot down questions and notes on a copy of the DLS Contract handout, and feel free to ask questions or add to the discussion.***
- It may be helpful to refer caregivers to the Tips for Creating a Successful DLS Contract handout (from Session 4) when discussing the goals on the DLS contract (e.g., clearly defining expectations, re-evaluating rewards regularly to ensure they are motivating, etc.).
- Points of discussion or questions to ask each caregiver include the following:
    - DLS contract
        - ***Did the teen make progress at becoming more independent with each of their goals – morning routine, cleaning the bedroom, laundry, and cooking?***
        - ***What went well?***
        - ***What was difficult?***
        - ***Did they receive a reward?***
        - ***Did they use any strategies to help them to learn the skill or become more independent?***
        - ***Any obstacles or barriers?***
        - ***Do you plan on modifying any goals on the current DLS contract?***
    - Making a list and purchasing items
        - ***Was your teen able to make a list of ingredients for a recipe that they want to cook?***
        - ***Was your teen able to find and purchase the items at the store?***
        - ***What went well?***
        - ***What skills still need to be practiced?***

- Ask: ***Any questions about the Real World Practice assignment?***

STRW Session 9 Goals (1 min)

- *The goal of today's session is to discuss how we will target the DLS goal of grocery shopping. We will also review how to build an effective system to help you and your teen achieve their DLS goals now and in the future.*
- *As we continue to build your teen's DLS, it may seem overwhelming to add in another goal. With grocery shopping, it will be helpful to keep in mind if there are ways that the teen can incorporate this into their daily or weekly schedule. For example:*
  - *Could the teen begin to add items to the grocery list instead of just telling you?*
  - *Could the teen go grocery shopping with you or another family member?*
  - *Could the teen put groceries away?*

- Ask and Discuss: *Any questions?*

Review Dyad Session 9 Content (36 mins)

- *Now we will briefly review the material that will be covered in the upcoming dyad session with your teen. This will allow you to have some time to prepare for the upcoming session. Please feel free to ask any questions as we go over the content of the dyad session, which will focus on building your teen's independence with grocery shopping.*
- *Before we review the dyad session content, let's all briefly share your teen's abilities to do the four main steps of grocery shopping:*
  - *Creating and adding to a grocery list.*
  - *Shopping for items at the grocery store – which may include navigating the grocery store, finding the items, comparing the prices of items, and choosing items to purchase.*
  - *Checking out and paying for items at the grocery store.*
  - *Putting items away at home in the fridge, freezer, or pantry.*

- The therapist should have each caregiver briefly share their teen's skill and level of involvement with the previous four steps of grocery shopping.
- The therapist should refer to the PowerPoint presentation slides for Dyad Session 9 while reviewing the content for the session.
- The therapist should have also prepared for the session by reviewing the Dyad Session 9 content discussed in the manual, which has detailed information about the content that will be covered.
- The important points to make while reviewing the Dyad Session 9 Content are:
  - We will do a Real World Practice Check-In, which will ask you and your teen specific questions about the goals on the DLS contract. This will be an opportunity to problem-solve any challenges and celebrate successes.
  - The elements of an effective system for achieving DLS goals will be reviewed with the teens as it relates to the goals on the DLS contract. This will be our main opportunity each session to revise the goals that are currently being targeted on the DLS contract before we add in a new goal at the end of the session.

- Grocery shopping consists of four main steps: (1) Creating and adding to a grocery list; (2) shopping for items at the grocery store; (3) checking out and paying for items at the grocery store; and (4) putting items away at home in the fridge, freezer, or pantry.
- The DLS Teaching Method will be used to teach the skill of grocery shopping by using the steps of learning, watching, practicing, and doing it independently.
- Other evidence strategies that will be discussed when learning how to grocery shop include video modeling, technology, visual supports, and clear rules and guidelines.
- Teens will practice determining if food items go in the fridge, freezer, or pantry.

♦ Ask: ***Any questions about the content for the upcoming dyad session?***

Prep for the Next Caregiver Session (3 mins)

♦ ***We will have our next caregiver group session on DAY and TIME. At this session, we will begin our sessions on money management and will talk about spending money. We will continue discussing how implementing the DLS contract went and discuss how to add a money management goal to your teen's DLS contract.***

♦ ***To prepare for the upcoming dyad session with your teen, please have your teen download any grocery shopping apps that you use and continue thinking about your teen's skills with creating and using a grocery list, finding items at the grocery store, purchasing items, and then helping to put groceries away at home.***

♦ ***After your dyad session with your teen, it will be important to prioritize working on the goals on the DLS contract and the Real World Practice assignment so that we can celebrate successes and also discuss any challenges or questions that arose in the caregiver group session.***

♦ Ask: ***Are there any questions before we end the session?***

Wrap-Up

♦ The therapist should send a calendar invite with the next caregiver group session's day/time to the caregiver.

♦ The therapist may also want to email caregivers a blank copy of the DLS contract or refer them to the STRW website.

Daily Living Skills Contract

Date ______________________

Goal	Expectations	Reward	MONDAY	TUESDAY	WEDNESDAY	THURSDAY	FRIDAY	SATURDAY	SUNDAY

______________________ Teen

______________________ Parent / Caregiver

Caregiver/Teen Dyad Session 9 Content (60 mins)

STRW Session 9 Schedule (1 min)

- The therapist should greet the caregiver and teen.
- *Let's get started! As a reminder, it will be helpful to sit together at a table so that we can all see each other and work together. Please pull out your STRW workbook that contains the handouts for all STRW sessions. This session is called Session 9 – Grocery Shopping. Please turn to that section in your workbook.*
- *Let's go over the session schedule so that you know what we will be doing. Please feel free to ask any questions about our schedule!*
- Briefly go over each item on the Session Schedule.

Real World Practice Check-In: Contract and Morning Routine (3 mins)

- Refer to the Session 8 Real World Practice handout and the DLS Contract handout.
- *Let's check in on how you are doing with each goal on your DLS contract. Please be honest, as this is an opportunity to talk about what is working and what is not working and do some brainstorming to address any challenges.*
- As needed, the therapist should spend time modifying the DLS contract and problem solving how to make a more effective system to target the DLS goal (e.g., make expectations more specific, change reward, increase/decrease number of prompts, modify the strategies being used to help with goals).
- If the therapist used a fillable PDF of the DLS Contract handout in the previous session, it may be helpful to share this on the screen so that the goal, expectations, and reward can be easily discussed.
- The following questions should be asked (if applicable), and the responses and any relevant notes should be entered into the Real World Practice Tracking Sheet:
    - *Did you use your DLS contract this week?*
    - *Did you work on your morning routine goal during the week?*
        - *What went well?*
        - *What was challenging?*
        - *How many days did you work on your morning routine goal?*
        - *Did you earn a reward for your morning routine goal?*
        - *How many days did you earn a reward?*

Real World Practice Check-In: Cleaning the Bedroom and Laundry (3 mins)

- The following questions should be asked (if applicable), and the responses and any relevant notes should be entered into the Real World Practice Tracking Sheet:

- *Did you work on your cleaning the bedroom goal during the week?*
  - *What went well?*
  - *What was challenging?*
  - *How many days did you work on your cleaning the bedroom goal?*
  - *Did you earn a reward for your cleaning the bedroom goal?*
- *Did you work on your laundry goal during the week?*
  - *What went well?*
  - *What was challenging?*
  - *How many days did you work on your laundry goal?*
  - *Did you earn a reward for your laundry goal?*

Real World Practice Check-In: Cooking and Money (4 mins)

- The following questions should be asked (if applicable), and the responses and any relevant notes should be entered into the Real World Practice Tracking Sheet:
  - *Did you work on your cooking goal or goals during the week?*
    - *What went well?*
    - *What was challenging?*
    - *How many days did you work on your cooking goal or goals?*
    - *Did you earn a reward for your cooking goal or goals?*
  - *For your Real World Practice, you were also given a money assignment.*
    - *Did you work on or complete a money assignment?*
    - *What did you do?*
    - *What went well?*
    - *What was challenging?*

- Ask: *Any questions or comments about your Real World Practice assignments?*
- If the caregiver/teen dyad struggled to complete the Real World Practice assignments, the therapist should spend some time discussing how to identify days/times that they could designate to commit to working on the assignments.
- If the therapist used a fillable PDF of the DLS Contract handout in the previous session, it may be helpful to share this on the screen so that the goal, expectations, and reward can be easily discussed.

Elements of an Effective System for Achieving DLS Goals (2 mins)

- Ask: *Are there any issues you want to discuss or troubleshoot related to the DLS contract?*
- Ask and Discuss: *Are we considering all of the important elements to increase the likelihood of you achieving your DLS goals by developing the most effective system?*
- If applicable, discuss how to modify any DLS goals to address (1) qualities of the teen and their caregiver; (2) use of evidence-based strategies to teach and master DLS; and (3) ensuring that goals are obvious, attractive, easy, and satisfying.

Grocery Shopping Steps (2 mins)

- *Today we are going to talk about learning how to do all the steps of grocery shopping which include the following:*
  - *Creating and adding items to a grocery list.*
  - *Shopping for items at the grocery store, which includes navigating the grocery store, finding the items, comparing the prices of items, and choosing items to purchase.*
  - *Checking out and paying for items at the grocery store.*
  - *Putting items away at home in the fridge, freezer, or pantry.*

- *We are going to talk about some proven strategies to help you become independent in doing all of the steps of grocery shopping, but first we want to get an understanding of your grocery shopping skills and how your family grocery shops.*

Your Experience with Grocery Shopping (5 mins)

- *Let's talk a little about your experience with grocery shopping so that we can get an understanding of your areas of strength and areas in which you may need some additional instruction or practice.*
- Ask the teen the following questions and briefly discuss their answers. Caregivers can also add to the discussion of their teen's experience with grocery shopping.
  - *Do you create or add to your family's grocery list?*
  - *Where does your family typically grocery shop?*
  - *Do you go with your caregiver to the grocery store (or help with online grocery shopping)?*
  - *Do you help get items at the store?*
  - *What items do you typically get?*
  - *How do you find items at the store?*
  - *Do you help with checking out at the grocery store?*
  - *Do you help put away the groceries at home?*

- Ask: *Is there anything else you want to discuss about your grocery shopping skills?*

Evidence-Based Strategy: DLS Teaching Method-Grocery Shopping (2 mins)

- Refer to the <u>DLS Teaching Method for Grocery Shopping</u> handout.
- *We will continue to use the DLS Teaching Method to build up your skills with grocery shopping. In session today, we will talk through various proven strategies and then set a DLS goal on your contract that incorporates one or more of the strategies to target your grocery shopping skills.*
- *The DLS Teaching Method is one of the most beneficial strategies for teaching grocery shopping skills to teens. It requires your caregiver to provide instruction, demonstration, and feedback to you as you do the various steps of grocery shopping together. This will then make it more likely that you will be able to independently do all of the steps of grocery shopping. For example, while a teen may not ever do all of the family's grocery shopping on their own, they may be able to go to the grocery store and purchase 10–12 items from a list, pay for the items, and then put them away when they get home.*

- *As part of your DLS contract in the coming weeks, you will have a grocery shopping goal. It can be helpful to make your grocery shopping goal related to the other goals on your DLS contract. For example, you could add items to the grocery list that are needed for meals that you are cooking or add personal hygiene items you need for your morning routine to the grocery list.*

Creating and Adding Items to a Grocery List-Evidence-Based Strategy: Technology (3 mins)

- *For creating and adding items to a grocery list, there are several strategies that you could use to make it more likely that you get everything that is needed at the grocery store.*
- *Before we talk about technology options, one "old fashioned" method is to keep a whiteboard or piece of paper in an easily accessible place, such as hanging it on the refrigerator. Anyone can then write down items that they need at the grocery store. This strategy is easy and simple!*
- *The use of technology through apps, computers/tablets, and smart speakers is also a strategy that can be particularly beneficial for a skill such as remembering to add items to a grocery list. If you think of a grocery item you need, it can be quick and easy to just add it to a list on your phone instead of trying to remember to tell your caregiver or write it on a list at home.*
- *It can also be helpful to organize the grocery list by category when making it. For example, some families may have categories such as breakfast, lunch, dinner, drinks, and snacks and then include the items that are needed under each category.*
- Ask and Discuss:
  - *Which of these strategies would be beneficial for you (or your family) to use to add items to a grocery list?*
  - *Are there other strategies you could use to keep a grocery list?*

Creating and Adding Items to a Grocery List-Evidence-Based Strategy: Grocery Store Apps (3 mins)

- *Another technology based strategy is to utilize the app of the grocery store that you shop at. This is an example of a grocery store app, which has a lot of features, including a shopping list, coupons, and an item locator feature that tells you the specific aisle an item is in. If your family uses a grocery store app, it can be helpful to become familiar with it and use its features when grocery shopping.*
- NOTE: The therapist should individualize the discussion of a grocery store app to be specific to the app that the caregiver and teen may use when they grocery shop.
- Ask and Discuss (if applicable):
  - *Does your family use a grocery shopping app?*
  - *How does your family use the grocery shopping app?*
    - The caregiver can demonstrate the features on their phone or their teen's phone if they had the teen download the grocery store app.
  - *How could you work on your grocery shopping skills using the app?*

Shopping at the Grocery Store-Evidence-Based Strategy: Visual Supports (3 mins)

- Refer to the Grocery Store Map handout.
- *This is a visual support that depicts the layout of most grocery stores, though it may look slightly different from yours. The back of the grocery store usually has dairy, eggs, and meat. The middle of the grocery store typically contains the frozen food aisles and also the aisles with items such as cereal, baking goods, snacks, drinks, and canned goods.*
- Ask and Discuss:
  - *Is the layout of your grocery store similar to this map? Why or why not?*
  - *Is it helpful for you to use visual supports like this one to better understand where things are?*
  - *How can you find items in a grocery store?*
    - *Once you are in a grocery store, there are typically signs hanging from the ceiling that indicate the aisle number and items contained in that aisle. For example, if you see that Aisle 19 has "cereal" listed, you will be able to find products such as cereal and oatmeal in that aisle.*
    - *Many grocery store apps allow you to look up an item in your designated "home" store that will tell you the exact location of an item.*
    - *You can also ask someone who works at the grocery store to help you find an item.*

Guidelines for Shopping at the Grocery Store (3 mins)

- Refer to the Guidelines for Shopping at the Grocery Store handout.
- *The guidelines for grocery shopping are not always communicated clearly. Many teens find it helpful to clearly define some rules so that they know what they need to do.*
- Have the caregiver and teen take turns reading the Guidelines for Shopping at the Grocery Store handout.
- Ask and Discuss: *Are there any other rules or tips to add based on your experiences?*

Shopping at the Grocery Store-Evidence-Based Strategy: DLS Teaching Method (3 mins)

- *When shopping at the grocery store, the DLS teaching method can be used to instruct and demonstrate skills such as finding specific items and comparing prices between two items. After caregivers instruct and demonstrate how to do this, you can then be given opportunities to practice the skills. For example, your caregiver can discuss the layout of your grocery store and then demonstrate how to find items. Then, you could practice finding specific items from your grocery list with support from your caregiver.*
- *The DLS teaching method can be done while shopping at the grocery store and does not take much additional time or effort. Grocery shopping will also go faster once you are able to practice your skills!*
- Ask and Discuss: *Any questions about using the DLS Teaching Method to learn about shopping for items at the grocery shop?*

Shopping at the Grocery Store – Evidence-Based Strategy: Video Modeling (1 min)

- Refer to the STRW Resources handout (from Session 1).
- *Watching videos to learn new skills is another evidence-based strategy that can be used to learn how to shop at the grocery store. On the* STRW Resources *handout, there is a video of a college student shopping at the grocery store and also checking out at the grocery store. It may be helpful to watch this video and some of the other videos on the* STRW Resources *handout to learn more about grocery shopping.*

Checking Out at the Grocery Store-Evidence-Based Strategy: DLS Teaching Method (2 mins)

- *When checking out and paying for items at the grocery store, caregivers can use the DLS Teaching Method to instruct and demonstrate skills such as unloading the grocery cart, paying with cash or credit/debit card, and using coupons. After these skills are instructed and demonstrated by the caregiver, you can then be given opportunities to practice.*
- Ask and Discuss: *Any questions about using the DLS Teaching Method to learn how to pay and check out at the grocery store?*

Putting Groceries Away-Evidence-Based Strategy: DLS Teaching Method (2 mins)

- *When putting groceries away at home, caregivers can also use the DLS Teaching Method to instruct and demonstrate skills such as prioritizing which items to put away first and where certain items go – such as which fruits and vegetables go in the pantry vs. in the refrigerator. After these skills are instructed and demonstrated by the caregiver, you can then be given opportunities to practice.*
- Ask and Discuss: *Any questions about using the DLS Teaching Method to learn how to put items away?*

Fridge, Freezer, or Pantry (7 mins)

- *After you buy groceries and bring them home, you then need to put them away in the right place – the refrigerator, the freezer, or the pantry. One helpful rule of thumb is that if you bought an item in the freezer section, it needs to go in the freezer at home. Similarly, if you buy an item that is refrigerated, it should likely go in the refrigerator at home. Items that are purchased off of grocery shelves such as cereal, pasta, chips, pretzels, and spaghetti sauce should likely be placed in your pantry.*
- *Let's do a quiz to see if you know whether food items should go in the fridge, freezer, or pantry.*
- NOTE: Caregivers can also gather actual items from their fridge, freezer, or pantry for this activity instead of the pictures of items on the PowerPoint slides.
- The therapist should click through the next 17 slides that contain pictures of common grocery items and have the teen state whether the item should go in the fridge, freezer, or pantry.

- The therapist can change the grocery items for this activity to be specific to items that are in the teen's fridge, freezer, or pantry.
- Caregivers may need to weigh in about where they put items in their home because some food items can be put away in more than one place (e.g., bread).
- This activity is meant to be a fun and engaging way to build up the teen's understanding of where food items should go after they are bought at the grocery store! If the teen is averse to playing the game, it can be skipped.
- NOTE: There is no Guess the Price activity for this session. If time allows, teens can also try to guess the prices of items after stating whether they go in the fridge, freezer, or pantry. The therapist would need to look up the prices of items prior to the start of the session.

Elements of an Effective System for Achieving DLS Goals (3 mins)

- The therapist should briefly ask each teen about each of the elements and then incorporate the responses to the discussion on developing the DLS contract.
- *As we work to add the goal of grocery shopping to the DLS contract, let's make sure we are thinking about all of the following elements to build an effective system for achieving DLS goals:*
  - *Teen – are we considering your strengths, challenges, preferred learning style, and commitment?*
    - *There are ways to make grocery shopping fun! For example, you could compete with your caregiver to guess the total price after checking out. You could also see who can get the grocery items on their list the fastest.*
  - *Caregiver – are we considering your parenting style, time and effort, and commitment?*
    - *Some caregivers find it easy to have teens help with grocery shopping while they are doing it. This might include finding items in the store, discussing what item to buy based on price, and putting the groceries away at home.*
  - *Are we using evidence-based strategies?*
    - *We are using the DLS Teaching Method to help you learn and become independent with all of the steps involved in grocery shopping.*
    - *We talked about how you could use strategies including technology, video modeling, visual supports, and clear guidelines to become more independent with grocery shopping.*
  - *Is the goal of grocery shopping obvious, attractive, easy, and satisfying?*
    - *Obvious – some ideas might be to have a shared grocery list posted on the fridge or shared via a phone app.*
    - *Attractive – some ideas might be to go to the store with your caregiver or listen to music or a podcast on the way to the grocery store.*
    - *Easy – some ideas might be to choose a specific day and time to go grocery shopping each week.*
    - *Satisfying – some ideas include choosing a favorite item to eat after you get home from grocery shopping.*

- Ask and Discuss: *Any questions or comments?*
- *Let's apply all of this information to creating your DLS contract!*

Developing Your DLS Contract (5 mins)

- Refer to the DLS Contract handout.
- ***Let's spend the remainder of our time in today's session modifying your DLS contract to continue working on your morning routine, cleaning your bedroom, laundry, and cooking goals and add in the goal of grocery shopping. This could include any or all of the steps of grocery shopping such as creating or adding to a list, shopping, checking out, or putting items away. This could even involve you helping your caregiver go grocery shopping one day this week. Use a blank copy of the DLS Contract. We will also keep in mind the importance of making sure the goal is Obvious, Attractive, Easy, and Satisfying so that you are more likely to achieve your goal. The DLS contract will have you track your progress and set up rewards for you to earn, which makes working on the goals satisfying!***
- The therapist should support the caregiver/teen dyad in creating the DLS contract by doing the following:
  - Incorporate all of the information from the last several sessions (e.g., rewards that are motivating for the teen, use of strategies and supports to build independence with certain steps) and the Real World Practice Check-In to create the DLS contract. The therapist should also consider the goals that the caregiver and teen collaboratively developed during the Preparing for STRW session.
  - Use the DLS Contract handout to specify the (1) Goal, (2) Expectations, and (3) Reward for Morning Routine, Cleaning the Bedroom, Doing Laundry, Cooking, and Grocery Shopping.
  - Encourage the caregiver/teen dyad to work together and model appropriate and supportive coaching as they develop the DLS contract.

- Possible discussion questions that may be helpful to ask and discuss when creating the contract for the Morning Routine, Cleaning the Bedroom, Laundry, Cooking, and Grocery Shopping goals include:
  - ***How often are you going to need to do the goal – every day, every weekday, every other day, or once per week?***
  - ***What steps of your goal do you need help with?***
  - ***What steps do you not know how to do?***
  - ***What steps are you doing independently?***
  - ***How easy/hard do you think it will be to meet your goal?***
  - ***What reward would you like to earn?***
  - ***Does the reward fit the goal? For example, earning 1 hour of screen time for doing your morning routine goal each day is a lot, but maybe earning 15–20 extra minutes of screen time would be a better fit.***
  - ***How will you check in about your goals daily to discuss if the goal was met?***
  - ***Where can you post your DLS contract so that you can track goals daily and remember to get your reward if it was earned?***

- The caregiver and teen should write each goal, expectation, and reward on the DLS Contract handout. It may be helpful for the therapist to share their screen and add/modify the goals, expectations, and rewards on a fillable PDF of the DLS Contract handout. The therapist can then email it to the caregiver and teen after the session.

- When the DLS contract has been completed, encourage the dyad to sign it and post it somewhere where they can easily see it so that the goals may be tracked.

Real World Practice (1 min)

- Refer to the Real World Practice handout.
- Discuss the details of the Real World Practice assignment.
  - *Work on your morning routine, cleaning the bedroom, laundry, cooking, and grocery shopping goals for the remainder of the week using your DLS contract.*
    - *Set aside a specific time such as on the way to school or after dinner to discuss how the morning routine went and how to problem-solve the next day.*
    - *Schedule a day/time to work on watching and/or practicing how to clean your bedroom, do laundry, cook, and grocery shop.*
    - *Make sure that if the teen earns the reward, they receive it immediately! This makes it more likely that they will continue to be motivated to meet their goal!*
  - *Complete the Money Questionnaire handout that is included in your Session 10 handouts.*

- Ask: *Any questions about your Real World Practice assignment?*

Preparing for the Next Dyad Session (2 mins)

- *We will have our next caregiver/teen dyad session on DAY and TIME. At this session, we will discuss your understanding of money and start talking about money basics such as spending and saving. You will need to prepare for the session by completing the Money Questionnaire handout that is found in your workbook under the Session 10 handouts. It will be important for you to fill this out on your own.*
- *I will check in with you by email in a few days to remind you to complete the Money Questionnaire handout.*
- *It will be important to complete your Real World Practice assignment before our next dyad session and come prepared to discuss it. We will spend a lot of time next session talking about how the DLS contract went!*
- Ask: *Are there any questions before we end the session?*

Wrap-Up

- The therapist should send a calendar invite with the next caregiver/teen dyad session's day/time to the caregiver and teen. The therapist may also want to send the caregiver/teen a copy of the DLS contract if they completed it using a fillable PDF. The therapist can attach a copy of the Money Questionnaire handout (see STRW website for a fillable PDF) as a reminder for the teen to complete it.

Evidence-Based Strategy: **Daily Life Skills Teaching Method**

Grocery Shopping

LEARN

Review the 4 steps for grocery shopping with your caregiver including (1) making a list, (2) going to the store, (3) checking out and paying, and (4) putting groceries away.

Discuss what your role will be in each of the 4 steps.

WATCH

Your parent/caregiver will demonstrate (as needed) how to complete specific grocery shopping steps.

PRACTICE

You will practice completing specific grocery shopping steps.
Your parent/caregiver will observe and give feedback and support after you complete each step.

DO IT INDEPENDENTLY

You will complete the grocery shopping steps on your own.

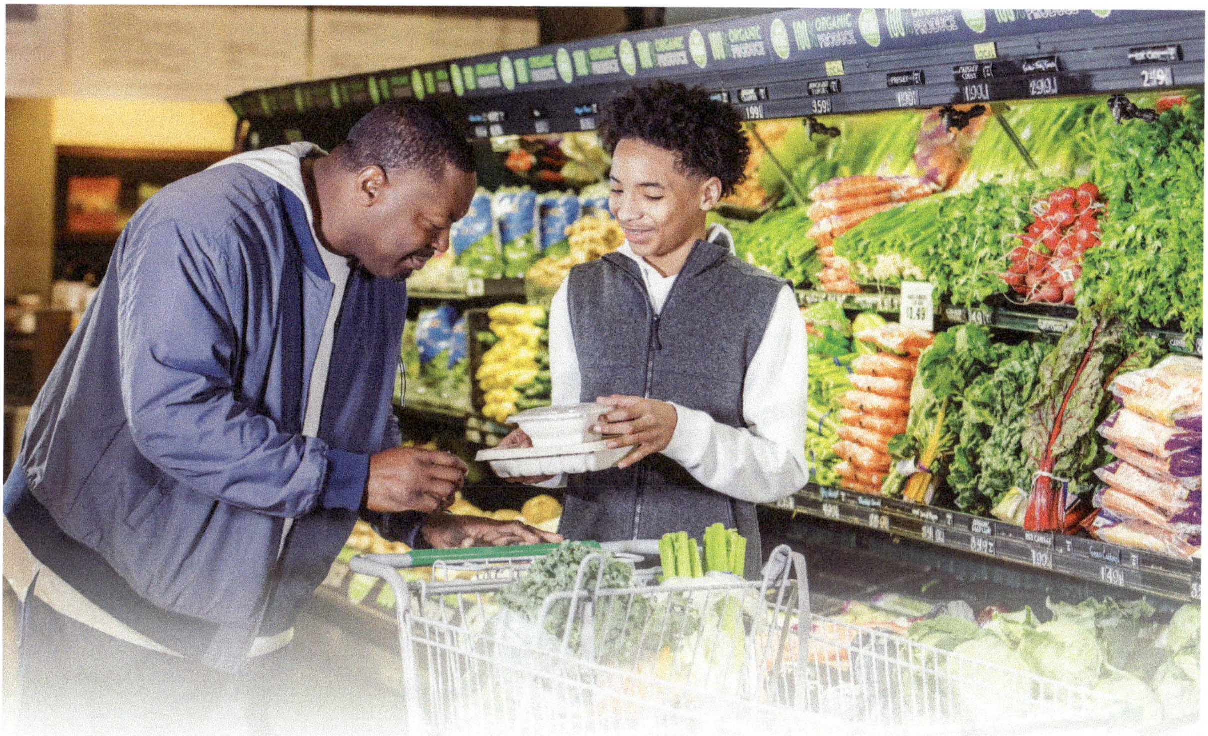

Map of a Typical Grocery Store

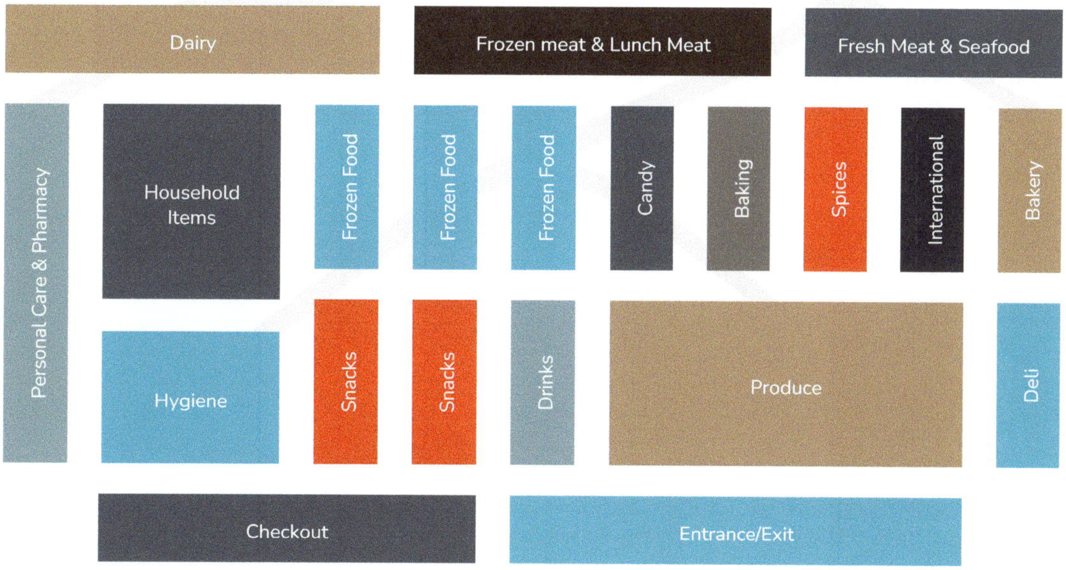

Guidelines for Shopping at the Grocery Store

- When pushing your grocery cart down the aisle, stay close to the right side so that others can pass you.
- Do not walk too closely behind others. Make sure to give some space between your cart and other people's carts.
- If you're on the phone or in the middle of a conversation while shopping, move your cart so that you're not in others' way.
- Pay attention while shopping. If you need to text, take a phone call, or look at your list, you should move to the side and out of the way of others.
- If you pick up an item and later decide you don't want it, put it back where you found it.
- If you accidentally drop or spill something, make sure to let an employee know.
- You should not eat any food without paying for it. If there are samples, take only one sample.
- Only use the express lane if you have fewer than the number of items that are stated on the sign.
- When you get in the checkout line, make sure to have your cash or credit/debit card ready so you don't hold up the line.
- If someone calls you on the phone while checking out, let it ring and call the person back later.
- After paying, move out of the way for the next person to check out.
- After unloading your groceries into your car, make sure to put your cart back in the corral where it belongs.

Daily Living Skills Contract

Date ______________________

Goal	Expectations	Reward	MONDAY	TUESDAY	WEDNESDAY	THURSDAY	FRIDAY	SATURDAY	SUNDAY

______________________ Teen

______________________ Parent / Caregiver

Surviving and Thriving in the Real World
Session 9 – Real World Practice

- Work on your (1) morning routine, (2) cleaning the bedroom, (3) doing laundry, (4) cooking, and (5) grocery shopping goals for the remainder of the week using your DLS contract.
    - Set aside a specific time (e.g., on the way to school, after dinner) to discuss how the morning routine went and how to problem-solve for the next day.
    - Schedule a day/time to work on watching and/or practicing how to clean the bedroom, do laundry, cook, and go grocery shopping.
    - Make sure that if a reward is earned, it is provided immediately!

- Complete the <u>Money Questionnaire</u> handout that is included in your Session 10 handouts before the next dyad session.

Surviving & Thriving in the Real World

Session 10

Money Basics

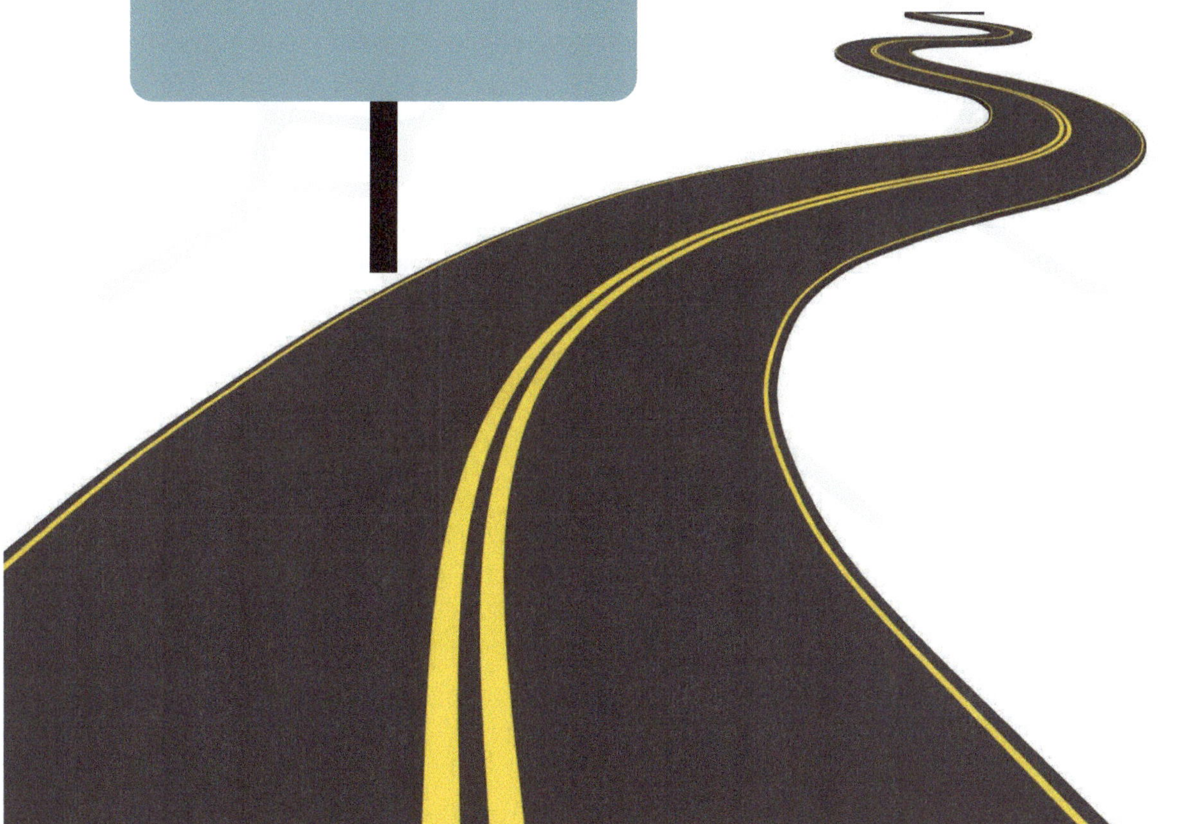

Session 10

Money Basics

Aims

- Continue to build rapport between caregiver group members and the therapist
- Continue to build rapport between the teen, caregiver, and therapist
- Further develop ability to use a DLS contract to set a DLS goal, define expectations, and identify a reward for meeting the goal
- Review the four elements for developing an effective system to achieve the teen's DLS goals
- Review the teen's current experience and skill level with managing their money
- Understand how to use the DLS Teaching Method to learn how to spend, save, and budget money
- Understand how to use a money diary to track spending
- Create and implement a DLS contract to target the goals of morning routine, cleaning the bedroom, doing laundry, cooking, grocery shopping, and money management

Structure

- Caregiver group session via telehealth
- Caregiver/teen dyad session via telehealth

Session Supplies

- Caregiver Group Handouts
    - DLS Contract

- Caregiver/Teen Dyad Handouts
    - Money Questionnaire
    - DLS Teaching Method for Money Management
    - Should I Buy It or Not?
    - Money Diary
    - DLS Contract
    - Session 10 – Real World Practice

DOI: 10.4324/9781003458838-13

- Other Supplies
  - STRW Budgeting Workbook (available on the STRW website)

Caregiver/Teen Preparation for Session

- The teen should complete the Money Questionnaire handout prior to the dyad session.

Therapist Preparation for Session

- The therapist should be familiar with using the STRW Budgeting Workbook as an option for how teens could track their income and expenses using a Money Diary. The therapist may want to email the caregiver a copy of the STRW Budgeting Workbook or refer them to the STRW website to download a copy to refer to or use during both the caregiver group session and dyad session.
- The therapist may want to review the Strategies Commonly Used to Target Goals on the DLS Contract handout (see appendix), which includes the evidence-based strategies, supports, and tools that teens utilize as they work on their DLS goals of morning routine, cleaning the bedroom, laundry, cooking, grocery shopping, and money management. It may be beneficial for therapists to review these prior to facilitating these sessions and developing the DLS contract with the caregiver/teen dyads.
- The therapist should use the Real World Practice Tracking Sheet for each caregiver/teen dyad in all subsequent STRW sessions to track progress on their DLS contract goals.
- A major goal of this session is to understand the money management skills that the teen needs to learn and develop, which will then allow the therapist to be mindful about individualizing the session for each dyad based on their experience with money management.
- The therapist should consider reviewing the Tips for STRW Therapists: How to Facilitate Achievement of DLS Goals handout prior to each caregiver group session or dyad session for tips and strategies on how to help teens achieve the goals on their DLS contract. Tips that may be beneficial for Session 10 include:
  - *Support caregivers if they need to modify expectations for earning rewards or privileges.* Caregivers may need to adjust or change their own behaviors, expectations, and boundaries in the home to effectively support their teen in building DLS. For example, if teens are able to access all of the things that are rewarding to them (e.g., video games, screen time, privileges) without doing "work" (e.g., laundry, cleaning their room, chores around the home), caregivers may need to edit these expectations so that they are now required to "earn" these rewards. The therapist can provide support and guidance by engaging in problem solving. It can often be helpful to discuss this during the caregiver group session to get ideas and support from other caregivers on how to do this.
  - *Label the teen's progress to instill a sense of pride.* Therapists should identify and describe the teen's progress with a goal to stimulate internal feelings of pride, accomplishment, and independence. Many teens may prefer this to the therapist

or caregiver praising them ("Great work!"), labeling emotions ("It must be exciting to make this much progress!"), or stating their own emotions ("I am so proud of you.").
- *Assess motivation continuously.* What is rewarding or motivating to a teen may change quickly, so it is important to regularly evaluate whether a reward for working towards a DLS goal is truly motivating them. The therapist should ask about the effectiveness of rewards at each session and brainstorm additional rewards as needed.

Session 10 Notes

- Fillable PDFs of handouts from this session (i.e., Should I Buy It or Not?, DLS Contract) are available on the STRW website.

- Caregiver Group Session
  - At this point in the STRW intervention, caregivers often benefit from a direct discussion and/or opportunity to reflect about how they are doing coaching their teen and supporting the goals on the DLS contract. Helpful points to address might include:
    - Caregivers are also putting a lot of time and effort into supporting their teen as they build their DLS.
    - It can feel overwhelming at times to be targeting many goals simultaneously, but the caregiver group can serve as a place for them to share their feelings and also engage in problem solving to decrease overwhelm.
    - Teens sometimes experience a sort of "honeymoon" period in the first few sessions after implementing the DLS contract, and then they may struggle to meet their goals. This is very normal and part of learning a new skill and making something a habit. Teens may need to incorporate additional strategies or may need to implement a previously used strategy to meet their goals.
    - Parenting neurodivergent teens can be challenging and takes a significant amount of time and effort, which can be exacerbated by working on new DLS goals, managing school and homework, balancing extracurricular activities, and managing relationships with family and friends.
  - The therapist should continue to devote the majority of the caregiver group session to reviewing how the DLS contract is progressing for each caregiver. This is an opportunity to identify any issues and brainstorm solutions prior to the dyad session.
  - The therapist should utilize the caregiver group session to get an understanding of how to individualize the dyad session content (e.g., the teen's experience with tracking the money they spend to determine how a money diary may be most effective).
  - The therapist should make an active effort to foster collaboration between the group members by encouraging active discussion and problem-solving of challenges or questions about the DLS contract.

- The therapist should have caregivers discuss how they build their teen's money management skills on a regular basis and get ideas from other caregivers (e.g., tracking how much money is spent on bills, demonstrating how to compare prices on an item at different stores or websites, looking up account balances for checking or savings accounts, getting money out of an ATM). Caregivers are likely doing various money management tasks daily or weekly, and it can be helpful to identify ways to include their teen in this process.

♦ Dyad Session
- This dyad session has less content, and it is meant to be a session for the therapist to spend additional time refining the current goals of the DLS contract prior to the teen adding their final money goal to the DLS contract.
- There will no longer be a money assignment given as part of the Real World Practice assignment. Instead, teens will be adding a money goal to their DLS contract, which will be very similar to the money assignments that they have been completing each week.
- Many caregivers and teens may be feeling overwhelmed by the goals on their DLS contract, so it may be beneficial to choose a money management goal that aligns with their other DLS contract goals (e.g., purchasing items from a list at the grocery store) or is something that the family or teen already does on a regular basis (e.g., tracking weekly spending, paying bills, making an online purchase, carrying a wallet whenever leaving the house).
- If teens are motivated by using apps on their phone, they could look into using an app or a spreadsheet program (e.g., Microsoft Excel) to track their spending instead of using the Money Diary handout. While not required, the therapist could show the teen an example of the money diary on the STRW Budgeting Workbook. The STRW Budgeting Workbook will also be used in Sessions 12 and 13.
- The STRW Resources handout also has various resources related to money management that may be helpful for the caregivers and teens.
- The caregiver and teen do not have to use a money diary for the money goal on the DLS contract and can instead choose another goal related to the session content (e.g., start using a wallet to store and carry money, look up the balance in their checking account, organize the money and gift cards they have in their room).
- When developing the DLS contract at the end of the dyad session, the therapist should continue to incorporate all of the information and knowledge gained from the past several sessions (e.g., issues that were brought up during the caregiver group session, task analysis steps, discussing how to incorporate the essential elements of an effective system for achieving DLS goals, identifying appropriate rewards, etc.).

Caregiver Group Session 10 Content (90 mins)

Review – Real World Practice Assignment (50 mins)

- The therapist should greet the caregivers and welcome them to the session.
- Discuss the Real World Practice assignment in detail by having all caregivers share how using the DLS contract to target the morning routine, cleaning the bedroom, laundry, cooking, and grocery shopping goals went with their teen. Encourage caregivers to jot down questions and notes on a blank copy of the DLS Contract handout that they may want to discuss or incorporate into their teen's contract at the next dyad session.
- ***We will have everyone share how using the DLS contract to target the morning routine, cleaning the bedroom, laundry, cooking, and grocery shopping goals went for their teen. This is an opportunity to celebrate successes and also problem-solve any challenges or obstacles that occurred. We will spend the majority of our session discussing each teen's progress with the DLS contract. It may be helpful to jot down questions and notes on a copy of the DLS Contract handout, and feel free to ask questions or add to the discussion.***
- It may be helpful to refer caregivers to the Tips for Creating a Successful DLS Contract handout (from Session 4) when discussing the goals on the DLS contract (e.g., clearly defining expectations, re-evaluating rewards regularly to ensure they are motivating, etc.).
- Points of discussion or questions to ask each caregiver include the following:
  - DLS contract
    - ***Did the teen make progress at becoming more independent with each of their goals – morning routine, cleaning the bedroom, laundry, cooking, and grocery shopping?***
    - ***What went well?***
    - ***What was difficult?***
    - ***Did they receive a reward?***
    - ***Did they use any strategies to help them to learn the skill or become more independent?***
    - ***Any obstacles or barriers?***
    - ***Do you plan on modifying any goals on the current DLS contract?***
  - Money Questionnaire
    - ***Was your teen able to complete the* Money Questionnaire *handout that will be discussed at the next dyad session?***

- Ask: ***Any questions about the Real World Practice assignment?***

STRW Session 10 Goals (1 min)

- *The goals of the next four sessions are to discuss the basics of spending, saving, and budgeting money, which are concepts that all teens should have an understanding of so that they can continue to build these skills gradually over time.*
- *In the upcoming dyad session, we will get an understanding of how much your teen knows about managing money and then talk about spending money including how to resist impulse buying and how to use a money diary to track spending. We will also review how to build an effective system to help you and your teen achieve their DLS goals now and in the future.*
- *As we continue to build your teen's DLS, it may seem overwhelming to add in another goal. However, money management is the last goal we are adding to the DLS contract and there are ways to incorporate these money goals into your daily or weekly schedule. For example:*
  - *Could the teen keep track of how they spend their own money?*
  - *Could the teen track spending in a specific category for themselves or the family in areas such as grocery shopping or eating out?*
  - *Could the teen review the bills you are paying that week such as water, electric, or cell phone?*

- Ask and Discuss: *Any questions?*

Review Dyad Session 10 Content (36 mins)

- *Now we will briefly review the material that will be covered in the upcoming dyad session with your teen. This will allow you to have some time to prepare for the upcoming session. Please feel free to ask any questions as we go over the content of the dyad session, which will focus on building basic money management skills including how to use a money diary to track spending. We will incorporate what we discuss today as a money goal on their DLS contract.*
- *Before we review the dyad session content, let's all briefly share your teen's abilities and experience with managing money:*
  - *Spending money – such as evaluating the quality and price of an item, tracking spending, and using a checking account.*
  - *Saving money – such as setting short-term and long-term savings goals, making a plan to save money, and using a savings account.*
  - *Budgeting money – such as making and sticking to a budget for an event or activity.*

- The therapist should have each caregiver briefly share their teen's experience and skill level with the previous money management concepts of spending, saving, and budgeting.
- The therapist should refer to the PowerPoint presentation slides for Dyad Session 10 while reviewing the content for the session.
- The therapist should have also prepared for the session by reviewing the Dyad Session 10 content discussed in the manual, which has detailed information about the content that will be covered.

- The important points to make while reviewing the Dyad Session 10 Content are:
  - We will do a Real World Practice Check-In, which will ask you and your teen specific questions about the goals on the DLS contract. This will be an opportunity to problem-solve any challenges and celebrate successes.
  - The elements of an effective system for achieving DLS goals will be reviewed with the teens as it relates to the goals on the DLS contract. This will be our main opportunity each session to revise the goals that are currently being targeted on the DLS contract before we add in a new goal at the end of the session.
  - The money questionnaire handout will increase our understanding of the teen's skill level with spending, saving, and budgeting money.
  - The DLS Teaching Method will be used to teach various skills related to money management. For example, if a money diary is used to track spending, the caregiver will provide instruction and demonstrate how to use it before the teen starts practicing using a money diary each day to track their spending or the family's spending.

- Ask: *Any questions about the content for the upcoming dyad session?*

Prep for the Next Caregiver Session (3 mins)

- *We will have our next caregiver group session on DAY and TIME. At this session, we will continue our sessions on money management and will talk in more detail about spending and saving money. We will continue discussing how implementing the DLS contract went and discuss how to change or add a money management goal to your teen's DLS contract.*
- *To prepare for the upcoming dyad session with your teen, please have your teen complete the Money Questionnaire handout on their own so that we have an understanding of their skills.*
- *After your dyad session with your teen, it will be important to prioritize working on the goals on the DLS contract and the Real World Practice assignment so that we can celebrate successes and also discuss any challenges or questions that arose in the caregiver group session.*
- Ask: *Are there any questions before we end the session?*

Wrap-Up

- The therapist should send a calendar invite with the next caregiver group session's day/time to the caregiver.
- The therapist may also want to email caregivers a blank copy of the DLS contract and can also email them the STRW Budgeting Workbook, which are both available on the STRW website.

Daily Living Skills Contract

Date ____________________

Goal	Expectations	Reward	MONDAY	TUESDAY	WEDNESDAY	THURSDAY	FRIDAY	SATURDAY	SUNDAY

____
Teen

____
Parent / Caregiver

Caregiver/Teen Dyad Session 10 Content (60 mins)

STRW Session 10 Schedule (1 min)

- The therapist should greet the caregiver and teen.
- *Let's get started! As a reminder, it will be helpful to sit together at a table so that we can all see each other and work together. Please pull out your STRW workbook that contains the handouts for all STRW sessions. This session is called Session 10 – Money Basics. Please turn to that section in your workbook.*
- *Let's go over the session schedule so that you know what we will be doing. Please feel free to ask any questions about our schedule!*
- Briefly go over each item on the Session Schedule.

Real World Practice Check-In: Contract and Morning Routine (3 mins)

- Refer to the Session 9 Real World Practice handout and the DLS Contract handout.
- *Let's check in on how you are doing with each goal on your DLS contract. Please be honest, as this is an opportunity to talk about what is working and what is not working and do some brainstorming to address any challenges.*
- As needed, the therapist should spend time modifying the DLS contract and problem solving how to make a more effective system to target the DLS goal (e.g., make expectations more specific, change reward, increase/decrease number of prompts, modify the strategies being used to help with goals).
- If the therapist used a fillable PDF of the DLS Contract handout in the previous session, it may be helpful to share this on the screen so that the goal, expectations, and reward can be easily discussed.
- The following questions should be asked (if applicable), and the responses and any relevant notes should be entered into the Real World Practice Tracking Sheet:
  - *Did you use your DLS contract this week?*
  - *Did you work on your morning routine goal during the week?*
    - *What went well?*
    - *What was challenging?*
    - *How many days did you work on your morning routine goal?*
    - *Did you earn a reward for your morning routine goal?*
    - *How many days did you earn a reward?*

Real World Practice Check-In: Cleaning the Bedroom and Laundry (3 mins)

- The following questions should be asked (if applicable), and the responses and any relevant notes should be entered into the Real World Practice Tracking Sheet:

- *Did you work on your cleaning the bedroom goal during the week?*
    - *What went well?*
    - *What was challenging?*
    - *How many days did you work on your cleaning the bedroom goal?*
    - *Did you earn a reward for your cleaning the bedroom goal?*
- *Did you work on your laundry goal during the week?*
    - *What went well?*
    - *What was challenging?*
    - *How many days did you work on your laundry goal?*
    - *Did you earn a reward for your laundry goal?*

Real World Practice Check-In: Cooking and Grocery Shopping (6 mins)

♦ The following questions should be asked (if applicable), and the responses and any relevant notes should be entered into the Real World Practice Tracking Sheet:
- *Did you work on your cooking goal or goals during the week?*
    - *What went well?*
    - *What was challenging?*
    - *How many days did you work on your cooking goal or goals?*
    - *Did you earn a reward for your cooking goal or goals?*
- *Did you work on a grocery shopping goal?*
    - *What went well?*
    - *What was challenging?*
    - *How many days did you work on your grocery shopping goal?*
    - *Did you earn a reward for working on your grocery shopping goal?*

Real World Practice Check-In: Money (2 mins)

♦ The following questions should be asked (if applicable), and the responses and any relevant notes should be entered into the Real World Practice Tracking Sheet:
- *For your Real World Practice, you were also given an assignment to complete the Money Questionnaire handout.*
    - *Did you work on or complete the Money Questionnaire handout?*
    - *What went well?*
    - *What was challenging?*

♦ Ask: *Any questions or comments about your Real World Practice assignments?*

♦ If the caregiver/teen dyad struggled to complete the Real World Practice assignments, the therapist should spend some time discussing how to identify days/times that they could designate to commit to working on the assignments.

♦ If the therapist used a fillable PDF of the DLS Contract handout in the previous session, it may be helpful to share this on the screen so that the goal, expectations, and reward can be easily discussed.

Elements of an Effective System for Achieving DLS Goals (2 mins)

- Ask: ***Are there any issues you want to discuss or troubleshoot related to the DLS contract?***
- Ask and Discuss: ***Are we considering all of the important elements to increase the likelihood of you achieving your DLS goals by developing the most effective system?***
- If applicable, discuss how to modify any DLS goals to address (1) qualities of the teen and their caregiver; (2) use of evidence-based strategies to teach and master DLS; and (3) ensuring that goals are obvious, attractive, easy, and satisfying.

Money Questionnaire (10 mins)

- ***We are going to be discussing how to manage money over the next several sessions and will be going over topics such as buying items, spending and saving money, using checking and savings accounts, and budgeting. We want to get an idea of how much experience you have with managing your money.***
- Refer to the Money Questionnaire handout.
- ***If you have filled out this questionnaire prior to session, we will discuss it now. If you have not completed it, we will discuss your responses now and have your caregiver add on to your answers as needed.***
- Go through the teen's response to each question on the Money Questionnaire handout in detail and encourage the caregiver to provide coaching/support as needed.
- Ask and Discuss: ***Now that we have discussed your experience with money, what are some skills that you could build in this area?***
- The caregiver can also provide their thoughts if the teen is having difficulty coming up with possible areas to work on.

Evidence-Based Strategy: DLS Teaching Method-Money Management (2 mins)

- Refer to the DLS Teaching Method for Money Management handout.
- ***Throughout STRW, we have utilized many different evidence-based strategies to build daily living skills. For this and the upcoming sessions that are focused on spending, saving, and budgeting money, we will mostly utilize the DLS Teaching Method so that you can get hands-on instruction, modeling, and practice with your caregiver. For example, your caregiver may talk about how they track what they are spending and show you how they do this by checking their bank statement regularly.***
- ***We will also talk about some helpful tools that will help you build your money management skills.***
- ***As you get older and need to spend, save, and budget your own money, you will be able to apply the things you learned from your caregiver. As part of your DLS contract in the coming weeks, you will have a money goal. It can be helpful to make your money goal related to the other goals on your DLS contract. For***

example, you could track how much money you spend on things you buy at the grocery store. As another example, your grocery shopping goal could be to find 8 items at the grocery store from a list and then your money management goal could be to pay for the items using a debit card.

Tips for Safely Storing Your Money (3 mins)

- *Let's first talk about how to safely store your money. You may have cash or a debit or credit card, but it is important to develop good habits so that you do not misplace or lose your wallet.*
- Ask and Discuss:
  - *Do you use a wallet to store your money and/or debit/credit cards?*
  - *What else do you keep in your wallet?*
  - *Where do you keep your wallet?*

- *Let's talk about these tips for safely storing your money and then we will think through how you can apply these tips to yourself.*
- Have the caregiver and teen take turns reading the tips on the slide for safely storing money. These tips include the following:
  - Use a wallet to store cash and debit/credit cards.
  - Keep your wallet in the same place (e.g., pocket, backpack, purse) and always put it back after you use it.
    - This is a good habit and makes it less likely you will lose your wallet!
  - Only keep a small amount of money in your wallet (e.g., $20 to be used for emergencies).
  - Make a list of what you have stored in your wallet (e.g., driver's license, school ID, debit card, etc.).
    - If you lose it, you will know exactly what has been lost.
  - If you lose your wallet, let your caregiver know immediately and they can help you make a plan (e.g., contact the bank to report your missing debit card).

- Ask and Discuss: *Which of these tips would be helpful for you to start using?*

Should I Buy It or Not? (7 mins)

- *For the remainder of the session, we will talk about spending money. It is important to be smart about spending your money – which will then allow you to have more of it to spend or save in the real world.*
- *Before you spend your money, you should stop and think about the item you want to purchase to make sure you are not impulse buying. There are some questions that you can ask yourself to make sure you are making a good purchase and spending your money wisely.*
- *Let's use these questions to think about whether an item you want to purchase is a smart decision! Think about an item that you want to purchase and then we will go through the questions about whether you should buy it or not.*
- Refer to the <u>Should I Buy It or Not?</u> handout.

- Have the teen identify an item that they want to purchase.
- The therapist should then ask the following questions and have the caregiver and teen write their responses down on the handout or the therapist can transcribe responses directly onto the slide or onto the fillable PDF of the handout:
  - *Do I NEED this item?*
    - *If YES – What do I need it for? Will I use it?*
    - *If NO – Why do I want this item?*
  - *Do I have the money to buy this item now?*
    - *If YES – Will buying this item now affect my ability to buy other things I need in the coming weeks or months?*
    - *If NO – Do I need to come up with a plan to save my money?*
  - *Do I have time to delay buying this item so that I can think about whether I need buy it now?*
    - *Is there a chance the item will go on sale?*
    - *Could I purchase this item somewhere else at a lower price?*
  - *Are there any other things to consider before I make my decision?*

- *Overall, now that we have gone through all of these questions, is this item a good purchase to make right now?*
- Ask and Discuss:
  - *How was it going through this process to determine if you really need to buy an item?*
  - *Would this be helpful in the future?*

Keeping a Money Diary (2 mins)

- *It can be helpful to keep track of your income or how much money you have coming in, which may include money from an allowance, part-time job, and gifts.*
- *You should also keep track of your expenses or how much money you are spending, which may include things such as buying lunch at school, a drink at a coffee shop, movie tickets, and your cell phone bill.*
- *Keeping track of your money helps you understand how much money is coming in, how much money is being spent, and how to save your money more effectively.*
- *A money diary is a helpful tool for tracking money because it can help you see how much money you are spending in certain categories. Once you know how you are spending your money, you can make a plan to decrease spending and increase saving.*
- *For example, if you are mostly spending your money on fast food, you could try to cut down on how often you are buying fast food so that you have more money to save up for the new laptop you want to buy.*
- *We often get into the habit of spending without thinking, so the money diary is a great tool for showing you how much you are spending in different categories so that you can make a plan to spend less and save more!*

Money Diary (5 mins)

- Refer to the Money Diary handout.
- Ask and Discuss:
  - *Have you ever used a money diary or another tool to track how much money you are spending?*
  - *Do you feel like you have an understanding of what money is coming in (your income) and what money is going out (your expenses)?*
    - *Why or why not?*

- *This is an example of a money diary that you can use to keep track of both your income, which is all of the money that you have coming in from an allowance or a job, and your expenses, which is all of the money that is going out.*
- *As you do this, you may find that some expenses are "fixed" in that they are the around the same cost each day, week, or month. For example, your cell phone bill is roughly the same amount each month. Your lunch at school may also be a fixed expense such that you usually spend $6 per day, so you need $30 per week for buying lunch at school. Other examples of fixed expenses might include music lessons, a music or television subscription, a car insurance payment, or a monthly bus pass. Many of the bills that your caregivers pay for each month, including a mortgage or rent for your home, the water and electric bill, car insurance, and internet, are examples of fixed expenses.*
- Ask and Discuss: *What are some other examples of fixed expenses in your family?*
- *Other expenses may be more variable such that they change or vary each day, week, or month. For example, you may need to purchase new shoes one week but may not have this expense again for several weeks or months. You may go to the movies one week but may not go to the movies again for several weeks or months. It is still important to be aware of these "variable expenses," but they are not as consistent.*
- Ask and Discuss: *What are some other examples of variable expenses in your family?*
- *It can be extremely helpful to build your awareness of your income and your fixed and variable expenses by keeping a money diary. It may be helpful to fill out a Money Diary for the money goal on your DLS contract. You can use a handout like this or you can also use an excel spreadsheet to keep track of your expenses and income.*
- If time allows and/or if there is interest, the therapist can show the caregiver and teen the Money Diary worksheet in the STRW Budgeting Workbook, which is identical to the Money Diary handout but allows for automatic calculation of expenses and income across different categories that can be changed based on the teen's individual expenses and incomes.

- *Schedule a day/time to work on watching and/or practicing how to clean your bedroom, do laundry, cook, and grocery shop.*
- *It may be helpful to fill out a money diary for the money goal on your DLS contract!*
- *Make sure that if the teen earns the reward, they receive it immediately! This makes it more likely that they will continue to be motivated to meet their goal!*

♦ Ask: *Any questions about your Real World Practice assignment?*

Guess the Price (3 mins) – OPTIONAL

♦ NOTE: This activity can be skipped if there is not enough time to complete it.
♦ *Let's play a quick round of Guess the Price, which is just meant to be a fun way to build up your understanding of how much things cost.*
♦ *Let's see if you know the prices of some common items even if they are not necessarily items that you use!*
♦ The therapist can have the teen guess the price or have the caregiver and teen compete against each other.
♦ The therapist should click through the next four slides that contain examples of common expenses. Prior to the session, the therapist will need to look up the prices to ensure that they are accurate.
  - Therapists can change the items for the Guess the Price game.
  - This activity is meant to be fun and engaging! If the teen is averse to playing the game, it can be skipped. However, it would be helpful for the caregiver and teen to find other ways to build up an understanding of what things cost (e.g., compare the cost of products at the grocery store, involve the teen when purchasing cleaning items).

Preparing for the Next Dyad Session (2 mins)

♦ *We will have our next caregiver/teen dyad session on DAY and TIME. At this session, we will talk in more detail about spending and saving money.*
♦ *It will be important to complete your Real World Practice assignment before our next dyad session and come prepared to discuss it. We will spend a lot of time next session talking about how the DLS contract went!*
♦ Ask: *Are there any questions before we end the session?*

Wrap-Up

♦ The therapist should send a calendar invite with the next caregiver/teen dyad session's day/time to the caregiver and teen. The therapist may also want to send the caregiver/teen a copy of the DLS contract if they completed it using a fillable PDF.

Money Questionnaire

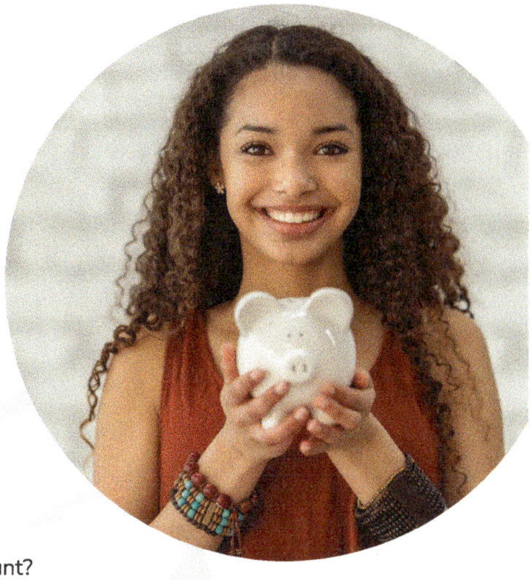

1. Where does your money come from?

2. What do you spend your money on?

3. Where do you keep or store your money?

4. Do you have a checking account? ☐ Yes ☐ No
If YES – do you know how to check to see how much money is in your account?

5. Do you have a debit card or ATM card? ☐ Yes ☐ No
If YES – do you know your pin or password?

6. Do you have a savings account? ☐ Yes ☐ No
If YES – do you know how to check to see how much money is in your account?

7. Do you have a credit card? ☐ Yes ☐ No
If YES – do you know how to check to see how much money you owe?

8. How do you buy things? (e.g., with cash, debit/ATM card, credit card)?

9. Have you ever saved up a small or large purchase? What was it?

10. Have you ever had to set a budget and stick to it?

Evidence-Based Strategy: **Daily Life Skills Teaching Method**

Money Management

LEARN

Learn how to spend, save, and budget money.

WATCH

Your parent/caregiver will demonstrate (as needed) how to spend, save, and budget money.

PRACTICE

You will practice how to spend, save, and budget money.
Your parent/caregiver will observe and give feedback and support as you practice.

DO IT INDEPENDENTLY

You will spend, save, and budget money on your own.

Should I Buy It or Not?

Directions: After identifying an item you may want to buy, it is a good idea to ask yourself these questions to make sure you are making a good purchase and spending your money wisely.

- Do I NEED this item?
  - If **YES** – What do I need it for? Will I use it?
  - If **NO** – Why do I want this item?
- Do I have the money to buy this item now?
  - If **YES** – Will buying this item now affect my ability to buy other things I need in the coming weeks or months?
  - If **NO** – Do I need to come up with a plan to save my money?
- Do I have time to delay buying this item so that I can think about whether I need buy it now?
  - Is there a chance the item will go on sale?
  - Could I purchase this item somewhere else at a lower price?
- Are there any other things to consider before I make my decision?

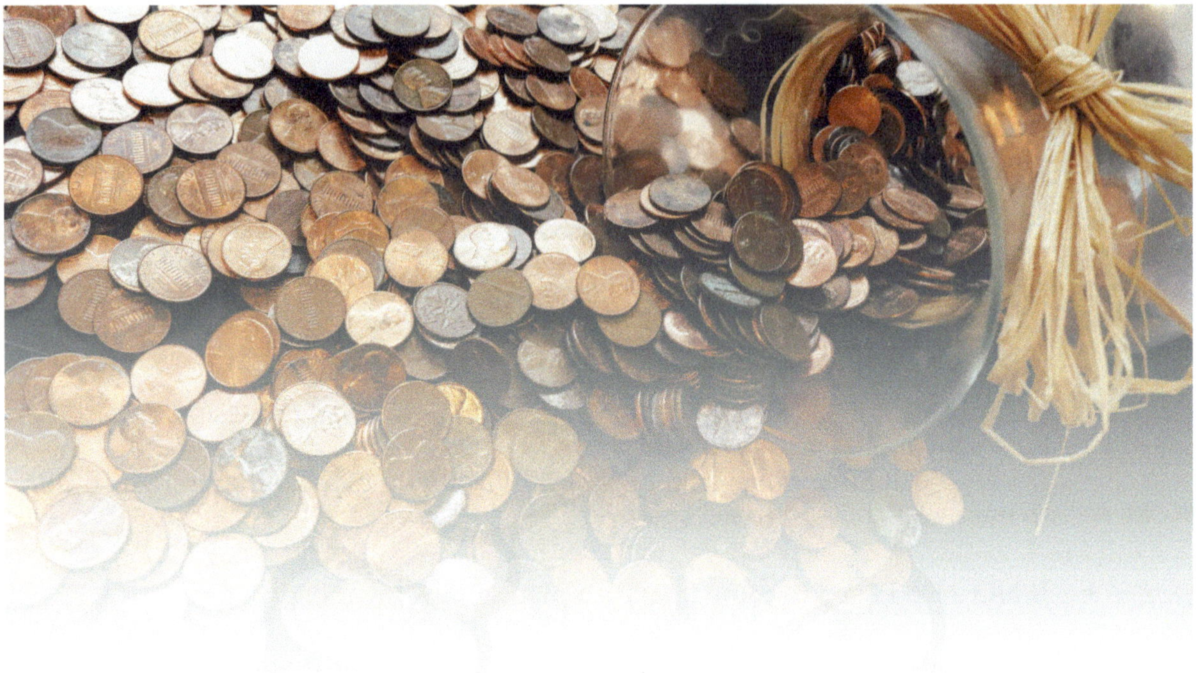

Money Diary

	Monday	Tuesday	Wednesday	Thursday	Friday	Saturday	Sunday
INCOME (ALL OF THE MONEY COMING IN)							
EXPENSES (ALL OF THE MONEY GOING OUT)							

Daily Living Skills Contract

Date ____________________

Goal	Expectations	Reward	MONDAY	TUESDAY	WEDNESDAY	THURSDAY	FRIDAY	SATURDAY	SUNDAY

____
Teen

____
Parent / Caregiver

Surviving and Thriving in the Real World
Session 10 – Real World Practice

- Work on your (1) morning routine, (2) cleaning the bedroom, (3) doing laundry, (4) cooking, (5) grocery shopping, and (6) money goals for the remainder of the week using your DLS contract.
  - Set aside a specific time (e.g., on the way to school, after dinner) to discuss how the morning routine went and how to problem-solve for the next day.
  - Schedule a day/time to work on watching and/or practicing how to clean the bedroom, do laundry, cook, go grocery shopping, and work on money management.
  - It may be helpful to fill out a money diary for the money goal on your DLS contract!
  - Make sure that if a reward is earned, it is provided immediately!

Surviving & Thriving in the Real World

Session 11

Saving and Spending Money

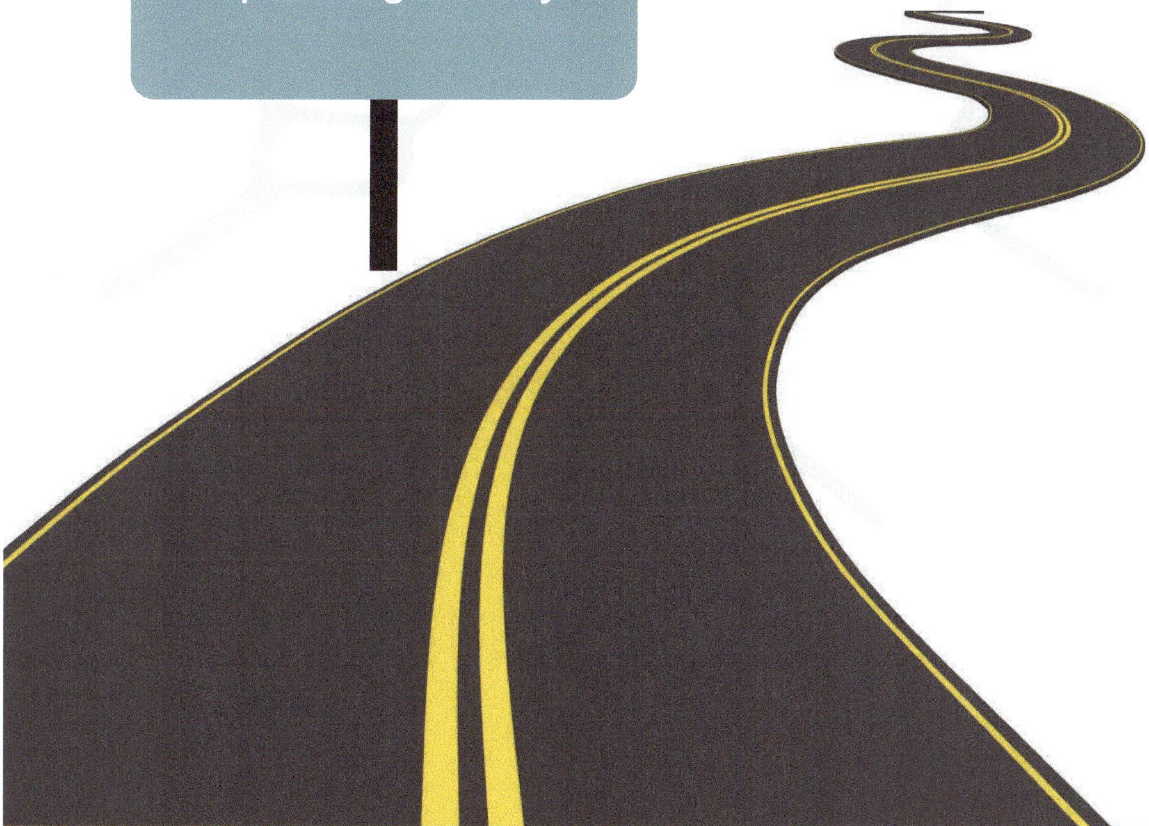

Session 11

Saving and Spending Money

Aims

- Continue to build rapport between caregiver group members and the therapist
- Continue to build rapport between the teen, caregiver, and therapist
- Further develop ability to use a DLS contract to set a DLS goal, define expectations, and identify a reward for meeting the goal
- Review the four elements for developing an effective system to achieve the teen's DLS goals
- Understand how to use the DLS Teaching Method to learn how to spend, save, and budget money
- Understand the difference between a checking account, a savings account, and a credit card
- Review the features of a checking and savings account and how it applies to the teen
- Demonstrate how to save up for a small and large purchase
- Understand how to use a savings contract to develop a plan to save money
- Discuss ways to keep personal information safe
- Create and implement a DLS contract to target the goals of morning routine, cleaning the bedroom, doing laundry, cooking, grocery shopping, and money management

Structure

- Caregiver group session via telehealth
- Caregiver/teen dyad session via telehealth

Session Supplies

- Caregiver Group Handouts
  - DLS Contract

- Caregiver/Teen Dyad Handouts
  - DLS Teaching Method for Money Management (from Session 10)
  - Saving Up Money for Purchases

DOI: 10.4324/9781003458838-14

- ❍ Savings Contract
- ❍ Example Savings Contract
- ❍ Keeping Your Personal Information Safe
- ❍ DLS Contract
- ❍ Session 11 – Real World Practice

Caregiver/Teen Preparation for Session

- ♦ None.

Therapist Preparation for Session

- ♦ The therapist may want to review the Possible Solutions to Common Challenges that Arise for STRW Therapists handout (see appendix), which includes ideas for how STRW therapists can address common challenges that arise when facilitating the caregiver group and dyad sessions including commitment, engagement, inattention, too much prompting, and family factors such as time, use of rewards, and caregiver/teen relationship.
- ♦ The therapist should use the Real World Practice Tracking Sheet for each dyad in all subsequent STRW sessions to track progress on their DLS contract goals.
- ♦ The therapist should consider reviewing the Tips for STRW Therapists: How to Facilitate Achievement of DLS Goals handout prior to each caregiver group session or dyad session for tips and strategies on how to help teens achieve the goals on their DLS contract. Tips that may be beneficial for Session 11 include:
  - *Fade support over time.* The therapist needs to be mindful of fading back their support during sessions and when creating and modifying the DLS contract. For example, during the last two to three sessions, the therapist should purposely facilitate the caregiver and teen's independence at creating DLS goals and modifying the DLS contract by letting them take the lead. In Session 14, the therapist will discuss how the caregiver can fade their support when identifying and targeting new DLS goals in the future.
  - *Normalize that all teens are different and will make progress at different rates.* Every teen, caregiver, and family environment is unique, and the therapist should consider the individual strengths and challenges when developing DLS goals to target. Additionally, teens will make progress at different rates depending on a range of factors (e.g., motivation, previous experience, commitment, etc.). It can be helpful for therapists to regularly normalize that progress takes time and looks different for everyone.

Session 11 Notes

- ♦ Fillable PDFs of handouts from this session (i.e., Saving Up Money for Purchases, DLS Contract) are available on the STRW website.

- ♦ Caregiver Group Session
  - The therapist should continue to devote the majority of the caregiver group session to reviewing how the DLS contract is progressing for each caregiver.

This is an opportunity to identify any issues and brainstorm solutions prior to the dyad session.

- The therapist should utilize the caregiver group session to get an understanding of how it may be necessary to personalize the dyad session content (e.g., the teen's experience with using a checking or savings account, the caregiver's interest in having the teen open a savings/checking account).
- The therapist should make an active effort to foster collaboration between the group members by encouraging active discussion and problem solving of challenges or questions about the DLS contract.
- The therapist should have caregivers discuss how they build their teen's money management skills on a regular basis and get ideas from other caregivers (e.g., specific checking account features that have been helpful in building teen's skills and experience with tracking their spending and saving). Caregivers are likely doing various money management tasks daily or weekly, and it can be helpful to identify ways to include their teen in this process (e.g., showing the teen how they look up their spending in their checking account app or website).

♦ Dyad Session

- Many caregivers and teens may be feeling overwhelmed by the goals on their DLS contract, so it may be beneficial to choose a money management goal that aligns with their other goals (e.g., purchasing items from a list at the grocery store) or is something that the family or teen already does on a regular basis (e.g., tracking weekly spending, paying bills, carrying a wallet whenever leaving the house).
- The STRW Resources handout also has various resources related to money management that may be helpful for the caregivers and teens.
- When doing the activity in the dyad session on short-term and long-term savings, the caregiver and teen can write their responses down on the handout or the therapist can transcribe responses directly onto the slide or onto the fillable PDF of the handout. It may also be beneficial to look up the actual price of an item, which could be done by having the therapist or the teen/caregiver share their computer screen as they do this.
- When developing the DLS contract at the end of the caregiver/teen dyad session, the therapist should continue to incorporate all of the information and knowledge gained from the past several sessions (e.g., issues that were brought up during the caregiver group session, task analysis steps, discussing how to incorporate the essential elements of an effective system for achieving DLS goals, identifying appropriate rewards, etc.).
- The Guess the Price activity in the dyad session provides an opportunity for the caregiver and teen to choose an item that they want to either learn or guess the price for. For example, the teen could choose to have their caregiver guess the price of a new video game that they want, and the caregiver could choose to have their teen guess the price of car insurance for when the teen starts driving.

Caregiver Group Session 11 Content (90 mins)

Review – Real World Practice Assignment (50 mins)

- The therapist should greet the caregivers and welcome them to the session.
- Discuss the Real World Practice assignment in detail by having all caregivers share how using the DLS contract to target the morning routine, cleaning the bedroom, laundry, cooking, grocery shopping, and money goals went with their teen. Encourage caregivers to jot down questions or notes on a blank copy of the DLS Contract handout that they may want to discuss or incorporate into their teen's contract at the next dyad session.
- ***We will have everyone share how using the DLS contract to target the morning routine, cleaning the bedroom, laundry, cooking, grocery shopping, and money goals went for their teen. This is an opportunity to celebrate successes and also problem-solve any challenges or obstacles that occurred. We will spend the majority of our session discussing each teen's progress with the DLS contract. It may be helpful to jot down questions or notes on a copy of the*** **DLS Contract** ***handout, and feel free to ask questions or add to the discussion.***
- It may be helpful to refer caregivers to the Tips for Creating a Successful DLS Contract handout (from Session 4) when discussing the goals on the DLS contract (e.g., clearly defining expectations, re-evaluating rewards regularly to ensure they are motivating, etc.).
- Points of discussion or questions to ask each caregiver include the following:
  - DLS contract
    - ***Did the teen make progress at becoming more independent with each of their goals – morning routine, cleaning the bedroom, laundry, cooking, grocery shopping, and money?***
    - ***What went well?***
    - ***What was difficult?***
    - ***Did they receive a reward?***
    - ***Did they use any strategies to help them to learn the skill or become more independent?***
    - ***Any obstacles or barriers?***
    - ***Do you plan on modifying any goals on the current DLS contract?***

- Ask: ***Any questions about the Real World Practice assignment?***

STRW Session 11 Goals (1 min)

- ***The goal of today's session is to continue discussing how to save and spend money. The specific aims are to increase the teen's understanding of how to use a checking*** *and savings account and then talk about how to save up for short-term and long-term purchases using tools such as a savings contract. We will also review how to build an effective system to help you and your teen achieve their DLS goals now and in the future.*

- *As we continue to build your teen's DLS, it may seem overwhelming to add in another goal. However, money management is the last goal we are adding to the DLS contract, and there are ways to incorporate these money goals into your weekly schedule. For example:*
  - *Could the teen track how they spend their own money?*
  - *Could the teen login to their checking or savings account app or website to see the balance or when a purchase is posted?*
  - *Could the teen create a plan to save up money for a purchase that they want to make using a savings contract?*

- Ask and Discuss: *Any questions?*

Review Dyad Session 11 Content (36 mins)

- *Now we will briefly review the material that will be covered in the upcoming dyad session with your teen. This will allow you to have some time to prepare for the upcoming session. Please feel free to ask any questions as we go over the content of the dyad session, which will focus on building their understanding of checking and savings accounts and how to use a savings contract to reach their savings goals. We will incorporate what we discuss today as a money goal on their DLS contract.*
- *Before we review the dyad session content, let's all briefly share your teen's experience with using a checking and/or savings account to manage their money.*
- The therapist should have each caregiver briefly share their teen's experience and skill level with using a checking and savings account.
- The therapist should refer to the PowerPoint presentation slides for Dyad Session 11 while reviewing the content for the session.
- The therapist should have also prepared for the session by reviewing the Dyad Session 11 content discussed in the manual, which has detailed information about the content that will be covered.
- The important points to make while reviewing the Dyad Session 11 Content are:
  - We will do a Real World Practice Check-In, which will ask you and your teen specific questions about the goals on the DLS contract. This will be an opportunity to problem-solve any challenges and celebrate successes.
  - The elements of an effective system for achieving DLS goals will be reviewed with the teens as it relates to the goals on the DLS contract. This will be our main opportunity each session to revise the goals that are currently being targeted on the DLS contract before we add in a new goal at the end of the session.
  - The DLS Teaching Method will be used to teach various skills related to money management. For example, if a savings contract is used to help the teen develop a plan for saving their money, the caregiver will provide instruction and demonstrate how to use it before the teen starts practicing with a savings contract.

- The features of a checking account, savings account, and credit card will be discussed so that they know the similarities and differences between the different types of accounts.
- We will discuss the benefits of opening up a checking and/or savings account and review the teen's experience with accessing their own checking or savings account.
- We will practice how to save up for a small purchase (less than $100) and a large purchase (more than $100).
- The features of a savings contract, which is a plan to help the teen identify their savings goals and how they can make progress towards meeting those goals, will be discussed.
- The importance of keeping personal information such as your Social Security number and debit card pin private will be reviewed.

♦ Ask: ***Any questions about the content for the upcoming dyad session?***

Prep for the Next Caregiver Session (3 mins)

♦ ***We will have our next caregiver group session on DAY and TIME. At this session, we will continue our sessions on money management and will talk in more detail about budgeting money. We will continue discussing how implementing the DLS contract went and discuss how to change or add a money goal to your teen's DLS contract.***

♦ ***After your dyad session with your teen, it will be important to prioritize working on the goals on the DLS contract and the Real World Practice assignment so that we can celebrate successes and also discuss any challenges or questions that arose in the caregiver group session.***

♦ Ask: ***Are there any questions before we end the session?***

Wrap-Up

♦ The therapist should send a calendar invite with the next caregiver group session's day/time to the caregiver.

♦ The therapist may also want to email caregivers a blank copy of the DLS contract or refer them to the STRW website.

Daily Living Skills Contract

Date ______________________

Goal	Expectations	Reward	MONDAY	TUESDAY	WEDNESDAY	THURSDAY	FRIDAY	SATURDAY	SUNDAY

______________________ Teen

______________________ Parent / Caregiver

Caregiver/Teen Dyad Session 11 Content (60 mins)

STRW Session 11 Schedule (1 min)

- The therapist should greet the caregiver and teen.
- *Let's get started! As a reminder, it will be helpful to sit together at a table so that we can all see each other and work together. Please pull out your STRW workbook that contains the handouts for all STRW sessions. This session is called Session 11 – Saving and Spending. Please turn to that section in your workbook.*
- *Let's go over the session schedule so that you know what we will be doing. Please feel free to ask any questions about our schedule!*
- Briefly go over each item on the Session Schedule.

Real World Practice Check-In: Contract and Morning Routine (3 mins)

- Refer to Session 10 Real World Practice handout and DLS Contract handout.
- *Let's check in on how you are doing with each goal on your DLS contract. Please be honest, as this is an opportunity to talk about what is working and what is not working and do some brainstorming to address any challenges.*
- As needed, the therapist should spend time modifying the DLS contract and problem solving how to make a more effective system to target the DLS goal (e.g., make expectations more specific, change reward, increase/decrease number of prompts, modify the strategies being used to help with goals).
- If the therapist used a fillable PDF of the DLS Contract handout in the previous session, it may be helpful to share this on the screen so that the goal, expectations, and reward can be easily discussed.
- The following questions should be asked (if applicable), and the responses and any relevant notes should be entered into the Real World Practice Tracking Sheet:
  - *Did you use your DLS contract this week?*
  - *Did you work on your morning routine goal during the week?*
    - *What went well?*
    - *What was challenging?*
    - *How many days did you work on your morning routine goal?*
    - *Did you earn a reward for your morning routine goal?*
    - *How many days did you earn a reward?*

Real World Practice Check-In: Cleaning the Bedroom and Laundry (3 mins)

- The following questions should be asked (if applicable), and the responses and any relevant notes should be entered into the Real World Practice Tracking Sheet:
  - *Did you work on your cleaning the bedroom goal during the week?*
    - *What went well?*
    - *What was challenging?*
    - *How many days did you work on your cleaning the bedroom goal?*
    - *Did you earn a reward for your cleaning the bedroom goal?*
  - *Did you work on your laundry goal during the week?*
    - *What went well?*
    - *What was challenging?*
    - *How many days did you work on your laundry goal?*
    - *Did you earn a reward for your laundry goal?*

Real World Practice Check-In: Cooking and Grocery Shopping (3 mins)

- The following questions should be asked (if applicable), and the responses and any relevant notes should be entered into the Real World Practice Tracking Sheet:
  - *Did you work on your cooking goal or goals during the week?*
    - *What went well?*
    - *What was challenging?*
    - *How many days did you work on your cooking goal or goals?*
    - *Did you earn a reward for your cooking goal or goals?*
  - *Did you work on a grocery shopping goal?*
    - *What went well?*
    - *What was challenging?*
    - *How many days did you work on your grocery shopping goal?*
    - *Did you earn a reward for working on your grocery shopping goal?*

Real World Practice Check-In: Money (3 mins)

- The following questions should be asked (if applicable), and the responses and any relevant notes should be entered into the Real World Practice Tracking Sheet:
  - *Did you work on a money goal?*
    - *What did you do?*
    - *What went well?*
    - *What was challenging?*
    - *How many days did you work on your money goal?*
    - *Did you earn a reward for working on your money goal?*

- Ask: *Any questions or comments about your Real World Practice assignments?*
- If the caregiver/teen dyad struggled to complete the Real World Practice assignments, the therapist should spend some time discussing how to identify days/times that they could designate to commit to working on the assignments.

- If the therapist used a fillable PDF of the DLS Contract handout in the previous session, it may be helpful to share this on the screen so that the goal, expectations, and reward can be easily discussed.

Elements of an Effective System for Achieving DLS Goals (2 mins)

- Ask: *Are there any issues you want to discuss or troubleshoot related to the DLS contract?*
- Ask and Discuss: *Are we considering all of the important elements to increase the likelihood of you achieving your DLS goals by developing the most effective system?*
- If applicable, discuss how to modify any DLS goals to address (1) qualities of the teen and their caregiver; (2) use of evidence-based strategies to teach and master DLS; and (3) ensuring that goals are obvious, attractive, easy, and satisfying.

Evidence-Based Strategy: DLS Teaching Method-Money Management (2 mins)

- Refer to the DLS Teaching Method for Money Management handout (from Session 10).
- *Today we will continue to use the DLS Teaching Method so that you can get hands-on instruction, modeling, and practice with your caregiver. We will also talk about some helpful tools that will help you build your money management skills.*
- *For example, today we will learn about checking and savings accounts and your caregiver will talk about how they use these accounts. We will then talk about how you can also open your own savings account and use the savings contract tool to make sure you are meeting your goals for saving money!*
- *As you get older and need to spend, save, and budget your own money, you will be able to apply the things you learned from your caregiver.*

Savings Account (3 mins)

- Ask and Discuss:
  - *Do you have a savings account?*
  - *What are some of the features of a savings account? What do you know about them?*

- Have caregiver and teen take turns reading the features of a savings account from the slide that include the following:
  - Allows you to keep and save money that you do not need to spend right away.
  - May be a way to save for a specific goal (e.g., college tuition, vacation, new laptop, car).
  - Pays you interest each month!
  - You deposit money into a savings account – at a bank, an ATM machine, or online.
  - It is recommended to save 10–20% of your income.
  - Some people have a regular savings account and an emergency savings account (e.g., car or home repairs).

- Ask: *Any questions or comments about using a savings account?*

Checking Account (3 mins)

- Ask and Discuss:
  - *Do you have a checking account?*
  - *What are some of the features of a checking account?*
  - *How does a checking account differ from a savings account?*

- Have caregiver and teen take turns reading the features of a checking account from the slide that include the following:
  - Allows easier access to money because you can use an ATM/debit card and/or write checks.
    - ATM/Debit Cards – Money is taken out of your account as soon as you make a purchase or withdrawal.
      - A debit card looks like a credit card but is NOT actually a credit card.
    - Checks – Paper "promises" of money that you give to a person or store.
      - Once you write a check, the money will be taken out of your account when the check is cashed. This could be days or weeks later, so it is important to keep track of the checks that you write.
      - Some banks allow you to send "electronic checks" from your checking account.
    - Helpful to have a checking account if you have money going into and out of your account often (e.g., regular paychecks, monthly bills, etc.).
    - May be easier to access your money quickly as compared to a savings account.
    - You may or may not earn interest.

- Ask: *Any questions or comments about using a checking account?*

Credit Card (3 mins)

- Ask and Discuss:
  - *Do you have a credit card?*
  - *What are some of the features of a credit card?*

- Have caregiver and teen take turns reading the features of a credit card from the slide that include the following:
  - You must apply for a credit card by submitting an application.
  - Using a credit card is basically taking out a loan from the credit card company.
  - You have a credit limit, which is a certain dollar amount set by the credit card company that you cannot go over.
  - Most credit cards have very high interest rates (>18%).
    - The longer it takes for you to pay it back, the more you pay in interest.
    - You should try pay your credit card balance every month to avoid paying very high interest rates.

- Ask: *Any questions or comments about using a credit card?*

Open Up a Checking or Savings Account (5 mins)

- *Now that we have talked about the differences between a savings account, checking account, and credit card – let's talk about how this applies to you.*
- *It can be very beneficial for teens to have a savings and/or checking account so that you can get experience with saving, spending, and budgeting your money. For example, if you earn money from babysitting or from an allowance, you could deposit this money into a checking or savings account instead of keeping the money in your wallet. If you put it into a savings account, you would earn interest on this money. If you put it into a checking account, you could get the money out at any time from an ATM or use your debit card to make purchases.*
- *There are also many no-fee teen checking and savings accounts that have features such as linking the teen's account to the caregiver's account, alerting caregivers when any money is spent, and preventing teens from spending more money than what is actually in their account.*
- Ask and Discuss:
  - *What are your thoughts about using a checking or savings account to manage your money?*
  - If the teen <u>DOES HAVE</u> a savings and/or checking account, discuss the following and then move to the next slide:
    - *What bank do you use?*
    - *Do you have a debit/ATM card?*
    - *Do you utilize the bank's app or log on to the bank's website to check your balance?*
    - *Do you know how to look up what your balance is?*
    - *Do you know how to look up a recent purchase?*
    - *How do you deposit your money?*
    - <u>If teen has a job:</u> ***Is your paycheck deposited directly or do you need to deposit it into an account?***
  - If teen <u>DOES NOT HAVE</u> a savings and/or checking account, discuss the following and then move to the next slide:
    - *Are you interested in possibly opening up a savings or checking account?*
    - *How would you use the checking or savings account to manage your money?*
    - *You can open up an account online or through a local bank in your community. Is there a specific bank that you would want to set up the teen's account through?*

- NOTE: The therapist's goal is to encourage the caregiver and teen to think about the advantages of using a savings or checking account to get experience with saving, spending, and budgeting money. If the caregiver/teen dyad is not interested or seems uncomfortable, the therapist should move on.

Short-Term Savings (5 mins)

- *We are now going to talk about saving money up for purchases.*
- Ask and Discuss:
  - *What is an item that you have saved up to purchase in the past?*
  - *How much did it cost?*
  - *How did you save up for the item?*
  - *How long did it take to save up for the item?*

- *It is important to understand how to save up for items because this is a skill that will make budgeting for expenses as an adult much easier. We are going to have you practice thinking through how you would save up for a short-term purchase (less than $100) and a long-term purchase (more than $100).*
- Refer to the Saving Up Money for Purchases handout.
- The therapist may also find it helpful to have the teen look up the price of an item (e.g., a laptop that they want, a new video game, etc.). The therapist can share their computer screen and look up the item or they can have the teen/caregiver share their computer screen or use their phone to look up the price of an item.
- The therapist should ask the following questions and have the caregiver and teen write their responses down on the handout or the therapist can transcribe responses directly onto the slide or onto the fillable PDF of the handout:
  - *What is the item you want to save up for?*
  - *What is the cost of the item?*
  - *How much money do you have to put towards an item? For example, do you have money in your checking or savings accounts you want to use?*
  - *When do you need to purchase the item?*
  - *How long do you have to save up for the item?*
  - *How much money do you need to save per week or month to purchase the item?*
  - *Where will you keep this money you are saving?*
  - *How will you pay for the item?*

Long-Term Savings (5 mins)

- *Now let's practice thinking through how you would save up for a long-term purchase that is greater than $100.*
- Refer to the Saving Up Money for Purchases handout.
- The therapist may also find it helpful to have the teen look up the price of an item (e.g., a laptop that they want, a new video game, etc.). The therapist can share their computer screen and look up the item, or they can have the teen/caregiver share their computer screen or use their phone to look up the price of an item.
- The therapist should ask the following questions and have the caregiver and teen write their responses down on the handout or the therapist can transcribe responses directly onto the slide or onto the fillable PDF of the handout:
  - *What is the item you want to save up for?*
  - *What is the cost of the item?*
  - *How much money do you have to put towards an item? For example, do you have money in your checking or savings accounts you want to use?*

- *When do you need to purchase the item?*
- *How long do you have to save up for the item?*
- *How much money do you need to save per week or month to purchase the item?*
- *Where will you keep this money you are saving?*
- *How will you pay for the item?*

Savings Contract (5 mins)

- Refer to the Savings Contract handout and Example Savings Contract handout.
- *Now that we have talked about things that you want to save up for, let's talk about how you can develop a solid plan to actually save up your money and how to stick to this plan!*
- *It can be helpful to use a savings contract, which is similar to the DLS contract you are using to work on DLS goals. A savings contract can first help you first identify what you are saving for and how much the items cost and then develop a plan for how to save up for these items. It is helpful to have rules or guidelines to make sure you stay on track with your saving goals. For example, if you have a job, it can be helpful to automatically put a certain amount of your earned money towards your savings goals – such as 30% – and deposit this money into a checking or savings account. It can be helpful to review your savings contract with your caregiver and make changes as needed.*
- The therapist should briefly review all sections of the savings contract and the rules.
- Ask and Discuss:
  - *Do you think this savings contract could be a useful strategy to help with saving your money?*
  - *Are there any rules that you would want to change or add to make sure you are meeting your savings goals?*

Keeping Your Personal Information Safe-3 mins (OPTIONAL)

- If time allows, refer to the Keeping Your Personal Information Safe handout.
- *This handout goes over some helpful tips and rules for making sure that you are keeping your personal information safe – which is especially important once you have a savings or checking account or credit card.*
- Have the caregiver and teen take turns reading the tips for keeping your personal information safe as listed on the handout.
- Ask and Discuss: *Do you have any other tips for keeping your personal information safe based on your own experiences?*

Elements of an Effective System for Achieving DLS Goals (3 mins)

- The therapist should briefly ask each teen about each of the elements and then incorporate the responses to the discussion on developing the DLS contract.

- *As we work to modify or keep working on the money goal to the DLS contract, let's make sure we are thinking about all of the following elements to build an effective system for achieving DLS goals:*
  - *Teen – are we considering your strengths, challenges, preferred learning style, and commitment?*
  - *Caregiver – are we considering your parenting style, time and effort, and commitment?*
    - *Some caregivers find it easy to have teens start checking their checking account after they make a purchase. Caregivers can also show teens the recent purchases that they have made in their checking account or discuss how they are saving up for an upcoming purchase or expense.*
  - *Are we using evidence-based strategies?*
    - *We are using the DLS Teaching Method to help you learn and become independent with managing your money.*
    - *We talked about how you could use tools such as a savings contract to make it more likely you will reach your savings goals.*
  - *Is the money management goal obvious, attractive, easy, and satisfying?*
    - *Obvious – some ideas might be to post your savings contract as a reminder of what you are saving up for.*
    - *Attractive – make a chart documenting your progress towards your goal or check your savings account weekly to review your progress.*
    - *Easy – some ideas might be to choose a specific day and time to review the savings contract.*
    - *Satisfying – some ideas include to think about how building these skills now will help you to be more independent in the future.*

- Ask and Discuss: *Any questions or comments?*
- *Let's apply all of this information to creating your DLS contract!*

Developing Your DLS Contract (5 mins)

- Refer to the DLS Contract handout
- *Let's spend the remainder of our time in today's session modifying your DLS contract to continue working on your morning routine, cleaning your bedroom, laundry, cooking, and grocery shopping goals and modify or keep working on the goal of money management. Your money goal could include opening a checking or savings account or using a savings contract. Use a blank copy of the DLS Contract. We will also keep in mind the importance of making sure the goal is Obvious, Attractive, Easy, and Satisfying so that you are more likely to achieve your goal. The DLS contract will have you track your progress and set up rewards for you to earn, which makes working on the goals satisfying!*
- The therapist should support the caregiver/teen dyad in creating the DLS contract by doing the following:
  - Incorporate all of the information from the last several sessions (e.g., rewards that are motivating for the teen, use of strategies and supports to build independence with certain steps) and the Real World Practice Check-In to create the DLS contract. The therapist should also consider the goals that the caregiver and teen collaboratively developed during the Preparing for STRW session.

  - Use the DLS Contract handout to specify the (1) Goal, (2) Expectations, and (3) Reward for Morning Routine, Cleaning the Bedroom, Doing Laundry, Cooking, Grocery Shopping, and Money.
  - Encourage the caregiver/teen dyad to work together and model appropriate and supportive coaching as they develop the DLS contract.

- Possible discussion questions that may be helpful to ask and discuss when creating the contract for the Morning Routine, Cleaning the Bedroom, Laundry, Cooking, Grocery Shopping, and Money goals include:
  - ***How often are you going to need to do the goal – every day, every weekday, every other day, or once per week?***
  - ***What steps of your goal do you need help with?***
  - ***What steps do you not know how to do?***
  - ***What steps are you doing independently?***
  - ***How easy/hard do you think it will be to meet your goal?***
  - ***What reward would you like to earn?***
  - ***Does the reward fit the goal? For example, earning 1 hour of screen time for doing your morning routine goal each day is a lot, but maybe earning 15–20 extra minutes of screen time would be a better fit.***
  - ***How will you check in about your goals daily to discuss if the goal was met?***
  - ***Where can you post your DLS contract so that you can track goals daily and remember to get your reward if it was earned?***

- The caregiver and teen should write each goal, expectation, and reward on the DLS Contract handout. It may be helpful for the therapist to share their screen and add/modify the goals, expectations, and rewards on a fillable PDF of the DLS Contract handout. The therapist can then email it to the caregiver and teen after the session.
- When the DLS contract has been completed, encourage the dyad to sign it and post it somewhere where they can easily see it so that the goals may be tracked.

Real World Practice (1 min)

- Refer to the Real World Practice handout.
- Discuss the details of the Real World Practice assignment.
  - ***Work on your morning routine, cleaning the bedroom, laundry, cooking, grocery shopping, and money goals for the remainder of the week using your DLS contract.***
    - ***Set aside a specific time such as on the way to school or after dinner to discuss how the morning routine went and how to problem-solve the next day.***
    - ***Schedule a day/time to work on watching and/or practicing how to clean your bedroom, do laundry, cook, and grocery shop.***
    - ***Some ideas for adding or modifying the money goal on your DLS contract include (1) open a savings or checking account, (2) develop a savings contract, or (3) use a money diary to keep track of your spending.***
    - ***Make sure that if the teen earns the reward, they receive it immediately! This makes it more likely that they will continue to be motivated to meet their goal!***

- Ask: ***Any questions about your Real World Practice assignment?***

Guess the Price (3 mins) – OPTIONAL

- NOTE: This activity can be skipped if there is not enough time to complete it.
- ***Let's play a quick round of Guess the Price, which is just meant to be a fun way to build up your understanding of how much things cost.***
- ***We are going to try something different and have both of you choose an item and then the other person will guess the price of the item.***
- The therapist should collaborate with the teen and caregiver to provide ideas of possible items to guess the price for (e.g., laptop, video game, car insurance, college tuition, etc.). The therapist can also assist with looking up the price of the item.
- The therapist should click through the next two slides.
  - This activity is meant to be fun and engaging! If the teen is averse to playing the game, it can be skipped. However, it would be helpful for the caregiver and teen to find other ways to build up an understanding of what things cost (e.g., compare the cost of products at the store, involve the teen when purchasing cleaning items).

Preparing for the Next Dyad Session (1 min)

- ***We will have our next caregiver/teen dyad session on DAY and TIME. At this session, we will talk about budgeting money.***
- ***It will be important to complete your Real World Practice assignment before our next dyad session and come prepared to discuss it. We will spend a lot of time next session talking about how the DLS contract went!***
- Ask: ***Are there any questions before we end the session?***

Wrap-Up

- The therapist should send a calendar invite with the next caregiver/teen dyad session's day/time to the caregiver and teen. The therapist may also want to send the caregiver/teen a copy of the DLS contract if they completed it using a fillable PDF.

Saving Up Money for Purchases

Directions: Identify items that you want to save up for. Answer the questions to help you come up with a plan for saving up for and then purchasing the item.

Short Term Savings Plan (item is < $100)

Item to Save Up For: ______________________________

- Cost of item:’
- How much money do you have to put towards the item?
- When do you need to purchase the item?
- How long do you have to purchase the item (e.g., weeks, months)?
- How much do you need to save up per week or month to purchase the item?
- Where will you keep the money as you are saving?
- How will you pay for the item?

Long Term Savings Plan (item is > $100)

- Item to Save Up For: ______________________________
- Cost of item:’
- How much money do you have to put towards the item?
- When do you need to purchase the item?
- How long do you have to purchase the item (e.g., weeks, months)?
- How much do you need to save up per week or month to purchase the item?
- Where will you keep the money as you are saving?
- How will you pay for the item?

Savings Contract

SHORT TERM GOALS (UNDER $100)

- ☐
- ☐
- ☐
- ☐
- ☐
- ☐

LONG TERM GOALS (OVER $100)

- ☐
- ☐
- ☐
- ☐
- ☐
- ☐

RULES

Teen Signature ______________________________ Date ______________

Caregiver Signature ______________________________ Date ______________

Savings Contract

SHORT TERM GOALS (UNDER $100)

- [ ] Set of colored pencils ($30)
- [ ] Sketchbook ($20)
- [ ] Concert ticket ($70)
- [ ]
- [ ]
- [ ]

LONG TERM GOALS (OVER $100)

- [ ] Gaming Laptop ($1000)
- [ ] Star Wars Lego Set ($180)
- [ ]
- [ ]
- [ ]
- [ ]

RULES

All money from my paycheck, gifts, and allowance will be divided up in the following way:
1. I will put 40% towards my long-term savings goals
2. I will put 30% towards my short-term savings goals.
3. I will put the remaining 30% in my checking account that can be used for spending money.

At the end of every month, I will meet with my mom to talk about my progress towards my goals and whether I need to change anything.

Teen Signature ______________________________ Date ______________

Caregiver Signature ______________________________ Date ______________

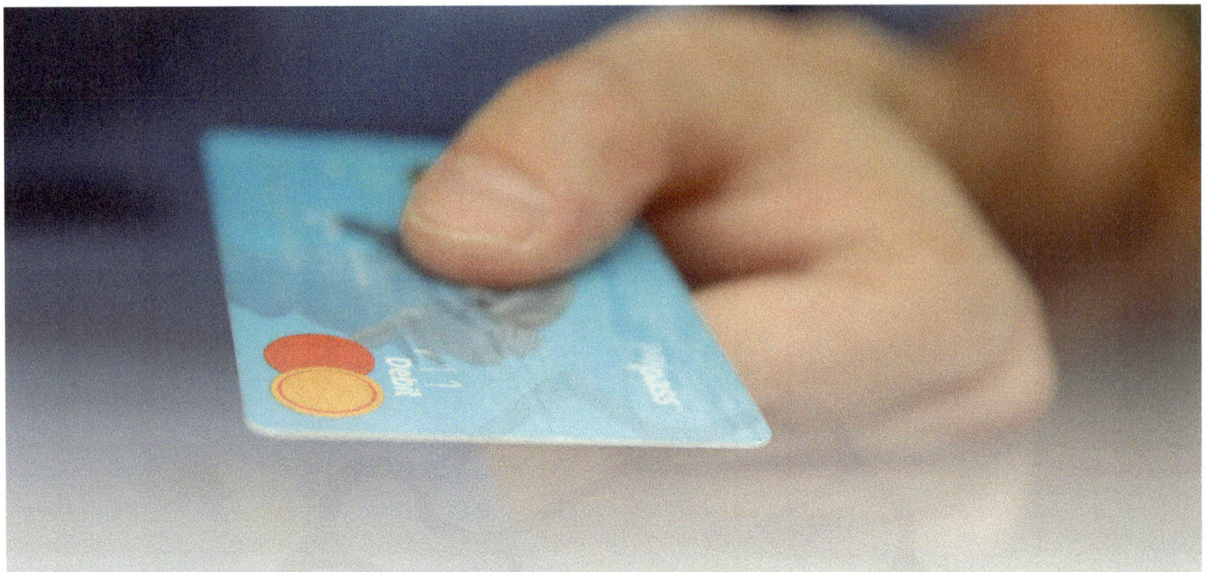

Keeping Your Personal Information Safe

Identify theft occurs when personal information (such as your full name, address, date of birth, social security number, credit card number, and/or checking or savings account number) is stolen, and others use this information to make purchases or apply for loans or credit cards.

STEPS TO KEEPING YOUR PERSONAL INFORMATION SAFE:

- Minimize who you give out your personal information to (e.g., parents, close family members).
- Be extremely careful about giving any personal information to someone over the phone (text or phone call) or over email.
  - » Banks do not call or email you to ask you to verify your account number or debit card pin.
  - » Credit card companies do not call or email you to ask you to verify your credit card number, expiration date, or 3 digit number on the signature panel.
- When you are using an ATM machine, do not let anyone see your pin.
- Keep your credit cards, debit card, and personal identification or driver's license in a safe place such as your wallet or purse.
- Keep track of what credit cards and debit cards you carry in case your wallet is lost or stolen.
- Do not carry your social security card, passport, or birth certificate in your wallet unless you need it for a very specific reason (e.g., traveling on an airplane).
- Don't throw away or recycle any documents that have your personal information (e.g., bank statement, credit card statement) written on them. Instead, shred any documents that you have personal information on it.
- Keep all documents from your work (e.g., W2 form, paystubs) and doctor (e.g., after visit summary, prescriptions) in a safe place, and shred them when you no longer need them.
- While you should be cautious of sharing your credit card information, you will need to provide this information if you order items online (e.g., Amazon) or order food to be delivered (e.g., local pizza place, food delivery service).
- Be careful of "open" wifi connections that are often at restaurants or stores. If you type in your credit card information while on an open wireless network connection, someone could steal your personal information.

Daily Living Skills Contract

Date ____________________

Goal	Expectations	Reward	MONDAY	TUESDAY	WEDNESDAY	THURSDAY	FRIDAY	SATURDAY	SUNDAY

____________________ Teen

____________________ Parent / Caregiver

Surviving and Thriving in the Real World
Session 11 – Real World Practice

- Work on your (1) morning routine, (2) cleaning the bedroom, (3) doing laundry, (4) cooking, (5) grocery shopping, and (6) money goals for the remainder of the week using your DLS contract.
    - Set aside a specific time (e.g., on the way to school, after dinner) to discuss how the morning routine went and how to problem-solve for the next day.
    - Schedule a day/time to work on watching and/or practicing how to clean the bedroom, do laundry, cook, go grocery shopping.
    - Some ideas for adding or modifying the money goal on your DLS contract include (1) open a savings/checking account, (2) develop a savings contract, or (3) use a money diary to keep track of your spending.
    - Make sure that if a reward is earned, it is provided immediately!

Surviving & Thriving in the Real World

Session 12

Budgeting Money

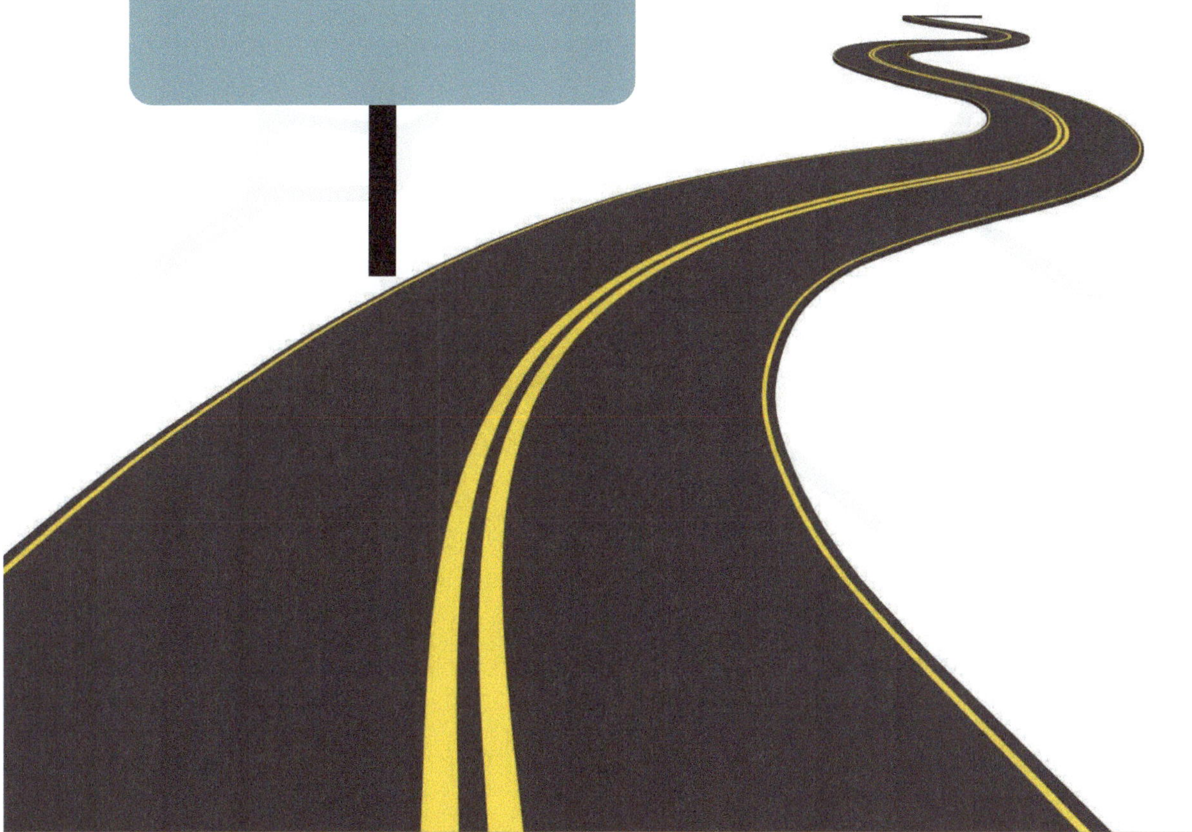

Session 12

Budgeting Money

Aims

- Continue to build rapport between caregiver group members and the therapist
- Continue to build rapport between the teen, caregiver, and therapist
- Further develop ability to use a DLS contract to set a DLS goal, define expectations, and identify a reward for meeting the goal
- Review the four elements for developing an effective system to achieve the teen's DLS goals
- Understand how to use the DLS Teaching Method to learn how to spend, save, and budget money
- Understand that a budget is a plan for one's money that considers income, expenses, and savings
- Understand the steps for developing a budget
- Review tips and guidelines for balancing a budget
- Create and implement a DLS contract to target the goals of morning routine, cleaning the bedroom, doing laundry, cooking, grocery shopping, and money management

Structure

- Caregiver group session via telehealth
- Caregiver/teen dyad session via telehealth

Session Supplies

- Caregiver Group Handouts
  - DLS Contract

- Caregiver/Teen Dyad Handouts
  - DLS Teaching Method for Money Management (from Session 10)
  - How to Develop a Monthly Budget
  - Monthly Budget
  - Example Monthly Budget
  - Sam's Monthly Budget

DOI: 10.4324/9781003458838-15

- Budget Tips
- Your Monthly Budget
- DLS Contract
- Session 12 – Real World Practice

- Other Supplies
  - STRW Budgeting Workbook (available on the STRW website)

Caregiver/Teen Preparation for Session

- None.

Therapist Preparation for Session

- The therapist should use the Real World Practice Tracking Sheet for each caregiver/teen dyad in all subsequent STRW sessions to track progress on their DLS contract goals.
- The therapist should be familiar with using the STRW Budgeting Workbook for the various activities in Session 12. The worksheets within the STRW Budgeting Workbook (i.e., Blank Monthly Budget, Example Monthly Budget, Sam's Monthly Budget, and Your Monthly Budget worksheets) directly correspond to the handouts discussed in the session. The therapist may want to email the caregiver a copy of the STRW Budgeting Workbook or refer them to the STRW website to download a copy to refer to or use during both the caregiver group session and dyad session. The therapist can also choose to use fillable PDFs of the handouts (i.e., Blank Monthly Budget, Your Monthly Budget) that are available on the STRW website or annotate directly on the slide.
- The therapist should consider reviewing the Tips for STRW Therapists: How to Facilitate Achievement of DLS Goals handout prior to each caregiver group session or dyad session for tips and strategies on how to help teens achieve the goals on their DLS contract. Tips that may be beneficial for Session 12 include:
  - *Explore future goals to build and maintain motivation.* In both the Preparing for STRW Session and Session 1, the caregiver and teen dyad are encouraged to identify future goals (e.g., going to college, getting a job, living in an apartment) and the specific DLS that are needed to reach these goals. The link between acquiring age-appropriate DLS and achieving future goals may increase motivation in both the caregiver and teen. It can also be helpful to revisit these goals over the course of the STRW intervention to remind the dyad of what they are working towards.
  - *Assist with building an effective system for reaching goals.* In *Atomic Habits* (2018) by James Clear, he stated the following: *Goals are good for setting a direction, but systems are best for making progress. You fall to the level of your systems.* The therapist will need to remind caregivers and teens that the key to achieving DLS goals that last is to build an effective system. Throughout STRW, the therapist will emphasize building an effective system that considers the teen, the caregiver and the family environment, use of evidence-based strategies, and the Four Laws of Behavior Change.

Session 12 Notes

- Fillable PDFs of handouts from this session (i.e., DLS Contract, Blank Monthly Budget) are available on the STRW website.

- Caregiver Group Session
    - The therapist should continue to devote the majority of the caregiver group session to reviewing how the DLS contract is progressing for each caregiver. This is an opportunity to identify any issues and brainstorm solutions prior to the dyad session.
    - The therapist should utilize the caregiver group session to get an understanding of how it may be necessary to personalize the dyad session content (e.g., the teen's experience with budgeting).
    - The therapist should make an active effort to foster collaboration between the group members by encouraging active discussion and problem solving of challenges or questions about the DLS contract.
    - The therapist should have caregivers discuss how they build their teen's money management skills on a regular basis and get ideas from other caregivers (e.g., involve teen in budgeting for birthday gifts, discuss how the caregiver tries to stay on budget with grocery shopping). Caregivers are likely doing various money management tasks daily or weekly, and it can be helpful to identify ways to include their teen in this process (e.g., involving teen in creating a budget for an upcoming trip).

- Dyad Session
    - Many caregivers and teens may be feeling overwhelmed by the goals on their DLS contract, so it may be beneficial to choose a money management goal that aligns with their other DLS contract goals (e.g., setting a budget for grocery shopping each month) or is something that the family or teen already does on a regular basis (e.g., review whether they are on track to stay on budget for specific monthly or weekly expenses).
    - The STRW Resources handout also has various resources related to money management that may be helpful for the caregivers and teens.
    - There are several options for completing various budgeting activities with the teen and caregiver. The STRW Budgeting Workbook contains all monthly budgets that directly correspond to the handouts used in Session 12. The therapist should download and use it for all activities in this session in conjunction with the handouts and slides. The therapist can share their computer screen and then directly enter information into the STRW Budgeting Workbook during the dyad session. Alternatively, the caregiver and teen can enter their responses on the STRW Budgeting Workbook instead of using the handouts. The therapist can email a copy of the STRW Budgeting Workbook, which is available on the STRW website, to caregivers and teens. As another option, the caregiver and teen can write their responses down on the handout or the therapist can transcribe responses directly onto the slide or onto the fillable PDF of the handout.

- The Monthly Budget activity allows the teen to develop an understanding of how budgeting applies to them now and in the future. While this activity may not be applicable for some teens if they have no income, the teen and caregiver could also discuss income, savings, and expenses for the future (e.g., when the teen gets a part-time job). This activity can also be assigned to the caregiver and teen dyad to complete before the next session or as part of the DLS contract money goal.
- When developing the DLS contract at the end of the dyad session, the therapist should continue to incorporate all of the information and knowledge gained from the past several sessions (e.g., issues that were brought up during the caregiver group session, task analysis steps, discussing how to incorporate the essential elements of an effective system for achieving DLS goals, identifying appropriate rewards, etc.).
- The Guess the Price activity in the dyad session provides an opportunity for the caregiver and teen to choose an item that they want to either learn or guess the price for. For example, the teen could choose to have their caregiver guess the price of a new video game that they want and the caregiver could choose to have their teen guess the price of car insurance for when the teen starts driving.
- In preparation for Session 13, the caregiver and teen should be encouraged to think of an event that they could make a budget for at the next dyad session. Examples of possible events/activities include the following: (1) a birthday party, (2) a graduation party, (3) a family vacation or trip, (4) going to a baseball game, (5) dinner and a movie with friends, and (6) planning and budgeting the ingredients for a family dinner. Ideally, the event or activity should be one that the caregiver and teen will actually do in the future.

Caregiver Group Session 12 Content (90 mins)

Review – Real World Practice Assignment (50 mins)

- The therapist should greet the caregivers and welcome them to the session.
- Discuss the Real World Practice assignment in detail by having all caregivers share how using the DLS contract to target the morning routine, cleaning the bedroom, laundry, cooking, grocery shopping, and money goals went with their teen. Encourage caregivers to jot down questions or notes on a blank copy of the DLS Contract handout that they may want to discuss or incorporate into their teen's contract at the next dyad session.
- ***We will have everyone share how using the DLS contract to target the morning routine, cleaning the bedroom, laundry, cooking, grocery shopping, and money goals went for their teen. This is an opportunity to celebrate successes and also problem-solve any challenges or obstacles that occurred. We will spend the majority of our session discussing each teen's progress with the DLS contract. It may be helpful to jot down questions or notes on a copy of the*** **DLS Contract** ***handout, and feel free to ask questions or add to the discussion.***
- It may be helpful to refer caregivers to the Tips for Creating a Successful DLS Contract handout (from Session 4) when discussing the goals on the DLS contract (e.g., clearly defining expectations, re-evaluating rewards regularly to ensure they are motivating, etc.).
- Points of discussion or questions to ask each caregiver include the following:
  - DLS contract
    - ***Did the teen make progress at becoming more independent with each of their goals – morning routine, cleaning the bedroom, laundry, cooking, grocery shopping, and money?***
    - ***What went well?***
    - ***What was difficult?***
    - ***Did they receive a reward?***
    - ***Did they use any strategies to help them to learn the skill or become more independent?***
    - ***Any obstacles or barriers?***
    - ***Do you plan on modifying any goals on the current DLS contract?***

- Ask: ***Any questions about the Real World Practice assignment?***

STRW Session 12 Goals (1 min)

- *The goal of today's session is to develop an understanding of how to create a monthly budget. Teens will learn about how income, savings, and spending categories are used to create a budget and determine if it is balanced. They will get practice creating budgets with the goal of working towards creating their own budget at next week's session. We will also review how to build an effective system to help you and your teen achieve their DLS goals now and in the future.*
- *As we continue to build your teen's DLS, it may seem overwhelming to add in another goal. However, money management is the last goal we are adding to the DLS contract and there are ways to incorporate these money goals into your weekly schedule. For example:*
  - *Could the teen get an understanding of the family's budget by creating a monthly family budget?*
  - *Could the teen use a money diary to track their spending or the family's spending for the week?*
  - *Could the teen login to their checking or savings account to see the balance or when a purchase has been posted?*
  - *Could the teen set up a plan to save up money for purchases that they want to make using a savings contract?*

- Ask and Discuss: *Any questions?*

Review Dyad Session 12 Content (36 mins)

- *Now we will briefly review the material that will be covered in the upcoming dyad session with your teen. This will allow you to have some time to prepare for the upcoming session. Please feel free to ask any questions as we go over the content of the dyad session, which will focus on understanding how to make a budget. We will incorporate what we discuss today as a money goal on their DLS contract.*
- *Before we review the dyad session content, let's all briefly share your teen's experience with making a budget.*
- The therapist should have each caregiver briefly share their teen's experience and skill level with budgeting.
- The therapist should refer to the PowerPoint presentation slides for Dyad Session 12 while reviewing the content for the session.
- The therapist should have also prepared for the session by reviewing the Dyad Session 12 content discussed in the manual, which has detailed information about the content that will be covered.
- The important points to make while reviewing the Dyad Session 12 Content are:
  - We will do a Real World Practice Check-In, which will ask you and your teen specific questions about the goals on the DLS contract. This will be an opportunity to problem-solve any challenges and celebrate successes.
  - The elements of an effective system for achieving DLS goals will be reviewed with the teens as it relates to the goals on the DLS contract. This will be our

main opportunity each session to revise the goals that are currently being targeted on the DLS contract before we add in a new goal at the end of the session.
- The DLS Teaching Method will be used to teach various skills related to money management. For example, if an example budget is used to help the teen develop their own monthly budget for saving and spending, the caregiver will provide instruction and demonstrate how to use it before the teen starts practicing on their own.
- A budget is a written plan for your money that considers your income, expenses, and savings.
- There are six steps to developing a monthly budget, and there are budget examples and templates to help with following these steps.
- We will practice how to make a monthly budget using tools such as an example budget handout and the STRW Budgeting Workbook.
- We will review some tips for making sure that your budget is balanced.

♦ Ask: *Any questions about the content for the upcoming dyad session?*

Prep for the Next Caregiver Session (3 mins)

♦ *We will have our next caregiver group session on DAY and TIME. At this session, we will continue our sessions on money management and will talk in more detail about budgeting money. We will continue discussing how implementing the DLS contract went and discuss how to change or add a money management goal to your teen's DLS contract.*

♦ *After your dyad session with your teen, it will be important to prioritize working on the goals on the DLS contract and the Real World Practice assignment so that we can celebrate successes and also discuss any challenges or questions that arose in the caregiver group session.*

♦ Ask: *Are there any questions before we end the session?*

Wrap-Up

♦ The therapist should send a calendar invite with the next caregiver group session's day/time to the caregiver.

♦ The therapist may also want to email caregivers a blank copy of the DLS contract and can also email them the STRW Budgeting Workbook, which are both available on the STRW website.

Daily Living Skills Contract

Date ____________________

Goal	Expectations	Reward	MONDAY	TUESDAY	WEDNESDAY	THURSDAY	FRIDAY	SATURDAY	SUNDAY

____
Teen

____
Parent / Caregiver

Caregiver/Teen Dyad Session 12 Content (60 mins)

STRW Session 12 Schedule (1 min)

- The therapist should greet the caregiver and teen.
- *Let's get started! As a reminder, it will be helpful to sit together at a table so that we can all see each other and work together. Please pull out your STRW workbook that contains the handouts for all STRW sessions. This session is called Session 12 – Budgeting Money. Please turn to that section in your workbook.*
- *Let's go over the session schedule so that you know what we will be doing. Please feel free to ask any questions about our schedule!*
- Briefly go over each item on the Session Schedule.

Real World Practice Check-In: Contract and Morning Routine (3 mins)

- Refer to Session 11 Real World Practice handout and DLS Contract handout.
- *Let's check in on how you are doing with each goal on your DLS contract. Please be honest, as this is an opportunity to talk about what is working and what is not working and do some brainstorming to address any challenges.*
- As needed, the therapist should spend time modifying the DLS contract and problem solving how to make a more effective system to target the DLS goal (e.g., make expectations more specific, change reward, increase/decrease number of prompts, modify the strategies being used to help with goals).
- If the therapist used a fillable PDF of the DLS Contract handout in the previous session, it may be helpful to share this on the screen so that the goal, expectations, and reward can be easily discussed.
- The following questions should be asked (if applicable), and the responses and any relevant notes should be entered into the Real World Practice Tracking Sheet:
  - *Did you use your DLS contract this week?*
  - *Did you work on your morning routine goal during the week?*
    - *What went well?*
    - *What was challenging?*
    - *How many days did you work on your morning routine goal?*
    - *Did you earn a reward for your morning routine goal?*
    - *How many days did you earn a reward?*

Real World Practice Check-In: Cleaning the Bedroom and Laundry (3 mins)

- The following questions should be asked (if applicable), and the responses and any relevant notes should be entered into the Real World Practice Tracking Sheet:
  - *Did you work on your cleaning the bedroom goal during the week?*
    - *What went well?*
    - *What was challenging?*
    - *How many days did you work on your cleaning the bedroom goal?*
    - *Did you earn a reward for your cleaning the bedroom goal?*
  - *Did you work on your laundry goal during the week?*
    - *What went well?*
    - *What was challenging?*
    - *How many days did you work on your laundry goal?*
    - *Did you earn a reward for your laundry goal?*

Real World Practice Check-In: Cooking and Grocery Shopping (3 mins)

- The following questions should be asked (if applicable), and the responses and any relevant notes should be entered into the Real World Practice Tracking Sheet:
  - *Did you work on your cooking goal or goals during the week?*
    - *What went well?*
    - *What was challenging?*
    - *How many days did you work on your cooking goal or goals?*
    - *Did you earn a reward for your cooking goal or goals?*
  - *Did you work on a grocery shopping goal?*
    - *What went well?*
    - *What was challenging?*
    - *How many days did you work on your grocery shopping goal?*
    - *Did you earn a reward for working on your grocery shopping goal?*

Real World Practice Check-In: Money (2 mins)

- The following questions should be asked (if applicable), and the responses and any relevant notes should be entered into the Real World Practice Tracking Sheet:
  - *Did you work on a money goal or goals during the week?*
    - *What did you do?*
    - *What went well?*
    - *What was challenging?*
    - *How many days did you work on your money goal or goals?*
    - *Did you earn a reward for working on your money goal or goals?*

- Ask: *Any questions or comments about your Real World Practice assignments?*
- If the caregiver/teen dyad struggled to complete the Real World Practice assignments, the therapist should spend some time discussing how to identify days/times that they could designate to commit to working on the assignments.

- If the therapist used a fillable PDF of the DLS Contract handout in the previous session, it may be helpful to share this on the screen so that the goal, expectations, and reward can be easily discussed.

Elements of an Effective System for Achieving DLS Goals (2 mins)

- Ask: ***Are there any issues you want to discuss or troubleshoot related to the DLS contract?***
- Ask and Discuss: ***Are we considering all of the important elements to increase the likelihood of you achieving your DLS goals by developing the most effective system?***
- If applicable, discuss how to modify any DLS goals to address (1) qualities of the teen and their caregiver; (2) use of evidence-based strategies to teach and master DLS; and (3) ensuring that goals are obvious, attractive, easy, and satisfying.

Evidence-Based Strategy: DLS Teaching Method-Money Management (2 mins)

- Refer to DLS Teaching Method for Money Management handout (from Session 10).
- ***Today we will continue to use the DLS Teaching Method so that you can get hands-on instruction, modeling, and practice with your caregiver. We will learn how to make a monthly budget by learning, watching, and practicing during session today.***
- ***The skill of budgeting becomes very important as you get older and you need to make sure that your expenses are not more than the income you have coming in from a job.***

What Is a Budget? (3 mins)

- Ask and discuss the following questions with the teen and have the caregiver also discuss their experiences with making and sticking to a budget:
  - ***Have you ever had to make a budget?***
    - If YES: ***How did you make the budget?***
    - If YES: ***Was it easy or hard to stick to the budget?***
  - ***Have you ever talked to your caregiver about the household budget, such as how much is spent on groceries each month or the cost of bills such as water and electric?***

- Have caregiver and teen take turns reading the important components of a budget on the slide that include the following:
  - A budget is a written plan for your money that considers your Income, Expenses, and Savings
    - Income: Money that is earned (e.g., paycheck, allowance)
    - Savings: Money put into a savings account
    - Expenses: Money that is spent (e.g., rent, cell phone bill, water bill, clothing, entertainment, etc.)

- Ask and Discuss: ***Any questions or comments about a budget?***

Steps for Developing a Monthly Budget (5 mins)

- Refer to How to Develop a Monthly Budget handout.
- *We are going to review the steps for developing a monthly budget before we practice creating a budget together.*
- Have caregiver and teen take turns reading the six steps for developing a monthly budget.
- Ask and Discuss: *Any questions before we move on to practicing how to make a budget?*

Example Monthly Budget (5 mins)

- Refer to the Monthly Budget handout, the Example Monthly Budget handout, and the STRW Budgeting Workbook (i.e., Monthly Budget and Example Monthly Budget worksheets).
- Allow the caregiver and teen to choose whether they want to use the handouts or the STRW Budgeting Workbook. The therapist can also choose to use fillable PDFs of the handouts (i.e., Monthly Budget) or annotate directly on the slide. If the teen/caregiver want to use the STRW Budgeting Workbook, the therapist should share their screen and fill in the teen's responses.
- NOTE: If they have the ability to share their screen during the session, the caregiver and teen can also fill in the information for each activity in the STRW Budgeting Workbook if they have downloaded it. This would be a nice opportunity for the teen to get hands-on practice creating a budget with feedback and support from their caregiver and therapist.
- *Here is an example of a monthly budget. Let's review the income, savings, and expenses to determine what the teen's balance is. The balance is how much money you have after subtracting expenses and savings from your income.*
- Ask and discuss the following questions:
  - *Where is the teen's income coming from?*
  - *How much is the total monthly income?*
  - *How much is the teen saving in total?*
  - *What are the fixed expenses?*
  - *How much are the total fixed expenses?*
  - *What are the variable expenses?*
  - *How much are the total variable expenses?*
  - *What is the teen's balance after you subtract savings and expenses from their income?*
    - *The teen has a positive balance of $70 at the end of the month, which means that they have an extra $70 that they can save or spend. If you have a negative balance, it means your expenses and savings are greater than your income and you will have to redo your budget to make it work!*
- Ask: *Any questions about this example monthly budget?*

Sam's Monthly Budget (3 mins)

- Refer to Sam's Monthly Budget handout and/or the STRW Budgeting Workbook (i.e., Sam's Monthly Budget worksheet).
- ***Let's create a budget for Sam based on his income and expenses. We can either write down this information on the** Sam's Monthly Budget **handout or we can fill this out on the STRW Budgeting Workbook. One advantage to using the STRW Budgeting Workbook is that it is set up to add and subtract the numbers in a budget automatically.***
- Allow the caregiver and teen to choose whether they want to use the handouts or the STRW Budgeting Workbook. The therapist should then choose to use a fillable PDF of the handout, annotate directly on the slide, or share their computer screen and fill in the information directly in the STRW Budgeting Workbook. The caregiver and teen can also fill in the information directly in the STRW Budgeting Workbook.
- NOTE: It may be easiest to continue using the STRW Budgeting Workbook or the handouts, rather than switching back and forth between the two options.

Sam's Monthly Budget-Activity (5 mins)

- Refer to the Sam's Monthly Budget handout and/or the STRW Budgeting Workbook. The teen will need to read over the information on the Sam's Monthly Budget handout to answer the questions for this activity.
- The therapist should then choose to use a fillable PDF of the handout, annotate directly on the slide, or share their computer screen and fill in the information directly in the STRW Budgeting Workbook. The dyad can also fill in the information directly in the STRW Budgeting Workbook.
- The teen should respond to the following questions while completing this activity and can refer to the Sam's Monthly Budget handout as needed:
    - ***How much is Sam's total income?***
    - ***How much is Sam's total savings?***
    - ***How much are his total fixed expenses?***
    - ***How much are his total variable expenses?***
    - ***What is Sam's balance after subtracting savings and expenses from his income?***

Sam's Monthly Budget-Answer Key (1 min)

- Refer to the slide and/or the STRW Budgeting Workbook for the answer key.
- ***Here is the completed monthly budget for Sam that we just discussed.***
- Ask: ***Any questions about Sam's monthly budget?***

Budget Tips (3 mins)

- Refer to the Budget Tips handout.
- Have teen and caregiver take turns reading through the tips on the handout.
- Ask and discuss the following questions:
    - ***Any questions about these budgeting tips?***
    - ***Are there any other tips that you would like to add?***

Your Monthly Budget (5 mins)

- Refer to the Your Monthly Budget handout and/or the STRW Budgeting Workbook (i.e., Your Monthly Budget worksheet).
- The therapist should then choose to use a fillable PDF of the handout, annotate directly on the slide, or share their computer screen and fill in the information directly in the STRW Budgeting Workbook. The dyad can also fill in the information directly in the STRW Budgeting Workbook.
- NOTE: If the teen does not have any income or expenses, it may be helpful to think about what the teen's budget would be if they had a part-time job and had to take on specific expenses (e.g., gas in the car, purchasing movie tickets on the weekend, etc.). The goal is to increase the teen's understanding of how a monthly budget could apply to them. If the teen/caregiver appear to be overwhelmed, this activity can be skipped or could be completed as part of the Real World Practice Assignment (i.e., the teen and caregiver complete the Your Monthly Budget handout as the money goal on their DLS contract).
- *Now that you have gotten a lot of practice on developing a monthly budget, we want you to think through what your own monthly budget is based on your income, savings, and expenses. You can either write down this information on the Your Monthly Budget handout, or we can fill this out in the STRW Budgeting Workbook.*
- The caregiver and therapist should provide support as needed.

Elements of an Effective System for Achieving DLS Goals (3 mins)

- The therapist should briefly ask each teen about each of the elements and then incorporate the responses to the discussion on developing the DLS contract.
- *As we work to modify or keep working on the money goal to the DLS contract, let's make sure we are thinking about all of the following elements to build an effective system for achieving DLS goals:*
  - *Teen – are we considering your strengths, challenges, preferred learning style, and commitment?*
  - *Caregiver – are we considering your parenting style, time and effort, and commitment?*
  - *Are we using evidence-based strategies?*
    - *We are using the DLS Teaching Method to help you learn and become independent with managing your money.*
    - *We talked about how you could use tools such as an example budget to help you create a monthly or weekly budget. Tools such as a savings contract or money diary are also helpful when budgeting.*
  - *Is the money management goal obvious, attractive, easy, and satisfying?*
    - *Obvious – some ideas might be to post your budget as a reminder of your income and expenses.*
    - *Attractive – check your checking and savings accounts weekly to review your progress with staying on budget.*

  - *Easy – some ideas might be to choose a specific day and time to review how you are doing with sticking to your budget.*
  - *Satisfying – some ideas include to think about how building these skills now will help you to be more independent in the future.*

- Ask and Discuss: *Any questions or comments?*
- *Let's apply all of this information to creating your DLS contract!*

Developing Your DLS Contract (5 mins)

- Refer to the DLS Contract handout
- *Let's spend the remainder of our time in today's session modifying your DLS contract to continue working on your morning routine, cleaning your bedroom, laundry, cooking, and grocery shopping goals and modify or keep working on the goal of money management. This could include implementing a budget or you could continue working on your previous money goals. Use a blank copy of the DLS Contract. We will also keep in mind the importance of making sure the goal is Obvious, Attractive, Easy, and Satisfying so that you are more likely to achieve your goal. The DLS contract will have you track your progress and set up rewards for you to earn, which makes working on the goals satisfying!*
- The therapist should support the caregiver/teen dyad in creating the DLS contract by doing the following:
  - Incorporate all of the information from the last several sessions (e.g., rewards that are motivating for the teen, use of strategies and supports to build independence with certain steps) and the Real World Practice Check-In to create the DLS contract. The therapist should also consider the goals that the caregiver and teen collaboratively developed during the Preparing for STRW session.
  - Use the DLS Contract handout to specify the (1) Goal, (2) Expectations, and (3) Reward for Morning Routine, Cleaning the Bedroom, Doing Laundry, Cooking, Grocery Shopping, and Money.
  - Encourage the caregiver/teen dyad to work together and model appropriate and supportive coaching as they develop the DLS contract.

- Possible discussion questions that may be helpful to ask and discuss when creating the contract for the Morning Routine, Cleaning the Bedroom, Laundry, Cooking, Grocery Shopping, and Money goals include:
  - *How often are you going to need to do the goal – every day, every weekday, every other day, or once per week?*
  - *What steps of your goal do you need help with?*
  - *What steps do you not know how to do?*
  - *What steps are you doing independently?*
  - *How easy/hard do you think it will be to meet your goal?*
  - *What reward would you like to earn?*
  - *Does the reward fit the goal? For example, earning 1 hour of screen time for doing your morning routine goal each day is a lot, but maybe earning 15–20 extra minutes of screen time would be a better fit.*

- *How will you check in about your goals daily to discuss if the goal was met?*
- *Where can you post your DLS contract so that you can track goals daily and remember to get your reward if it was earned?*

- The caregiver and teen should write each goal, expectation, and reward on the DLS Contract handout. It may be helpful for the therapist to share their screen and add/modify the goals, expectations, and rewards on a fillable PDF of the DLS Contract handout. The therapist can then email it to the caregiver and teen after the session.
- When the DLS contract has been completed, encourage the dyad to sign it and post it somewhere where they can easily see it so that the goals may be tracked.

Real World Practice (1 min)

- Refer to the Real World Practice handout.
- Discuss the details of the Real World Practice assignment.
  - *Work on your morning routine, cleaning the bedroom, laundry, cooking, grocery shopping, and money goals for the remainder of the week using your DLS contract.*
    - *Set aside a specific time such as on the way to school or after dinner to discuss how the morning routine went and how to problem-solve the next day.*
    - *Schedule a day/time to work on watching and/or practicing how to clean your bedroom, do laundry, cook, and grocery shop.*
    - *Some ideas for adding or modifying the money goal on your DLS contract include (1) develop a monthly or weekly budget and stick to it; (2) develop a savings contract, or (3) use a money diary to keep track of your spending.*
    - *Make sure that if the teen earns the reward, they receive it immediately! This makes it more likely that they will continue to be motivated to meet their goal!*

- Ask: *Any questions about your Real World Practice assignment?*

Guess the Price (3 mins) – OPTIONAL

- NOTE: This activity can be skipped if there is not enough time to complete it.
- *Let's play a quick round of Guess the Price, which is just meant to be a fun way to build up your understanding of how much things cost.*
- *We are going to try something different and have both of you choose an item, and then the other person will guess the price of the item.*
- The therapist should collaborate with the teen and caregiver to provide ideas of possible items to guess the price for (e.g., laptop, video game, car insurance, college tuition, etc.). The therapist can also assist with looking up the price of the item.

- The therapist should click through the next two slides.
  - This activity is meant to be fun and engaging! If the teen is averse to playing the game, it can be skipped. However, it would be helpful for the caregiver and teen to find other ways to build up an understanding of what things cost (e.g., compare the cost of products at the store, involve the teen when purchasing cleaning items).

Preparing for the Next Dyad Session (1 min)

- *We will have our next caregiver/teen dyad session on DAY and TIME. At this session, we will practice budgeting for an event. We will need you to work together to come up with an event or activity that we could create a budget for.*
- *It will be important to complete your Real World Practice assignment before our next dyad session and come prepared to discuss it. We will spend a lot of time next session talking about how the DLS contract went!*
- Ask: *Are there any questions before we end the session?*

Wrap-Up

- The therapist should send a calendar invite with the next caregiver/teen dyad session's day/time to the caregiver and teen.
- The therapist may also want to send the caregiver/teen a copy of the DLS contract if they completed it using a fillable PDF.

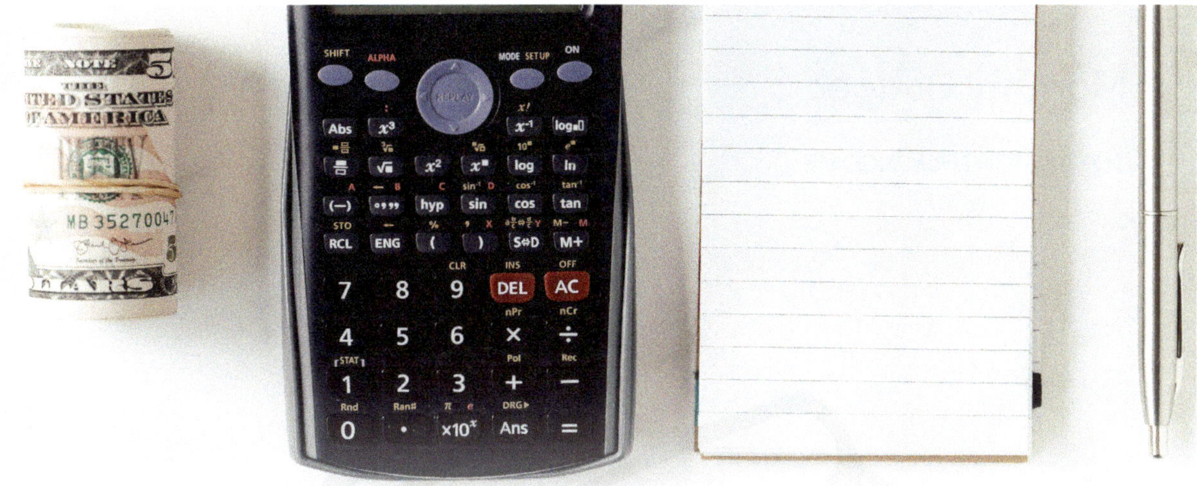

How to Develop a Monthly Budget

A budget is a written plan for your money that considers your Income, Expenses, and Savings. The following steps will help you develop a monthly budget:

1 Before you make a budget, it can be helpful to get an understanding of how much money you are spending. For example, you could use a money diary to track expenses.

2 Figure out your Income, which is how much money you are earning. Your income may depend on whether you have a job, whether you get an allowance, and if it is near your birthday or a holiday that you may get money or gifts for.

3 Determine how much money you want to put into Savings. Ideally, you should try to save a certain percentage of your money each month and you can use a savings contract to help you stick to your savings goals!

- A good rule of thumb is to deposit 20-50% of your income into a savings account that can be used for your savings goals (e.g., college, car, new laptop or video game) or emergency expenses (e.g., car repairs).

4 Deposit your remaining money into a checking account for Expenses, which can then be used to pay for:

- Fixed expenses – expenses that are consistent each week/month such as a cell phone bill, car payment, or rent
- Variable expenses – expenses that change each week/month such as going out to eat with friends and buying clothing

5 Do the math. Your Savings + Expenses should be less than or equal to your Income. Any money that is left is your Balance and can be used for other expenses or savings.

6 Adjust your budget and make changes as needed.

Monthly Budget

TOTAL MONTHLY INCOME ______________

TOTAL SAVINGS ______________

TOTAL FIXED EXPENSES ______________

TOTAL VARIABLE EXPENSES ______________

TOTAL MONTHLY EXPENSES (FIXED + VARIABLE) ______________

Income		Savings		Expenses		Balance
______	–	______	–	______	=	______

Example Monthly Budget

TOTAL MONTHLY INCOME $200

Allowance: $40

Job: $160

Other:

TOTAL SAVINGS $30

Savings: $20

Emergency Fund: $10

Other:

TOTAL FIXED EXPENSES $130

Guitar Class: $80

Car Insurance: $50

Other:

Other:

TOTAL VARIABLE EXPENSES $30

Eating Out: $20

Video Games: $10

Other:

Other:

Other:

TOTAL MONTHLY EXPENSES (FIXED + VARIABLE) $160

Income		Savings		Expenses		Balance
$200	−	$30	−	$160	=	$10

Sam's Monthly Budget

Sam needs help creating his monthly budget. Sam makes $120 from his part-time job bussing tables at a restaurant. He also gets a monthly allowance of $40 from his parents and also makes $40 each month by doing yardwork for his neighbors.

Sam wants to put 10% of his income in an emergency savings account. He also wants to put 10% of his income into a regular savings account.

He will put the remainder of his money into his checking account to pay for fixed expenses and variable expenses. As far as fixed expenses go, Sam sometimes buys his lunch at school ($40 per month) and is responsible for putting gas in the car he drives ($30 per month). Sam also has to pay $60 per month for the karate class he takes. He wants to budget $25 for entertainment (e.g., buying books, going to the movies, going to restaurants).

Total Monthly Income: _______

-
-
-

Total Savings: _______

-
-
-

Total Fixed Expenses: _______

-
-
-

Total Variable Expenses: _______

-
-

Total Monthly Expenses (Fixed + Variable): _______

Income	–	Savings	–	Expenses	=	Balance
_______		_______		_______		_______

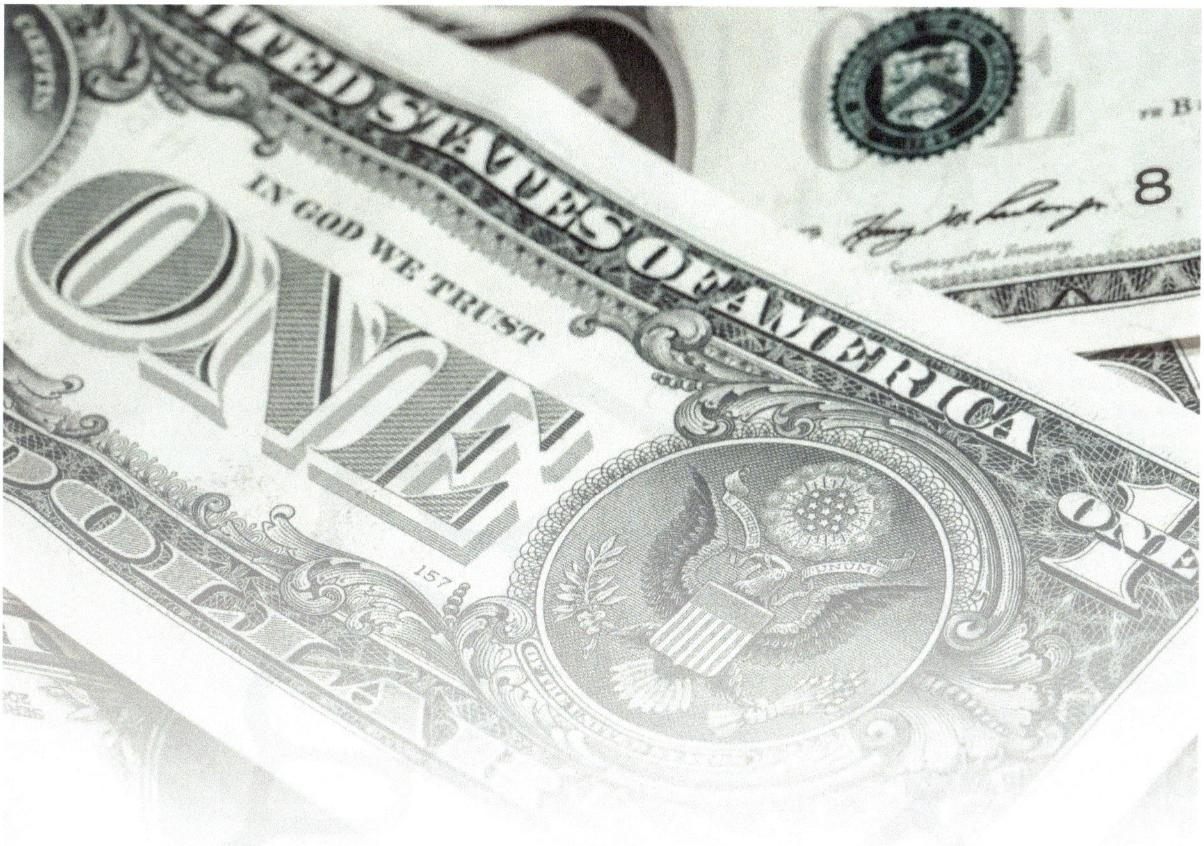

Budget Tips

- Don't panic if your budget does not balance (i.e., your savings and expenses are more than your income). You may have to revise your budget regularly depending on how income, expenses, and savings change over time!
- Revising your budget when you have MORE INCOME than EXPENSES and SAVINGS:
  - » Make sure you are listing all of your expenses accurately.
  - » Figure out if you can add more money to your savings.
  - » Determine if you want to add money to expenses (e.g., increase your clothing budget, purchase something you have been wanting to buy)
- Revising your budget when you have MORE EXPENSES and SAVINGS than INCOME:
  - » Examine where you might be able to cut back on expenses, such as buying fewer coffees at coffeeshops or spending less on music or video games.
  - » Figure out a way to increase your income.
- Using tools such as a savings contract and money diary can be helpful as you develop and revise your budget!

Monthly Budget

TOTAL MONTHLY INCOME ______________

TOTAL SAVINGS ______________

TOTAL FIXED EXPENSES ______________

TOTAL VARIABLE EXPENSES ______________

TOTAL MONTHLY EXPENSES (FIXED + VARIABLE) ______________

Income		Savings		Expenses		Balance
______	–	______	–	______	=	______

Surviving and Thriving in the Real World STRW.org

Daily Living Skills Contract

Date ____________________

Goal	Expectations	Reward	MONDAY	TUESDAY	WEDNESDAY	THURSDAY	FRIDAY	SATURDAY	SUNDAY

____________________ Teen

____________________ Parent / Caregiver

Surviving and Thriving in the Real World Session 12 – Real World Practice

- Work on your (1) morning routine, (2) cleaning the bedroom, (3) doing laundry, (4) cooking, (5) grocery shopping, and (6) money goals for the remainder of the week using your DLS contract.
  - Set aside a specific time (e.g., on the way to school, after dinner) to discuss how the morning routine went and how to problem-solve for the next day.
  - Schedule a day/time to work on watching and/or practicing how to clean the bedroom, do laundry, cook, go grocery shopping, and work on money management.
  - Some ideas for adding or modifying the money goal on your DLS contract include (1) develop a monthly or weekly budget and stick to it, (2) develop a savings contract, or (3) use a money diary to keep track of your spending.
  - Make sure that if a reward is earned, it is provided immediately!

Surviving & Thriving in the Real World

Session 13

Practicing Budgeting Money

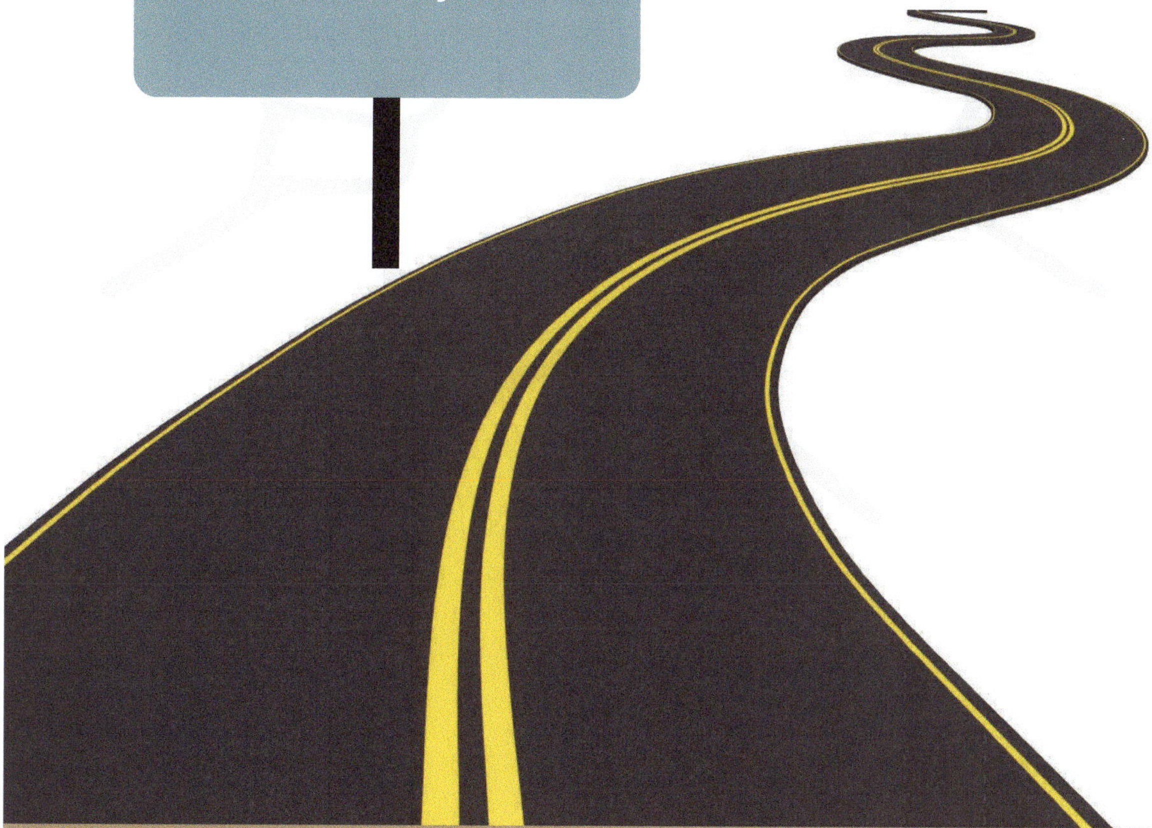

Session 13

Practicing Budgeting Money

Aims

- Continue to build rapport between caregiver group members and the therapist
- Continue to build rapport between the teen, caregiver, and therapist
- Further develop ability to use a DLS contract to set a DLS goal, define expectations, and identify a reward for meeting the goal
- Review the four elements for developing an effective system to achieve the teen's DLS goals
- Understand how to use the DLS Teaching Method to learn how to spend, save, and budget money
- Understand that a budget is a written plan for one's money that considers income, expenses, and savings
- Understand and practice the steps for developing a budget for an activity or event
- Practice applying knowledge about spending money in real-world situations
- Create and implement a DLS contract to target the goals of morning routine, cleaning the bedroom, doing laundry, cooking, grocery shopping, and money management

Structure

- Caregiver group session via telehealth
- Caregiver/teen dyad session via telehealth

Session Supplies

- Caregiver Group Handouts
  - DLS Contract

- Caregiver/Teen Dyad Handouts
  - DLS Teaching Method for Money Management (from Session 10)
  - Budgeting for an Activity
  - How Savvy Are Your Spending Skills?

DOI: 10.4324/9781003458838-16

  - DLS Contract
  - Session 13 – Real World Practice

- Other Supplies
  - STRW Budgeting Workbook (available on the STRW website)

Caregiver/Teen Preparation for Session

- The Caregiver and teen should have identified an activity that they can budget for in the dyad session. Examples of possible events or activities include the following: (1) a birthday party, (2) a graduation party, (3) a family vacation or trip, (4) going to a baseball game, (5) dinner and a movie with friends, and (6) planning and budgeting the ingredients for a family dinner. Ideally, the event or activity should be one that the caregiver and teen will actually do in the future.

Therapist Preparation for Session

- The therapist should use the Real World Practice Tracking Sheet for each caregiver/teen dyad in all subsequent STRW sessions to track progress on their DLS contract goals.
- The therapist should be familiar with using the STRW Budgeting Workbook for the budgeting activity in Session 13. The worksheets within the STRW Budgeting Workbook (i.e., Example Budgeting for an Activity and Budgeting for an Activity worksheets) directly correspond to the handouts discussed in the session. The therapist may want to email the caregiver a copy of the STRW Budgeting Workbook or refer them to the STRW website to download a copy to refer to or use during both the caregiver group session and dyad session. The therapist can also choose to use a fillable PDF of the handout (i.e., Budgeting for an Activity) or annotate directly on the slide.
- The therapist should consider reviewing the Tips for STRW Therapists: How to Facilitate Achievement of DLS Goals handout prior to each caregiver group session or dyad session for tips and strategies on how to help teens achieve the goals on their DLS contract. Tips that may be beneficial for Session 13 include:
  - *Encourage the caregiver to find an accountability partner after the STRW intervention ends.* Many caregivers have reported that meeting with the STRW therapist in both the caregiver group session and the dyad session provides a level of accountability that motivates them to "do the work" in supporting their teen to build their DLS. It can be beneficial to help the caregiver identify someone (e.g., spouse, partner, family member, friend, another STRW caregiver from the group session) that will check in with them (e.g., via text, email, or in person) as they move forward with targeting their teen's goals on the DLS contract.
  - *Identify the individual strategies that work best for a teen.* For many teens, there are likely four to five strategies that they can use over and over again to successfully meet their DLS goals. It is critical for therapists to assist with identifying successful strategies that can be used for current and future DLS goals. The therapist should regularly discuss what strategies work and do not work with the dyad.

Session 13 Notes

- Fillable PDFs of handouts from this session (i.e., DLS Contract, Budgeting for an Activity, How Savvy Are Your Spending Skills?) are available on the STRW website.
- Caregiver Group Session
  - The therapist should continue to devote the majority of the caregiver group session to reviewing how the DLS contract is progressing for each caregiver. This is an opportunity to identify any issues and brainstorm solutions prior to the dyad session.
  - The therapist should utilize the caregiver group session to get an understanding of how it may be necessary to personalize the dyad session content (e.g., the teen's experience with budgeting).
  - The therapist should make an active effort to foster collaboration between the group members by encouraging active discussion and problem solving of challenges or questions about the DLS contract.
  - The therapist should have caregivers discuss how they build their teen's money management skills on a regular basis and get ideas from other caregivers (e.g., involve teen in budgeting for birthday gifts, discuss ways that a caregiver tries to stay on budget with grocery shopping). Caregivers are likely doing various money management tasks daily or weekly, and it can be helpful to identify ways to include their teen in this process (e.g., involving teen in creating a budget for an upcoming trip).

- Dyad Session
  - Many caregivers and teens may be feeling overwhelmed by the goals on their DLS contract, so it may be beneficial to choose a money management goal that aligns with their other DLS contract goals (e.g., setting a budget for grocery shopping each month) or is something that the family or teen already does on a regular basis (e.g., review whether they are on track to stay on budget for specific monthly or weekly expenses).
  - In preparation for the final session, caregivers should be encouraged to think about any questions that they have about continuing to target DLS goals using the DLS contract after the STRW intervention ends.
  - The STRW Resources handout also has various resources related to money management that may be helpful for the caregivers and teens.
  - If the caregiver and teen are unable to come up with an actual event or activity to practice budgeting for, they can choose a hypothetical example (e.g., family night out, trip to a museum, graduation party, birthday party).
  - There are several options for completing the budget for an event or activity with the teen and caregiver. The STRW Budgeting Workbook contains the budget for planning an event or activity in Session 13. The therapist should download and use it in conjunction with the handout and slides. The therapist can share their computer screen and then directly enter information into the STRW Budgeting Workbook during the dyad session. Alternatively, the caregiver and teen can enter their responses on the STRW Budgeting Workbook instead of using the handouts. The therapist can email a copy of the STRW Budgeting Workbook, which is available on the STRW website, to caregivers and teens. As another

option, the caregiver and teen can write their responses down on the Budgeting for an Activity handout or the therapist can transcribe responses directly onto the slide or onto the fillable PDF of the handout.

- Therapists should either share their screen or have the dyad share their screen when looking up the cost of items for the activity (e.g., cost of food, cost of movie tickets, etc.). It is often easiest and most time-efficient to have the therapist enter the information in the STRW Budgeting Workbook while the caregiver/teen work together to look up the prices of items.
- When developing the DLS contract at the end of the caregiver/teen dyad session, the therapist should continue to incorporate all of the information and knowledge gained from the past several sessions (e.g., issues that were brought up during the caregiver group session, task analysis steps, discussing how to incorporate the essential elements of an effective system for achieving DLS goals, identifying appropriate rewards, etc.).
- The Guess the Price activity in the dyad session provides an opportunity for the caregiver and teen to choose an item that they want to either learn or guess the price for. For example, the teen could have their caregiver guess the price of a TV, and the caregiver could have their teen guess the price of a season pass to an amusement park.

Caregiver Group Session 13 Content (90 mins)

Review – Real World Practice Assignment (50 mins)

- The therapist should greet the caregivers and welcome them to the session.
- Discuss the Real World Practice assignment in detail by having all caregivers share how using the DLS contract to target the morning routine, cleaning the bedroom, laundry, cooking, grocery shopping, and money goals went with their teen. Encourage caregivers to jot down questions or notes on a blank copy of the DLS Contract handout that they may want to discuss or incorporate into their teen's contract at the next dyad session.
- ***We will have everyone share how using the DLS contract to target the morning routine, cleaning the bedroom, laundry, cooking, grocery shopping, and money goals went for their teen. This is an opportunity to celebrate successes and also problem-solve any challenges or obstacles that occurred. We will spend the majority of our session discussing each teen's progress with the DLS contract. It may be helpful to jot down questions or notes on a copy of the* DLS Contract *handout, and feel free to ask questions or add to the discussion.***
- It may be helpful to refer caregivers to the Tips for Creating a Successful DLS Contract handout (from Session 4) when discussing the goals on the DLS contract (e.g., clearly defining expectations, re-evaluating rewards regularly to ensure they are motivating, etc.).
- Points of discussion or questions to ask each caregiver include the following:
  - DLS contract
    - *Did the teen make progress at becoming more independent with each of their goals – morning routine, cleaning the bedroom, laundry, cooking, grocery shopping, and money?*
    - *What went well?*
    - *What was difficult?*
    - *Did they receive a reward?*
    - *Did they use any strategies to help them to learn the skill or become more independent?*
    - *Any obstacles or barriers?*
    - *Do you plan on modifying any goals on the current DLS contract?*

- Ask: *Any questions about the Real World Practice assignment?*

STRW Session 13 Goals (1 min)

- ***The goal of today's session is further develop your teen's understanding of how to budget by practicing how to budget for an activity. Your teen will get hands-on practice on setting a budget, identifying items needed for an activity, looking up*** *the cost of items, and determining whether one is under or over budget. We will also review how to build an effective system to help you and your teen achieve their DLS goals now and in the future.*

- *As we continue to build your teen's DLS, it may seem overwhelming to add in another goal. However, money management is the last goal we are adding to the DLS contract, and there are ways to incorporate these money goals into your weekly schedule. For example:*
  - *Could the teen help with budgeting for an upcoming family event or activity?*
  - *Could the teen help with budgeting for grocery shopping?*
  - *Could the teen get an understanding of the family's budget by creating a monthly family budget?*

- Ask and Discuss: *Any questions?*

Review Dyad Session 13 Content (36 mins)

- *Now we will briefly review the material that will be covered in the upcoming dyad session with your teen. This will allow you to have some time to prepare for the upcoming session. Please feel free to ask any questions as we go over the content of the dyad session, which focuses on making a budget for an activity. We will incorporate what we discuss today as a money goal on their DLS contract.*
- *Before we review the dyad session content, let's spend some time brainstorming what events or activities your teens could practice making a budget for. For example, some ideas include an upcoming family vacation, going to dinner and a movie, a graduation or birthday party, an outing to an amusement park or sporting event, getting take-out on the weekend for the family, or planning the ingredients for a dinner. Another idea might be making a budget for groceries for an entire week or month. Ideally, we just want your teen to get practice budgeting for an actual event or activity.*
- The therapist should have each caregiver briefly share their ideas for what activity/event their teen could budget for.
- The therapist should refer to the PowerPoint presentation slides for Dyad Session 13 while reviewing the content for the session.
- The therapist should have also prepared for the session by reviewing the Dyad Session 13 content discussed in the manual, which has detailed information about the content that will be covered.
- The important points to make while reviewing the Dyad Session 13 Content are:
  - We will do a Real World Practice Check-In, which will ask you and your teen specific questions about the goals on the DLS contract. This will be an opportunity to problem-solve any challenges and celebrate successes.
  - The elements of an effective system for achieving DLS goals will be reviewed with the teens as it relates to the goals on the DLS contract. This will be our main opportunity each session to revise the goals that are currently being targeted on the DLS contract before we add in a new goal at the end of the session.
  - The DLS Teaching Method will be used to teach various skills related to money management. For example, if an example budget is used to help the teen

develop their own monthly budget for saving and spending, the caregiver will provide instruction and demonstrate how to use it before the teen starts practicing on their own.
- Briefly review what a budget is and the steps for developing a budget.
- We will practice how to make a budget for an upcoming event or activity using tools such as an example budget handout and an Excel worksheet.
- We will practice applying what your teen has learned about spending money.

- Ask: *Any questions about the content for the upcoming dyad session?*

Prep for the Next Caregiver Session (3 mins)

- ***We will have our next caregiver group session on DAY and TIME. Please come to the session with any questions you have about continuing to work on DLS goals after STRW intervention has ended. We will continue discussing how implementing the DLS contract went and how to continue to use the DLS contract in the future.***
- ***After your dyad session with your teen, it will be important to prioritize working on the goals on the DLS contract and the Real World Practice assignment so that we can celebrate successes and also discuss any challenges or questions that arose in the caregiver group session.***
- Ask: ***Are there any questions before we end the session?***

Wrap-Up

- The therapist should send a calendar invite with the next caregiver group session's day/time to the caregiver.
- The therapist may also want to email caregivers a blank copy of the DLS contract and can also email them the STRW Budgeting Workbook, which are both available on the STRW website.

Daily Living Skills Contract

Date ______________________

Goal	Expectations	Reward	MONDAY	TUESDAY	WEDNESDAY	THURSDAY	FRIDAY	SATURDAY	SUNDAY

______________________ Teen

______________________ Parent / Caregiver

Caregiver/Teen Dyad Session 13 Content (60 mins)

STRW Session 13 Schedule (1 min)

- The therapist should greet the caregiver and teen.
- *Let's get started! As a reminder, it will be helpful to sit together at a table so that we can all see each other and work together. Please pull out your STRW workbook that contains the handouts for all STRW sessions. This session is called Session 13 – Practicing Budgeting Money. Please turn to that section in your workbook.*
- *Let's go over the session schedule so that you know what we will be doing. Please feel free to ask any questions about our schedule!*
- Briefly go over each item on the Session Schedule.

Real World Practice Check-In: Contract and Morning Routine (3 mins)

- Refer to the Session 12 Real World Practice handout and the DLS Contract handout.
- *Let's check in on how you are doing with each goal on your DLS contract. Please be honest, as this is an opportunity to talk about what is working and what is not working and do some brainstorming to address any challenges.*
- As needed, the therapist should spend time modifying the DLS contract and problem solving how to make a more effective system to target the DLS goal (e.g., make expectations more specific, change reward, increase/decrease number of prompts, modify the strategies being used to help with goals).
- If the therapist used a fillable PDF of the DLS Contract handout in the previous session, it may be helpful to share this on the screen so that the goal, expectations, and reward can be easily discussed.
- The following questions should be asked (if applicable), and the responses and any relevant notes should be entered into the Real World Practice Tracking Sheet:
  - *Did you use your DLS contract this week?*
  - *Did you work on your morning routine goal during the week?*
    - *What went well?*
    - *What was challenging?*
    - *How many days did you work on your morning routine goal?*
    - *Did you earn a reward for your morning routine goal?*
    - *How many days did you earn a reward?*

Real World Practice Check-In: Cleaning the Bedroom and Laundry (3 mins)

- The following questions should be asked (if applicable), and the responses and any relevant notes should be entered into the Real World Practice Tracking Sheet:

- *Did you work on your cleaning the bedroom goal during the week?*
  - *What went well?*
  - *What was challenging?*
  - *How many days did you work on your cleaning the bedroom goal?*
  - *Did you earn a reward for your cleaning the bedroom goal?*
- *Did you work on your laundry goal during the week?*
  - *What went well?*
  - *What was challenging?*
  - *How many days did you work on your laundry goal?*
  - *Did you earn a reward for your laundry goal?*

Real World Practice Check-In: Cooking and Grocery Shopping (3 mins)

- The following questions should be asked (if applicable), and the responses and any relevant notes should be entered into the Real World Practice Tracking Sheet:
  - *Did you work on your cooking goal or goals during the week?*
    - *What went well?*
    - *What was challenging?*
    - *How many days did you work on your cooking goal or goals?*
    - *Did you earn a reward for your cooking goal or goals?*
  - *Did you work on a grocery shopping goal?*
    - *What went well?*
    - *What was challenging?*
    - *How many days did you work on your grocery shopping goal?*
    - *Did you earn a reward for working on your grocery shopping goal?*

Real World Practice Check-In: Money (2 mins)

- The following questions should be asked (if applicable), and the responses and any relevant notes should be entered into the Real World Practice Tracking Sheet:
  - *Did you work on a money goal or goals during the week?*
    - *What did you do?*
    - *What went well?*
    - *What was challenging?*
    - *How many days did you work on your money goal or goals?*
    - *Did you earn a reward for working on your money goal or goals?*

- Ask: *Any questions or comments about your Real World Practice assignments?*
- If the caregiver/teen dyad struggled to complete the Real World Practice assignments, the therapist should spend some time discussing how to identify days/times that they could designate to commit to working on the assignments.

Elements of an Effective System for Achieving DLS Goals (2 mins)

- Ask: *Are there any issues you want to discuss or troubleshoot related to the DLS contract?*
- Ask and Discuss: *Are we considering all of the important elements to increase the likelihood of you achieving your DLS goals by developing the most effective system?*
- If applicable, discuss how to modify any DLS goals to address (1) qualities of the teen and their caregiver; (2) use of evidence-based strategies to teach and master DLS; and (3) ensuring that goals are obvious, attractive, easy, and satisfying.

Evidence-Based Strategy: DLS Teaching Method-Money Management (2 mins)

- Refer to the DLS Teaching Method for Money Management handout (from Session 10).
- *Today we will continue to use the DLS Teaching Method so that you can get hands-on instruction, modeling, and practice with your caregiver. We will learn how to make a budget when planning an activity by learning, watching, and practicing today.*
- *As you get older, it will be important to understand and plan for the cost of planning activities such as having friends over, going to a baseball game, going on a weekend trip to visit a college, or going on a family vacation.*

Budget Review (1 min)

- *As we discussed at the last session, a budget is a written plan for your money that considers your income, expenses, and savings. Last session, we also went through the steps for creating a monthly budget that involve figuring out your income and expenses.*
- Ask and Discuss: *Any questions about a budget?*

Example Budget for a Birthday Party (3 mins)

- Refer to the Budgeting for an Activity handout and/or the STRW Budgeting Workbook (i.e., Example Budgeting for an Activity and Budgeting for an Activity worksheets).
- Allow the caregiver and teen to choose whether they want to use the handout or the STRW Budgeting Workbook. It may be easiest to continue using the STRW Budgeting Workbook or the handout, rather than switching back and forth between the two options.
- *As you can see, this is an example of a budget that was created for a teen's birthday party. The following sections were completed to determine whether the teen was staying on budget for their birthday party.*
  - *Description: This section specifies what the activity is and may include details such as number of people attending, location, and supplies needed.*

- ***Budget:*** ***This section indicates the total budget for the event or activity.***
- ***Expenses: This section lists out each item, the cost, quantity, and total cost. All expenses need to be listed and it is possible you may need to make a good estimate if you are not sure of the actual cost of an item.***
- ***Balance: This section subtracts the total cost of expenses from the total budget. You will be able to determine if you are over budget or under budget. You may need to adjust your budget after determining if you are over or under budget.***
- ***We will be using this format to plan and budget for the event or activity that you have chosen.***

♦ Ask and Discuss: ***Any questions before we move on to practicing how to make a budget for an event or activity?***

Practicing Budgeting for an Activity (15 mins)

♦ Refer to the Budgeting for an Activity handout and/or the Budgeting for an Activity worksheet in the STRW Budgeting Workbook.
♦ Allow the caregiver and teen to choose whether they want to use the handout or the STRW Budgeting Workbook.
♦ ***We are now going to practice the skill of making a budget by having you choose an event or activity you would like to budget for. We will complete the categories for description of the activity, budget, expenses, and balance on the handout or workbook. We can look up the cost of items as we complete the budget.***
♦ Using an activity of the teen's choosing, practice budgeting by identifying the total budget, cost of items, and the balance to determine if the teen is over or under budget for the activity. The therapist should encourage the teen to take the lead on this and the caregiver and therapist should provide coaching and support as needed.
♦ If the cost of items needs to be looked up (e.g., the price of movie tickets, the price of food items), the therapist can share their computer screen, have the caregiver/teen dyad share their computer screen, or have the caregiver/teen dyad use their phone/computer to look up the cost of items.
♦ The therapist could share their computer screen and fill in the information directly in the Budgeting for an Activity worksheet in the STRW Budgeting Workbook. The caregiver and teen could also write their responses down on the Budgeting for an Activity handout or the therapist can transcribe responses directly onto the slide or onto the fillable PDF of the handout. Alternatively, the caregiver and teen could also fill in the information directly in the STRW Budgeting Workbook.

How Savvy Are Your Spending Skills? (12 mins)

♦ Refer to the STRW Savvy Spending handout.
♦ ***We are going to through a few hypothetical scenarios to see how savvy you are at knowing how to (1) use cash to purchase items – including making sure you give the right amount of money and then also get the correct amount of change, (2) use a debit card to purchase items, and (3) use a credit card to purchase items.***

- The therapist should do the following for the next six slides:
  - Have the teen read each scenario aloud before providing an answer.
  - For each spending scenario, the therapist can either have the teen answer the questions verbally, record their responses on the fillable PDF of the handout, or annotate the teen's responses directly on to the slides while sharing their computer screen.
  - Provide support and answer questions, but the teen should be encouraged to work out the answers to the purchasing scenarios. The therapist may need to coach caregivers on how to provide the optimal level of support.
  - Encourage the teen to use a calculator on their phone because this is something that they could use while making a purchase at a store. The therapist can also use the calculator on their computer to demonstrate how to arrive at the correct answer.
  - The therapist can also modify these scenarios as needed to individualize the content for the teen.

Elements of an Effective System for Achieving DLS Goals (3 mins)

- The therapist should briefly ask each teen about each of the elements and then incorporate the responses to the discussion on developing the DLS contract.
- *As we work to modify or keep working on the money goal to the DLS contract, let's make sure we are thinking about all of the following elements to build an effective system for achieving DLS goals:*
  - *Teen – are we considering your strengths, challenges, preferred learning style, and commitment?*
  - *Caregiver – are we considering your parenting style, time and effort, and commitment?*
  - *Are we using evidence-based strategies?*
    - *We are using the DLS Teaching Method to help you learn and become independent with managing your money.*
    - *We talked about how you could use tools such as an example budget to help you create a budget for an event or activity. Tools such as a savings contract or money diary are also helpful when budgeting.*
  - *Is the money management goal obvious, attractive, easy, and satisfying?*
    - *Obvious – some ideas might be to post your budget as a reminder of your income and expenses.*
    - *Attractive – check your checking and savings accounts weekly to review your progress with staying on budget.*
    - *Easy – some ideas might be to choose a specific day and time to review how you are doing with sticking to your budget.*
    - *Satisfying – some ideas include to think about how building these skills now will help you to be more independent in the future.*

- Ask and Discuss: *Any questions or comments?*
- *Let's apply all of this information to creating your DLS contract!*

Developing Your DLS Contract (5 mins)

- Refer to the DLS Contract handout
- ***Let's spend the remainder of our time in today's session modifying your DLS contract to continue working on your morning routine, cleaning your bedroom, laundry, cooking, and grocery shopping goals and modify or keeping working on the goal of money management. This could be creating a monthly budget, developing a budget for an upcoming activity, or continuing to use a money diary to track what you are spending on your own or what your family spends over the course of a week. Use a blank copy of the DLS Contract. We will also keep in mind the importance of making sure the goal is Obvious, Attractive, Easy, and Satisfying so that you are more likely to achieve your goal. The DLS contract will have you track your progress and set up rewards for you to earn, which makes working on the goals satisfying!***
- The therapist should support the caregiver/teen dyad in creating the DLS contract by doing the following:
    - Incorporate all of the information from the last several sessions (e.g., rewards that are motivating for the teen, use of strategies and supports to build independence with certain steps) and the Real World Practice Check-In to create the DLS contract. The therapist should also consider the goals that the caregiver and teen collaboratively developed during the Preparing for STRW session.
    - Use the DLS Contract handout to specify the (1) Goal, (2) Expectations, and (3) Reward for Morning Routine, Cleaning the Bedroom, Doing Laundry, Cooking, Grocery Shopping, and Money.
    - Encourage the caregiver/teen dyad to work together and model appropriate and supportive coaching as they develop the DLS contract.

- Possible discussion questions that may be helpful to ask and discuss when creating the contract for the Morning Routine, Cleaning the Bedroom, Laundry, Cooking, Grocery Shopping, and Money goals include:
    - ***How often are you going to need to do the goal – every day, every weekday, every other day, or once per week?***
    - ***What steps of your goal do you need help with?***
    - ***What steps do you not know how to do?***
    - ***What steps are you doing independently?***
    - ***How easy/hard do you think it will be to meet your goal?***
    - ***What reward would you like to earn?***
    - ***Does the reward fit the goal? For example, earning 1 hour of screen time for doing your morning routine goal each day is a lot, but maybe earning 15–20 extra minutes of screen time would be a better fit.***
    - ***How will you check in about your goals daily to discuss if the goal was met?***
    - ***Where can you post your DLS contract so that you can track goals daily and remember to get your reward if it was earned?***

- The caregiver and teen should write each goal, expectation, and reward on the DLS Contract handout. It may be helpful for the therapist to share their screen and add/modify the goals, expectations, and rewards on a fillable PDF of the DLS Contract handout. The therapist can then email it to the caregiver and teen after the session.

- When the DLS contract has been completed, encourage the dyad to sign it and post it somewhere where they can easily see it so that the goals may be tracked.

Real World Practice (1 min)

- Refer to the Real World Practice handout.
- Discuss the details of the Real World Practice assignment.
    - *Work on your morning routine, cleaning the bedroom, laundry, cooking, grocery shopping, and money goals for the remainder of the week using your DLS contract.*
        - *Set aside a specific time such as on the way to school or after dinner to discuss how the morning routine went and how to problem-solve the next day.*
        - *Schedule a day/time to work on watching and/or practicing how to clean your bedroom, do laundry, cook, and grocery shop.*
        - *Some ideas for adding or modifying the money goal on your DLS contract include (1) develop a monthly or weekly budget and stick to it, (2) develop a budget for an upcoming activity or event, (3) develop a savings contract, or (4) use a money diary to keep track of your spending for an entire week.*
        - *Make sure that if the teen earns the reward, they receive it immediately! This makes it more likely that they will continue to be motivated to meet their goal!*
- Ask: *Any questions about your Real World Practice assignment?*

Guess the Price (3 mins) – OPTIONAL

- NOTE: This activity can be skipped if there is not enough time to complete it.
- *Let's play a quick round of Guess the Price, which is just meant to be a fun way to build up your understanding of how much things cost.*
- *We are going to try something different and have both of you choose an item and then the other person will guess the price of the item.*
- The therapist should collaborate with the teen and caregiver to provide ideas of possible items to guess the price for (e.g., laptop, video game, car insurance, college tuition, etc.). The therapist can also assist with looking up the price of the item.
- The therapist should click through the next two slides.
    - This activity is meant to be fun and engaging! If the teen is averse to playing the game, it can be skipped. However, it would be helpful for the caregiver and teen to find other ways to build up an understanding of what things cost (e.g., compare the cost of products at the store, involve the teen when purchasing cleaning items).

Preparing for the Next Dyad Session (1 min)

- *We will have our last caregiver/teen dyad session on DAY and TIME. At this session, we will celebrate your successes over the last few months and also talk about next steps for your DLS goals.*
- *It will be important to complete your Real World Practice assignment before our next dyad session and come prepared to discuss it. We will spend a lot of time next session talking about how the DLS contract went and planning for the future!*
- Ask: *Are there any questions before we end the session?*

Wrap-Up

- The therapist should send a calendar invite with the next caregiver/teen dyad session's day/time to the caregiver and teen. The therapist may also want to send the caregiver/teen a copy of the DLS contract if they completed it using a fillable PDF.

Daily Living Skills Contract

Date ______________________

Goal	Expectations	Reward	MONDAY	TUESDAY	WEDNESDAY	THURSDAY	FRIDAY	SATURDAY	SUNDAY

______________________ Teen

______________________ Parent / Caregiver

Surviving and Thriving in the Real World
Session 13 – Real World Practice

- Work on your (1) morning routine, (2) cleaning the bedroom, (3) doing laundry, (4) cooking, (5) grocery shopping, and (6) money goals for the remainder of the week using your DLS contract.
  - Set aside a specific time (e.g., on the way to school, after dinner) to discuss how the morning routine went and how to problem-solve for the next day.
  - Schedule a day/time to work on watching and/or practicing how to clean the bedroom, do laundry, cook, go grocery shopping, and work on money management.
  - Some ideas for adding or modifying the money goal on your DLS contract include (1) develop a monthly or weekly budget and stick to it, (2) develop a budget for an upcoming activity or event, (3) develop a savings contract, or (4) use a money diary to keep track of your spending for an entire week.
  - Make sure that if a reward is earned, it is provided immediately!

Surviving & Thriving in the Real World

Session 14

Graduation

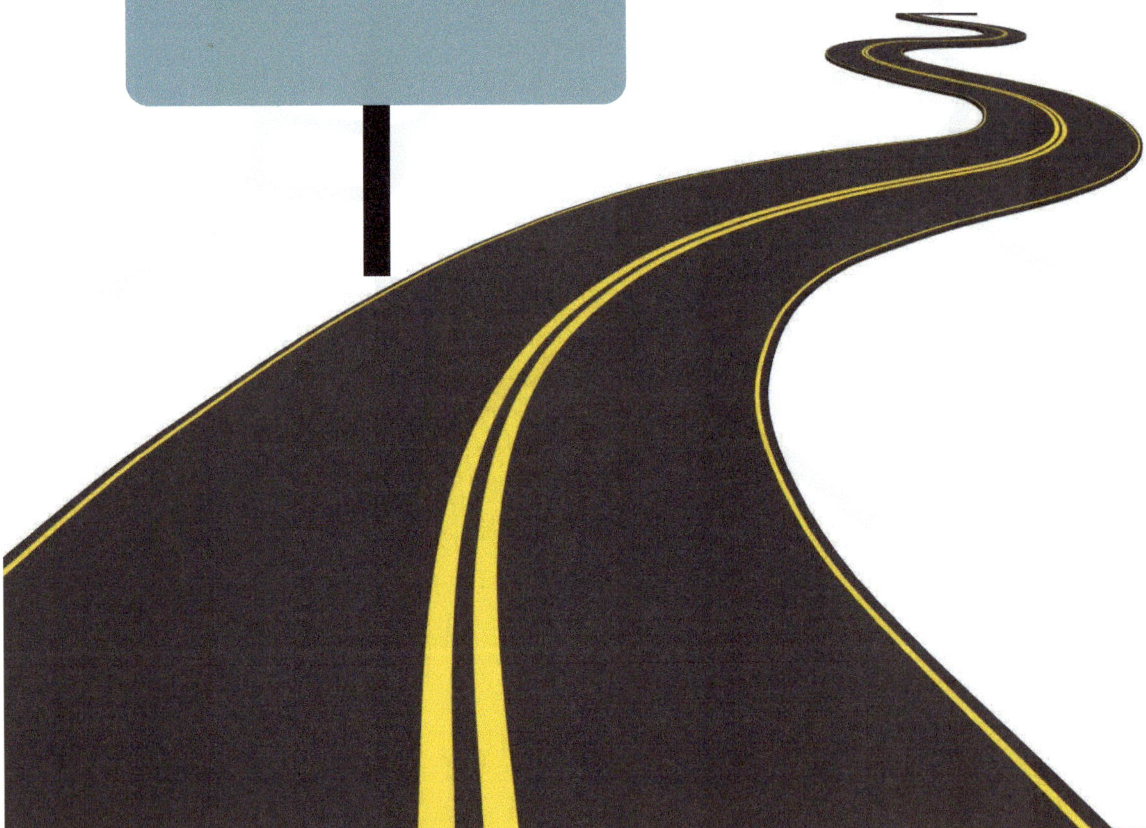

Session 14

Graduation

Aims

- Further develop ability to use a DLS contract to set a DLS goal, define expectations, and identify a reward for meeting the goal
- Review the four elements for developing an effective system to achieve the teen's DLS goals
- Discuss how to continue to target DLS goals by using a DLS contract
- Discuss how to fade rewards for goals that are being targeted on the DLS contract
- Review the progress that teens made on their individualized DLS goals
- Celebrate the successes of both the teen and their caregiver as they worked towards achieving the teen's individualized DLS goals over the last 15 weeks
- Identify future DLS to learn, practice, and master
- Create and implement a DLS contract to target the goals of morning routine, cleaning the bedroom, doing laundry, cooking, grocery shopping, and money management

Structure

- Caregiver group session via telehealth
- Caregiver/teen dyad session via telehealth

Session Supplies

- Caregiver Group Handouts
  - Moving Forward After STRW
  - DLS Contract
  - Individualized DLS Goals (from the Preparing for STRW Session)
  - STRW Resources (from Session 1)

- Caregiver/Teen Dyad Handouts
  - Future Daily Living Skills Goals
  - DLS Contract

DOI: 10.4324/9781003458838-17

- ❍ Session 14 – Real World Practice
- ❍ Individualized DLS Goals (from the Preparing for STRW Session)

Caregiver/Teen Preparation for Session

- ♦ None.

Therapist Preparation for Session

- ♦ The therapist may want to review the Strategies Commonly Used to Target Goals on the DLS Contract handout (see appendix), which includes the evidence-based strategies, supports, and tools that teens utilize as they work on their DLS goals of morning routine, cleaning the bedroom, laundry, cooking, grocery shopping, and money management. It may be beneficial for therapists to review these prior to facilitating these sessions and developing the DLS contract with the caregiver/teen dyads.
- ♦ The therapist should use the Real World Practice Tracking Sheet for each caregiver/teen dyad in the current STRW session to track progress on their DLS contract goals.
- ♦ The therapist can choose to administer a DLS assessment to the caregiver and teen prior to Session 14 to get an understanding of the progress that they have made and to assist with developing future DLS goals in Session 14. It would be most beneficial to use the same DLS assessment that was discussed in the Preparing for STRW session with the caregiver and teen.
- ♦ The therapist should prepare for the dyad session by identifying some of the specific successes of the teen in building their DLS that can be discussed at the end of the session. The therapist can also share favorite stories or funny memories.
- ♦ The therapist should individualize the STRW Graduation Certificate in the dyad session (final slide) with the teen's name and/or also email and/or send them a copy of the STRW Graduation Certificate (see "Therapist Resources" in the manual and also the STRW website).
- ♦ The therapist should consider reviewing the Tips for STRW Therapists: How to Facilitate Achievement of DLS Goals handout prior to the caregiver group session or dyad session for tips and strategies on how to help teens achieve the goals on their DLS contract.

Session 14 Notes

- ♦ Fillable PDFs of handouts from this session (i.e., DLS Contract, Future DLS Goals) are available on the STRW website.

- ♦ Caregiver Group
  - The therapist should continue to devote a large portion of the caregiver group session to reviewing how the DLS contract is progressing for each caregiver. This is the final opportunity to identify any issues and brainstorm solutions prior to the dyad session.

- The therapist should plan on spending a large portion of the caregiver group session discussing how to move forward after the STRW intervention. Caregivers often have specific questions related to identifying future DLS goals, continuing to use the DLS contract, and fading back rewards. A thorough discussion will likely be beneficial to all caregivers, and it can be helpful to brainstorm ideas for the questions or issues that the caregivers bring up.
- The therapist should make an active effort to foster collaboration between the group members by encouraging active discussion and problem solving of challenges or questions about the DLS contract.
- The STRW Resources handout also has various resources related to DLS (e.g., articles, books, resources for building specific DLS using evidence-based strategies) and it may be helpful for the therapist to briefly go over some of these resources in the caregiver group session.

♦ Dyad Session
- The therapist should be encouraging and positive throughout the caregiver/teen dyad session as the teen's progress towards their DLS goals are discussed in detail. The therapist should also encourage collaboration as the caregiver and teen work together to identify future DLS goals to target using the DLS contract.
- When developing the DLS contract at the end of the caregiver/teen dyad session, the therapist should continue to incorporate all of the information and knowledge gained from the past several sessions (e.g., issues that were brought up during the caregiver group session, task analysis steps, discussing how to incorporate the essential elements of an effective system for achieving DLS goals, identifying appropriate rewards, etc.).

Caregiver Group Session 14 Content (90 mins)

Review – Real World Practice Assignment (30 mins)

- The therapist should greet the caregivers and welcome them to the session.
- Discuss the Real World Practice assignment in detail by having all caregivers share how using the DLS contract to target the morning routine, cleaning the bedroom, laundry, cooking, grocery shopping, and money goals went with their teen. Encourage caregivers to jot down questions or notes on a blank copy of the DLS Contract handout that they may want to discuss or incorporate into their teen's contract at the next dyad session.
- ***We will have everyone share how using the DLS contract to target the morning routine, cleaning the bedroom, laundry, cooking, grocery shopping, and money goals went for their teen. This is our final opportunity to celebrate successes together and also problem-solve any challenges or obstacles that occurred. It may be helpful to jot down questions or notes on a copy of the DLS Contract handout, and feel free to ask questions or add to the discussion.***
- It may be helpful to refer caregivers to the Tips for Creating a Successful DLS Contract handout (from Session 4) when discussing the goals on the DLS contract (e.g., clearly defining expectations, re-evaluating rewards regularly to ensure they are motivating, etc.).
- Points of discussion or questions to ask each caregiver include the following:
  - DLS contract
    - ***Did the teen make progress at becoming more independent with each of their goals – morning routine, cleaning the bedroom, laundry, cooking, grocery shopping, and money?***
    - ***What went well?***
    - ***What was difficult?***
    - ***Did they receive a reward?***
    - ***Did they use any strategies to help them to learn the skill or become more independent?***
    - ***Any obstacles or barriers?***
    - ***Do you plan on modifying any goals on the current DLS contract?***

- Ask: ***Any questions about the Real World Practice assignment?***

STRW Session 14 Goals (1 min)

- ***The goal of today's session is to discuss how to continue to build your teen's age-appropriate DLS after the STRW intervention is over. You have all of the tools*** *needed to support your teen as they work on learning, practicing, and mastering the DLS needed for adulthood. We will also discuss the final dyad session in which we will celebrate your teen's progress and gains over the last 15 weeks and identify possible DLS goals to work on over the next several months. Last, we will review how to build an effective system to help you and your teen achieve their DLS goals now and in the future.*

- Ask and Discuss: *Any questions?*

Moving Forward After STRW: Continue to Use the DLS Contract (15 mins)

- Refer to the Moving Forward After STRW handout.
- *Let's spend some time discussing how to continue to work on current DLS goals and add in new DLS goals when you are no longer attending weekly STRW sessions. Before we start, we want to emphasize that you truly have all of the tools that you need to continue working with your teen on building daily living skills!*
- *Let's go over three specific recommendations that have been found to be successful for families after completing STRW. Please feel free to ask questions throughout, and we will make sure to save some time after we review these recommendations for any additional questions or comments.*
- *The first recommendation is to continue to use the DLS contract. This is a highly effective strategy that will keep both you and your teen accountable for working on both current and new DLS goals and making sure previously targeted DLS goals continue to be maintained and mastered.*
- *An easy way to continue to make sure you are using the DLS contract is to have weekly check-ins that will allow you to:*
    - *Discuss overall progress with DLS goals*
    - *Discuss any obstacles and brainstorm how to address these obstacles or challenges*
    - *Discuss whether specific evidence-based strategies need to be added or changed to increase the likelihood of meeting a DLS goal*
    - *Discuss whether rewards need to be changed*
    - *Celebrate the successes*

- *It can be particularly helpful to have weekly check-ins at the same day/time as the dyad sessions were held and to schedule these in your calendar so that you remember to do this. It can also be helpful to post the DLS contract where you and your teen can see it.*
- *Another tip is to have an accountability partner who will check in with you as you work towards continuing to use the DLS contract to target your teen's DLS. This could be another caregiver from this group, a partner or spouse, or a family member or friend.*
- Ask and discuss: *What questions do you have about continuing to use the DLS contract?*

Moving Forward After STRW: Identify and Add New Goal(s) to the DLS Contract (15 mins)

- *The second recommendation is to identify and add a new goal or goals to the DLS contract as needed. We are going to identify some specific DLS that you and your teen may want to work on over the next year, and these are likely the goals that you would eventually want to add in to the DLS contract.*
- *If you and your teen would like to add a new goal to the DLS contract, think about the following things to ensure you and your teen are ready to do this:*
    - *Has the teen mastered some or all of the goals on their DLS contract?*
        - *A goal is mastered when it is done the majority of the time without any help or reminders from caregivers. For example, the morning routine goal is likely mastered if the teen is doing all of the steps on Monday through Friday with only an occasional reminder from you.*
        - *Depending on the frequency of the DLS, it could take weeks or months for a DLS to be mastered. For example, it may take longer to master the goal of laundry because it may only be done once per week as opposed to the morning routine goal that is done multiple times per week.*
        - *Mastery also depends on the complexity and difficulty of the DLS goal. For example, while the morning routine goal is done multiple times per week, it does consist of many steps, so it may actually take several months for teens to master this DLS.*
    - *Does the teen have the necessary evidence-based strategies and supports in place for their current DLS goals? If specific strategies are working, these will likely be the ones that you use when adding in any new goals to the DLS contract. For example, if a task analysis was a successful strategy for meeting the DLS goals of doing laundry and cleaning one's bedroom, it could be used to teach the teen how to clean a bathroom.*
    - *Do the caregiver and teen have the time and energy to commit to working on another goal on the DLS contract? It can take time to learn, practice, and then work on mastering a DLS so it is important to ask this question before adding in a new goal.*

- *Once you and your teen have decided you are ready to add a new goal to the DLS contract, you should work with your teen to identify the new DLS to target by thinking through the following questions:*
    - *What DLS would be beneficial right now?*
        - *It can be helpful to identify chores that will build on the teen's independence or autonomy. For example, it may be helpful to learn to use a checking account because the teen is getting a job over the summer.*
    - *What DLS would be beneficial for their goals in the next 6–12 months?*
        - *Teens may be more motivated to work on DLS that are relevant to their life and need to be done in adulthood. For example, the teen may need to learn how to budget money and navigate a college campus before they start college.*

- *What DLS have they almost mastered? These are DLS that may require some prompting or support, but they may be easier to master than a new skill. Teens may be more motivated if you work up from the least amount of effort to the most amount of effort.*
  - *For example, if they can clean the sink in the bathroom, it may be a good idea to teach the teen how to clean the other parts of a bathroom such as the toilet, shower, or bathtub.*
- *What DLS would decrease arguing or stress between the caregiver and teen?*
  - *These are often skills such as the afternoon routine or nighttime routine that may lead to arguments or frustration between the caregiver and teen. Thus, it may be beneficial to tackle having the teen become independent in these routines in the same way that the morning routine was targeted.*
- *What DLS would the teen be most motivated to work on?*
  - *If the teen enjoys cooking, it may be a good idea to target making meals for the family or planning meals for the week.*
  - *It can also be helpful to make some DLS part of the entire family's routine and set aside time to do it together. For example, everyone pitches in to clean up after dinner or everyone cleans a room on Sunday afternoon.*

- *By thinking through the previous questions, you are more likely to get increased buy-in and commitment from both you and your teen.*
- Ask: *What questions do you have about identifying new goals to add to the DLS contract?*

Moving Forward After STRW: Fading Rewards (16 mins)

- *An area that can be challenging for caregivers is fading rewards once a DLS is mastered. It is important to note that you should not remove or decrease rewards until a teen has truly mastered a DLS goal.*
- Ask and Discuss:
  - *For those of you who have faded rewards, how did you know it was the right time to do this?*
  - *How did you have this conversation with your teen?*

- *Rewards are often faded somewhat naturally. Many of us likely rewarded our children for skills such as learning how to use the toilet, but we no longer reward them and it is likely not something we thought about when we faded the rewards. As our child mastered the skill of using the toilet and became increasingly independent, they no longer needed a reward. It can be helpful to discuss how becoming more independent and skilled in DLS will allow your teen to become more independent and meet their goals as an adult.*
- *Let's talk through the steps of fading rewards. I will go through all of the steps and feel free to ask questions throughout.*

- *Schedule a specific time to have a conversation about their DLS goals and rewards. For example, you could discuss this during the weekly check-in about the DLS contract.*
- *Remain calm and neutral during the discussion with your teen. Emphasize that it is a big deal that they have mastered a DLS, and that they now have several strategies that can help them learn other DLS!*
- *Allow the teen to ask questions – especially if this is the first time a reward has been faded!*
- *Discuss the progress that the teen has made with their DLS goal and how this relates to their future goals in adulthood such as working, going to college, and living on their own.*
- *State that they seem like they are now ready to start doing DLS on their own without earning a reward.*
- *Discuss that it is still expected that teen do the DLS even though they are not being rewarded.*
  - *Provide examples of other DLS the teen does without being rewarded such as doing homework, feeding the dog, taking vitamins, or making a snack for themselves. Also provide examples of DLS that the caregiver does without being rewarded such as cooking meals, paying bills, mopping the floor, and cutting the grass.*
  - *Discuss that as they get older and become more independent, teens will be expected to do things that they do not receive a reward for. Examples include cleaning their dorm room at college, washing the uniform that they wear to work, and making dinner for themselves.*
- *Encourage teens to use self-rewards when they complete a DLS. Self-rewards are a way to stay motivated by rewarding oneself for making progress towards or achieving a goal. Examples of self-rewards are watching a TV show after cleaning their room, taking a nap after finishing laundry, or having a dessert after doing the dishes.*
- *Discuss how to make sure the teen continues to be successful with mastered DLS they are not being rewarded for. For example, they could continue to use the strategies that work for them and continue to have weekly check-ins to discuss mastered goals on the DLS contract.*
- *Discuss any new goals that can be added to the DLS contract and the reward that the teen can earn.*
- *Talk to the teen about incentives that they can earn for continuing to work on mastered DLS. For example, many caregivers allow teens to earn a flat allowance for continuing to complete all mastered DLS goals, which will also build up their money management skills.*

♦ Ask and Discuss:
  - *What questions do you have about fading rewards?*
  - *Are there any guidelines you would like to discuss in more detail?*

Review Dyad Session 14 Content (10 mins)

♦ *Now we will briefly review the material that will be covered in the upcoming dyad session with your teen. This will allow you to have some time to prepare for the*

upcoming session. Please feel free to ask any questions as we go over the content of the final dyad session.

- The therapist should refer to the PowerPoint presentation slides for Dyad Session 14 while reviewing the content for the session.
- The therapist should have also prepared for the session by reviewing the Dyad Session 14 content discussed in the manual, which has detailed information about the content that will be covered.
- The important points to make while reviewing the Dyad Session 14 Content are:
  - We will do a Real World Practice Check-In, which will ask you and your teen specific questions about the goals on the DLS contract. This will be an opportunity to problem-solve any challenges and celebrate successes.
  - The elements of an effective system for achieving DLS goals will be reviewed with the teens as it relates to the goals on the DLS contract. This will be our main opportunity to revise the goals that are currently being targeted on the DLS contract.
  - We will review progress towards the individualized DLS goals that teens set in the Preparing for STRW session at the beginning of the STRW intervention.
  - We will discuss other DLS that teens learned during STRW and identify the evidence-based strategies that led to them achieving their goals.
  - The success and perseverance of the teens over the last 15 weeks will be celebrated.
  - Specific DLS to target in the next 3–12 months will be identified to continue the momentum from the STRW intervention.

- Ask: ***Any questions about the content for the upcoming dyad session?***

Conclusion (3 mins)

- ***While this is our final caregiver group session, please feel free to reach out if you have any questions or concerns. For the upcoming dyad session, it would be helpful to think about whether there are specific DLS goals you would like your teen to work on in the next 3 months, 6 months, and 12 months. You should also be ready to celebrate your teen's progress by talking through some of their successes over the last 15 weeks as they worked on their DLS. After your dyad session with your teen, it will be important to continue to work on the goals on the DLS contract so that they build the necessary skills to survive and thrive in the real world!***
- ***Finally, you are welcome to exchange contact information with one another before the session ends and I can also send out that information with your permission. We have found that some caregivers in STRW continue to stay in touch because of how they connected during these sessions but also as a way to continue to have accountability partners as they work on building their teen's DLS.***
- The therapist can spend a few minutes thanking the caregivers for their time, energy, and enthusiasm as they worked on building their teen's DLS.
- Ask: ***Are there any questions before we end the session?***

Moving Forward After STRW

1. **Continue to Use the Daily Living Skills Contract**
   - The DLS contract is meant to be a tool that you can continue to use after STRW to monitor and modify goals, expectations, and rewards.
   - Have weekly check-ins (similar to the dyad sessions) to:
     - Discuss overall progress with DLS goals
     - Discuss any obstacles to meeting DLS goals and brainstorm how to address them (e.g., change reward, modify expectations)
     - Discuss whether specific evidence-based strategies need to added or modified
     - Discuss whether any rewards need to be changed
     - Celebrate successes

2. **Identify and Add New Goal(s) to the DLS Contract**
   - Think about adding a new goal to the DLS contract when:
     - Teen has mastered some or all of the current goals on the DLS contract
       - A DLS is mastered when teen is doing it the majority of the time without any help or reminders from the caregiver. Depending on frequency of goal (daily vs. weekly), it could take weeks or months for a DLS to be mastered
       - Teen has necessary evidence-based strategies and appropriate supports in place with current DLS goals
       - Caregiver and teen have the time and energy to commit to working on another DLS goal
     - Work with teen to identify and prioritize new DLS goal(s) by thinking through the following:
       - What DLS would be beneficial right now?
       - What DLS would be beneficial for their goals in the next 6–12 months?
       - What DLS have they almost mastered?
       - These are DLS that may require some prompting or support, but they may be easy to master
       - What DLS would decrease arguing or stress between the caregiver and teen?
       - What DLS would the teen be most motivated to work on?

3. **Fade Rewards**
    - You should not remove or decrease any rewards your teen has been earning until they have truly mastered a DLS goal.
    - When your teen has mastered a DLS and you feel it is time to start fading a reward, here are some helpful steps:
        - Schedule a specific time to have a conversation about their DLS goals and rewards (e.g., during the weekly check-in).
        - Remain calm and neutral during the discussion with your teen – it is a big deal that they have mastered a DLS!
        - Allow the teen to ask questions (especially if this is the first time a reward has been faded!).
        - Discuss the progress that the teen has made with their DLS goal and how this relates to their future goals in adulthood such as working, going to college, and living on their own.
        - State that they seem like they are now ready to start doing DLS on their own without earning a reward.
        - Discuss that it is still expected that the teen do the DLS even though they are not being rewarded.
            - Provide examples of other DLS the teen (e.g., doing HW, feeding the dog, taking vitamins) or caregiver (e.g., cooking meals, paying bills, cutting grass) does without being rewarded.
        - Discuss that as they get older and become more independent – teens will be expected to do things that they do not receive a reward for. Examples include cleaning their dorm room, washing their work uniform, and making dinner for themselves.
    - Encourage teens to use self-rewards when they complete a DLS. Self-rewards are a way to stay motivated by rewarding oneself for making progress towards or achieving a goal. Examples of self-rewards are watching a TV show after cleaning their room, taking a nap after finishing laundry, or having a dessert after doing the dishes.
    - Discuss how to make sure the teen continues to be successful with mastered DLS they are not being rewarded for (e.g., use of specific strategies, discuss mastered DLS in weekly check-ins, continue to track mastered goals on DLS contract).
    - Discuss any new goals that will be added to the DLS contract and the reward that can be earned.
    - Discuss any additional incentives for mastered DLS.
        - Can earn a weekly bonus if teen meets all goals on contract (including mastered DLS).
        - Teen earns a flat allowance for doing all mastered DLS goals, which can assist with goals of spending, saving, and budgeting.

Daily Living Skills Contract

Date ____________________

Goal	Expectations	Reward	MONDAY	TUESDAY	WEDNESDAY	THURSDAY	FRIDAY	SATURDAY	SUNDAY

____________________ Teen

____________________ Parent / Caregiver

Caregiver/Teen Dyad Session 14 Content (60 mins)

STRW Session 14 Schedule (1 min)

- The therapist should greet the caregiver and teen.
- ***Let's get started! As a reminder, it will be helpful to sit together at a table so that we can all see each other and work together. Please pull out your STRW workbook that contains the handouts for all STRW sessions. This session is called Session 14 – Graduation. Please turn to that section in your workbook.***
- ***Let's go over the session schedule so that you know what we will be doing. Please feel free to ask any questions about our schedule!***
- Briefly go over each item on the Session Schedule.

Real World Practice Check-In: Contract and Morning Routine (3 mins)

- Refer to the Session 13 Real World Practice handout and the DLS Contract handout.
- ***Let's check in on how you are doing with each goal on your DLS contract. Please be honest, as this is an opportunity to talk about what is working and what is not working and do some brainstorming to address any challenges.***
- As needed, the therapist should spend time modifying the DLS contract and problem solving how to make a more effective system to target the DLS goal (e.g., make expectations more specific, change reward, increase/decrease number of prompts, modify the strategies being used to help with goals).
- If the therapist used a fillable PDF of the DLS Contract handout in the previous session, it may be helpful to share this on the screen so that the goal, expectations, and reward can be easily discussed.
- The following questions should be asked (if applicable), and the responses and any relevant notes should be entered into the Real World Practice Tracking Sheet:
  - ***Did you use your DLS contract this week?***
  - ***Did you work on your morning routine goal during the week?***
    - ***What went well?***
    - ***What was challenging?***
    - ***How many days did you work on your morning routine goal?***
    - ***Did you earn a reward for your morning routine goal?***
    - ***How many days did you earn a reward?***

Real World Practice Check-In: Cleaning the Bedroom and Laundry (3 mins)

- The following questions should be asked (if applicable), and the responses and any relevant notes should be entered into the Real World Practice Tracking Sheet:
  - *Did you work on your cleaning the bedroom goal during the week?*
    - *What went well?*
    - *What was challenging?*
    - *How many days did you work on your cleaning the bedroom goal?*
    - *Did you earn a reward for your cleaning the bedroom goal?*
  - *Did you work on your laundry goal during the week?*
    - *What went well?*
    - *What was challenging?*
    - *How many days did you work on your laundry goal?*
    - *Did you earn a reward for your laundry goal?*

Real World Practice Check-In: Cooking and Grocery Shopping (3 mins)

- The following questions should be asked (if applicable), and the responses and any relevant notes should be entered into the Real World Practice Tracking Sheet:
  - *Did you work on your cooking goal or goals during the week?*
    - *What went well?*
    - *What was challenging?*
    - *How many days did you work on your cooking goal or goals?*
    - *Did you earn a reward for your cooking goal or goals?*
  - *Did you work on a grocery shopping goal?*
    - *What went well?*
    - *What was challenging?*
    - *How many days did you work on your grocery shopping goal?*
    - *Did you earn a reward for working on your grocery shopping goal?*

Real World Practice Check-In: Money (2 mins)

- The following questions should be asked (if applicable), and the responses and any relevant notes should be entered into the Real World Practice Tracking Sheet:
  - *Did you work on a money goal or goals during the week?*
    - *What did you do?*
    - *What went well?*
    - *What was challenging?*
    - *How many days did you work on your money goal or goals?*
    - *Did you earn a reward for working on your money goal or goals?*
- Ask: *Any questions or comments about your Real World Practice assignments?*

- If the caregiver/teen dyad struggled to complete the Real World Practice assignments, the therapist should spend some time discussing how to identify days/times that they could designate to commit to working on the assignments.
- If the therapist used a fillable PDF of the DLS Contract handout in the previous session, it may be helpful to share this on the screen so that the goal, expectations, and reward can be easily discussed.

Elements of an Effective System for Achieving DLS Goals (2 mins)

- Ask: *Are there any issues you want to discuss or troubleshoot related to the DLS contract?*
- Ask and Discuss: *Are we considering all of the important elements to increase the likelihood of you achieving your DLS goals by developing the most effective system?*
- If applicable, discuss how to modify any DLS goals to address (1) qualities of the teen and their caregiver; (2) use of evidence-based strategies to teach and master DLS; and (3) ensuring that goals are obvious, attractive, easy, and satisfying.

STRW Session Content (2 mins)

- *Over the last 15 weeks, you have learned, practiced, and independently worked on building your DLS in the areas of personal hygiene and self-care, cleaning the bedroom, doing laundry and putting it away, cooking in the microwave, stovetop, and oven, going grocery shopping, and spending, saving, and budgeting money!*
- *You have also learned how to use many evidence-based strategies including a task analysis; the DLS Teaching Method of learn, watch, practice, and do it independently; a DLS contract with specific goals, expectations, and rewards; technology such as apps, alarms, reminders, and smart speakers; and video modeling.*
- *But most importantly, you have made progress in learning DLS that will help you to become more independent in adulthood as you strive to meet your goals with college, work, and living on your own.*

Individualized DLS Goals (14 mins)

- Refer to the previously completed Individualized DLS Goals handout (from Preparing for STRW Session).
- *In the first session we had together, we set six DLS goals based on your specific strengths and challenges and the DLS that you were going to be learning in STRW. Let's briefly revisit these goals and see how you did with making progress towards achieving them.*
- Ask and Discuss:
  - *Did you make progress toward your goals in:*
    - *Personal hygiene and self-care?*
    - *Cleaning?*
    - *Doing laundry?*
    - *Cooking?*
    - *Grocery shopping?*
    - *Managing money, including spending, saving, and budgeting?*

- The therapist should be positive and encouraging throughout this discussion and encourage the caregiver to also discuss progress that they saw in the teen. Many teens may not have made progress in all of the individualized goals that they set if they did not align with aspects of the STRW curriculum. However, these goals could be incorporated into the discussions later on in this session when thinking about future DLS goals.

The Road to Success: Evaluating Progress (5 mins)

- Ask and Discuss:
  - *What other DLS have you learned or mastered during STRW?*
  - *How did it feel as you made progress and gained new DLS?*
  - *What strategies seem to work best for you for learning and practicing DLS?*

- The therapist should be positive and encouraging throughout this discussion and encourage the caregiver to also discuss the teen's progress and use of effective strategies.

The Road to Success: Future DLS Goals (12 mins)

- Refer to the Future Daily Living Skills Goals handout.
- ***Let's talk about some of the DLS goals you want to keep working on and other DLS goals you may need to learn and work on in the future. We can work together to identify these DLS goals and then write them down on the Future DLS Goals handout. It can be helpful to post this handout somewhere where you see it regularly so that you are reminded of your current DLS goals and the future DLS goals that you are working towards.***
- Have the caregiver/teen collaborate to complete the handout by (1) identifying DLS goals to continue working on and (2) identifying DLS goals to target in the next 3 months, 6 months, and 12 months. The caregiver and teen can write their goals down on the handout or the therapist can transcribe responses directly onto the slide or onto the fillable PDF of the handout
- The therapist should be positive and encouraging during this discussion as the caregiver and teen work together. The therapist can also suggest possible goals based on what they know about the teen and the skills they have worked on throughout the STRW intervention.

Elements of an Effective System for Achieving DLS Goals (3 mins)

- The therapist should briefly ask each teen about each of the elements and then incorporate the responses to the discussion on developing the DLS contract.
- ***As we get ready to create you final DLS contract during STRW, let's think through the following to make sure we are including all of the elements to build an effective system for achieving DLS goals:***
  - ***Teen – are we considering your strengths, challenges, preferred learning style, and commitment?***

- *Caregiver – are we considering your parenting style, time and effort, and commitment?*
- *Are we using evidence-based strategies such as the DLS contract, task analysis, technology, the DLS Teaching Method, or video modeling?*
- *Is the goal obvious, attractive, easy, and satisfying?*

♦ Ask and Discuss: *Any questions or comments?*

♦ *These elements will also be important to remember to include in your future DLS contracts so that you are more likely to meet your goals!*

Developing Your DLS Contract (5 mins)

♦ Refer to the DLS Contract handout

♦ *Even though STRW is ending, it is still important to keep working on your DLS goals. Let's spend the remainder of our time in today's session modifying your DLS contract to continue working on your morning routine, cleaning your bedroom, laundry, cooking, grocery shopping, and managing money goals. You could also add in a DLS goal that we just talked about wanting to work on. Use a blank copy of the DLS Contract. We will also keep in mind the importance of making sure the goal is Obvious, Attractive, Easy, and Satisfying so that you are more likely to achieve your goal. The DLS contract will have you track your progress and set up rewards for you to earn, which makes working on the goals satisfying!*

♦ The therapist should support the caregiver/teen dyad in creating the DLS contract by doing the following:
  - Incorporate all of the information from the last several sessions (e.g., rewards that are motivating for the teen, use of strategies and supports to build independence with certain steps) and the Real World Practice Check-In to create the DLS contract. The therapist should also consider the goals that the caregiver and teen collaboratively developed during the Preparing for STRW session and the goals for the future that were discussed in the current session.
  - Use the DLS Contract handout to specify the (1) Goal, (2) Expectations, and (3) Reward for Morning Routine, Cleaning the Bedroom, Doing Laundry, Cooking, Grocery Shopping, and Money.
  - Encourage the caregiver/teen dyad to work together and model appropriate and supportive coaching as they develop the DLS contract.

♦ Possible discussion questions that may be helpful to ask and discuss when creating the contract for the Morning Routine, Cleaning the Bedroom, Laundry, Cooking, Grocery Shopping, and Money goals include:
  - *How often are you going to need to do the goal – every day, every weekday, every other day, or once per week?*
  - *What steps of your goal do you need help with?*
  - *What steps do you not know how to do?*
  - *What steps are you doing independently?*
  - *How easy/hard do you think it will be to meet your goal?*
  - *What reward would you like to earn?*

Surviving and Thriving in the Real World Session 14 – Real World Practice

- Continue working on your DLS goals in the areas of (1) morning routine, (2) cleaning the bedroom, (3) doing laundry, (4) cooking, (5) grocery shopping, and (6) managing money using your DLS contract.
  - Make sure that if a reward is earned, it is provided immediately!
- Continue to set aside a specific day/time each week to review the DLS contract in the same way that we have been doing during our STRW sessions.
  - Schedule an appointment in your calendar to review the DLS contract.
- Review the DLS goals you want to work on in the future and add to your DLS contract over time.

Surviving & Thriving in the Real World

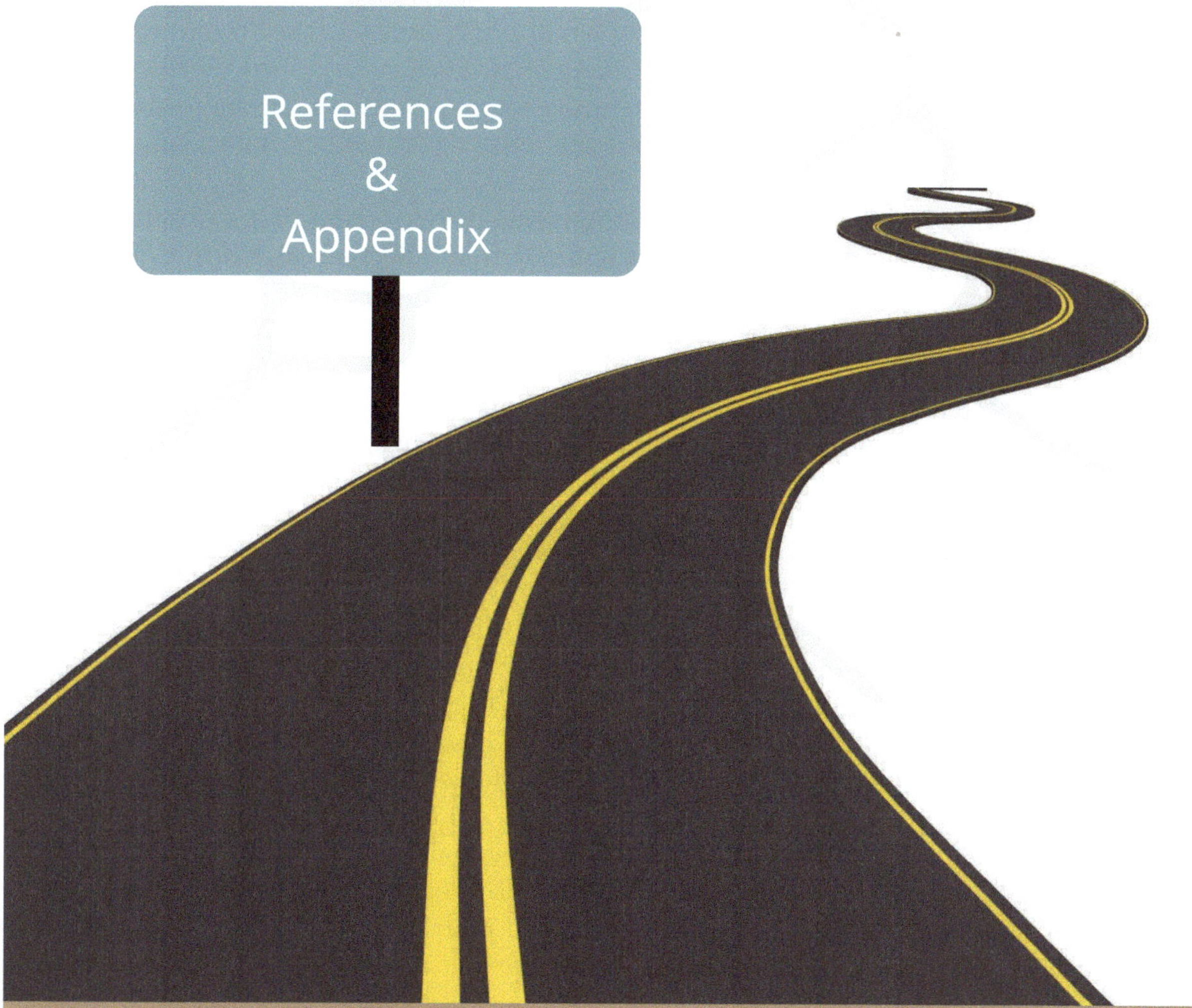

References

Armstrong, T. (2010). *Neurodiversity: Discovering the extraordinary gifts of autism, ADHD, dyslexia, and other brain differences*. ReadHowYouWant.com.

Bennett, K. D., & Dukes, C. (2014). A systematic review of teaching daily living skills to adolescents and adults with autism spectrum disorder. *Review Journal of Autism and Developmental Disorders, 1*, 2–10.

Clear, J. (2018). *Atomic habits: An easy & proven way to build good habits & break bad ones*. Penguin.

Cullen, J. M., & Alber-Morgan, S. R. (2015). Technology mediated self-prompting of daily living skills for adolescents and adults with disabilities: A review of the literature. *Education and Training in Autism and Developmental Disabilities*, 43–55.

Duncan, A., & Bishop, S. L. (2015). Understanding the gap between cognitive abilities and daily living skills in adolescents with autism spectrum disorders with average intelligence. *Autism, 19*(1), 64–72.

Duncan, A., Liddle, M., & Stark, L. J. (2021). Iterative development of a daily living skills intervention for adolescents with autism without an intellectual disability. *Clinical Child and Family Psychology Review*, 1–21. https://doi.org/10.1007/s10567-021-00360-6

Duncan, A., Meinzen-Derr, J., Ruble, L. A., Fassler, C., & Stark, L. J. (2022). A pilot randomized controlled trial of a daily living skills intervention for adolescents with autism. *Journal of Autism and Developmental Disorders, 52*, 938–949.

Duncan, A., Meinzen-Derr, J., Ruble, L. A., Fassler, C., & Stark, L. J. (2023). A randomized clinical trial targeting daily living skills in autistic adolescents without an intellectual disability prior to the transition to adulthood. *Journal of Developmental & Behavioral Pediatrics, 44*(9), 590–596.

Duncan, A., Meinzen-Derr, J., Ruble, L. A., Fassler, C., & Stark, L. J. (2025). Closing the gap: A pilot randomized clinical trial of a daily living skills intervention for autistic adolescents. *Focus on Autism and Other Developmental Disabilities*. https://doi.org/10.1177/10883576251355188.

Duncan, A., Ruble, L. A., Meinzen-Derr, J., Thomas, C. L., & Stark, L. J. (2017). Preliminary efficacy of a daily living skills intervention for adolescents with high-functioning autism spectrum disorder. *Autism*. https://doi.org/10.1177/1362361317716606

Duncan, A., Stark, L. J., Ruble, L., Fassler, C., & Meinzen-Derr, J. (2026). Maintenance of gains in autistic teens receiving a daily living skills intervention at a 6-month follow-up. *Research in Autism*. https://doi.org/10.1016/j.reia.2026.202790.

Erickson, A. G., Clark, G. M., & Patton, J. R. (2013). *Informal assessments for transition planning*. Pro-Ed.

Gardner, S., & Wolfe, P. (2013). Use of video modeling and video prompting interventions for teaching daily living skills to individuals with autism spectrum disorders: A review. *Research and Practice for Persons with Severe Disabilities, 38*(2), 73–87.

Harrison, P., & Oakland, T. (2015). *Adaptive behavior assessment system, third edition (ABAS-III)*. Western Psychological Services.

Hong, E. R., Ganz, J. B., Morin, K., Davis, J. L., Ninci, J., Neely, L., & Boles, M. B. (2017). Functional living skills and adolescents and adults with autism spectrum disorder: A meta-analysis. *Education and Training in Autism and Developmental Disabilities*, *52*(3), 268–279.

Hrabal, J. M., Davis, T. N., & Wicker, M. R. (2023). The use of technology to teach daily living skills for adults with autism: A systematic review. *Advances in Neurodevelopmental Disorders*, *7*(3), 443–458.

Hume, K., Boyd, B. A., Hamm, J. V., & Kucharczyk, S. (2014). Supporting independence in adolescents on the autism spectrum. *Remedial and Special Education*, *35*(2), 102–113. https://doi.org/10.1177/0741932513514617

Hume, K., Loftin, R., & Lantz, J. (2009). Increasing independence in autism spectrum disorders: A review of three focused interventions. *Journal of Autism and Developmental Disorders*, *39*(9), 1329–1338. https://doi.org/10.1007/s10803-009-0751-2

Lord, C., Rutter, M., DiLavore, P. C., Risi, S., Gotham, K., & Bishop, S. L. (2012). *Autism diagnostic observation schedule, second edition (ADOS-2) modules 1–4*. Western Psychological Services.

Lythcott-Haims, J. (2015). *How to raise an adult: Break free of the overparenting trap and prepare your kid for success*. Henry Holt and Company.

McCauley, J. B., Pickles, A., Huerta, M., & Lord, C. (2020). Defining positive outcomes in more and less cognitively able autistic adults. *Autism Research*, *13*(9), 1548–1560. https://doi.org/https://doi.org/10.1002/aur.2359

Miller, W. R., & Rollnick, S. (2012). *Motivational interviewing: Helping people change*. Guilford Press.

Myles, B. S., & Simpson, R. L. (2001). Understanding the hidden curriculum: An essential social skill for children and youth with Asperger syndrome. *Intervention in School and Clinic*, *36*(5), 279–286.

Odom, S. L., Hall, L. J., Morin, K. L., Kraemer, B. R., Hume, K. A., McIntyre, N. S., Nowell, S. W., Steinbrenner, J. R., Tomaszewski, B., & Sam, A. M. (2021). Educational interventions for children and youth with autism: A 40-year perspective. *Journal of Autism and Developmental Disorders*, 1–16.

Palmen, A., Didden, R., & Lang, R. (2012). A systematic review of behavioral intervention research on adaptive skill building in high-functioning young adults with autism spectrum disorder. *Research in Autism Spectrum Disorders*, *6*(2), 602–617.

Reaven, J., Blakeley-Smith, A., Culhane-Shelburne, K., & Hepburn, S. (2012, April). Group cognitive behavior therapy for children with high-functioning autism spectrum disorders and anxiety: A randomized trial. *Journal of Child Psychology and Psychiatry*, *53*(4), 410–419.

Saulnier, C. A., & Klaiman, C. (2022). Assessment of adaptive behavior in autism spectrum disorder. *Psychology in the Schools*, *59*(7), 1419–1429.

Sparrow, S., Cicchetti, D. V., & Balla, D. (2005). *Vineland adaptive behavior scales, second edition (Vineland-II)*. Circle Pines: American Guidance Service.

Sparrow, S., Cicchetti, D. V., & Saulnier, C. A. (2016). *Vineland adaptive behavior scales, third edition (Vineland-3)*. Pearson.

Steinbrenner, J. R., Hume, K., Odom, S. L., Morin, K. L., Nowell, S. W., Tomaszewski, B., Szendrey, S., McIntyre, N. S., Yücesoy-Özkan, S., & Savage, M. N. (2020). *Evidence-based practices for children, youth, and young adults with autism*. FPG Child Development Institute.

Taylor, J. L., Henninger, N. A., & Mailick, M. R. (2015). Longitudinal patterns of employment and postsecondary education for adults with autism and average-range IQ. *Autism, 19*(7), 785–793. https://doi.org/10.1177/1362361315585643

Taylor, J. L., & Seltzer, M. M. (2011). Employment and post-secondary educational activities for young adults with autism spectrum disorders during the transition to adulthood. *Journal of Autism and Developmental Disorders, 41*(5), 566–574. https://doi.org/10.1007/s10803-010-1070-3

Vaillant, G. E. (2012). *Triumphs of experience: The men of the Harvard grant study*. Harvard University Press.

Appendix

- Example DLS Contracts
- Example Task Analyses for Morning Routine, Nighttime Routine, Cleaning the Bedroom, and Laundry
- Strategies Commonly Used to Target Goals on the DLS Contract
- Motivating Rewards Identified by Teens in the STRW Intervention
- Recipe Ideas for the STRW Cooking Sessions
- Tips for STRW Therapists: How to Facilitate Achievement of DLS Goals
- Possible Solutions to Common Challenges that Arise for STRW Therapists

Daily Living Skills Contract

Date ______________________

Goal	Expectations	Reward	MONDAY	TUESDAY	WEDNESDAY	THURSDAY	FRIDAY	SATURDAY	SUNDAY
Morning Routine	Complete 10 of 11 steps on checklist without a reminder from mom or dad on 4 out of 5 days (Monday-Friday). Check in with Mom/Dad when done.	Choice of dinner on the weekend							
Cleaning Bedroom	Clean room on Sunday using cleaning checklist. Tell Mom/Dad that this was completed in person.	30 minutes of extra screen time							
Laundry	Do 1 load from start to finish by Wed at 9pm. Put a reminder on whiteboard to start laundry. Use iPad alarm to switch load. Show Mom when done.	30 minutes of extra screen time							
Cooking	Help Mom/Dad cook dinner from start to finish on Wednesday nights.	Choice of dinner to cook and then eat							
Nighttime Routine	Complete 6 of 7 steps on checklist without a reminder from mom or dad on 4 out of 5 days (Sunday-Thursday). Check in with Mom/Dad when done.	Choice of movie rental on weekend							

______________________ ______________________

Teen **Parent / Caregiver**

Daily Living Skills Contract

Date ______________________

Goal	Expectations *(How often, Level of)*	Reward	MONDAY	TUESDAY	WEDNESDAY	THURSDAY	FRIDAY	SATURDAY	SUNDAY
Morning Routine	For 4 out of 5 days, complete all steps of my routine independently including getting out of bed at 6:45am on my own with an alarm and washing face.	$5 to buy lunch on Saturday at work							
Cleaning Bedroom	Complete 7 steps on my checklist. Have Grandma check in with me after each step to check I did it correctly by Sunday at 8pm.	Choice of snack at the grocery store							
Laundry	Complete 1 entire load of laundry (sort, wash, dry, fold, and put away) using the steps on the Laundry Task Analysis. Check in with Grandma that all steps were done on Thurs by 8pm.	Stay up 1 hour later on Friday night							
Cooking	Cook 1 recipe in the oven for dinner. Cook 1 recipe in the microwave for lunch at work on Sunday.	Choice of meal to cook and then eat							
Money	Create a money diary of my income and expenses for the last 2 weeks	Invite a friend over on the weekend							

______________________ ______________________

Teen **Parent / Caregiver**

Daily Living Skills Contract

Date ______________________

Goal	Expectations	Reward	MONDAY	TUESDAY	WEDNESDAY	THURSDAY	FRIDAY	SATURDAY	SUNDAY
Morning Routine	Complete 7 out of 8 steps in my morning routine with one reminder from Mom. Use morning routine task analysis and reminders on phone.	$1 per day							
Cleaning Bedroom	Put all of my laundry away in the correct place after doing laundry on Thursday by 9pm.	Choice of movie to watch/rent on the weekend							
Laundry	Complete one load of my laundry from start to finish on Thur. Use phone alarm to remember to start loads and switch from washer to dryer.	$2 towards a season pass at amusement park							
Cooking	Make breakfast every weekday on my own and put dishes in the dishwasher with one reminder. Help Mom cook 1 meal on Wed	Choice of breakfast food Choice of meal to cook and then eat							
Money & Grocery Shopping	Help Mom set a weekly grocery budget. Assist Mom with grocery shopping (make list, find items, check out) and see if we stayed on budget.	1 extra hour of video games							

______________________ Teen

______________________ Parent / Caregiver

Daily Living Skills Contract

Date ____________________

Goal	Expectations	Reward	MONDAY	TUESDAY	WEDNESDAY	THURSDAY	FRIDAY	SATURDAY	SUNDAY
Morning Routine	Wake up on own with alarm clock and out of bed by 7:15am for 4 out of 5 days.	$1 per day							
Cleaning Bedroom	Throw away all trash in room. Vacuum floor. Put dirty clothes in hamper. Check in with Mom on Sunday night.	$2							
Laundry	Complete 2 loads of my laundry without any help. Work with my Mom to put laundry away by Sunday night at 8pm.	$2							
Cooking	Cook spaghetti and garlic bread for dinner with 1 prompt. Pack my lunch each day using the checklist of items to pack.	Extra dessert Choice of snack items for lunch							
Money & Grocery Shopping	Purchase 5-10 items from a list at the grocery store and pay for it with Mom's debit card.	Choice of candy at the grocery store							

____________________ Teen

____________________ Parent / Caregiver

Daily Living Skills Contract

Date ______________________

Goal	Expectations	Reward	MONDAY	TUESDAY	WEDNESDAY	THURSDAY	FRIDAY	SATURDAY	SUNDAY
Morning Routine	Wake up on own (with 2 different alarms) at 7:30am. Put dirty clothes in hamper and put on clean clothes. Text Mom a picture of myself by 8:15am	Extra time to practice driving on the way to/from school							
Cleaning Bedroom	Complete cleaning room checklist (8 steps) on my own with 2 prompts. Have Mom check each step.	$5							
Laundry	Complete 1 load of laundry. Complete 1 load of towels.	$2 $2							
Cooking	Cook a dessert in the oven.	Eat the dessert							
Money	Set a budget for a family dinner at a restaurant and then pay with Mom's debit card and calculate the tip.	Ice cream on the way home from the restaurant							

______________________ Teen

______________________ Parent / Caregiver

Daily Living Skills Contract

Date ______________________

Goal	Expectations	Reward	MONDAY	TUESDAY	WEDNESDAY	THURSDAY	FRIDAY	SATURDAY	SUNDAY
Morning Routine	Complete 6 of 6 steps in morning routine with no reminders for 5 out of 5 days. Use checklist on my whiteboard.	$1 towards new laptop							
Cleaning Bedroom	Complete cleaning room checklist on Saturday mornings. Clean out backpack on Sunday night	$2 towards new laptop $1 towards new laptop							
Laundry	Do a complete load of laundry from start to finish (includes putting it away). Set alarms to get started, switch loads, and get out of dryer.	$3 towards new laptop							
Cooking	Make breakfast for myself on the weekend. Make dinner for family one day per week (can have help as needed).	Eat the food that I make Choice of dinner to cook							
Money	Research the quality and prices of laptop computer I will need for college. Discuss with my parents by Sunday evening.	Will make a plan for buying a computer based on my research. My earnings on DLS contract will go towards laptop.							

______________________ ______________________

Teen **Parent / Caregiver**

Daily Living Skills Contract

Date ____________________

Goal	Expectations	Reward	MONDAY	TUESDAY	WEDNESDAY	THURSDAY	FRIDAY	SATURDAY	SUNDAY
Morning Routine	Complete 9 out of 10 steps of my morning routine without help using a checklist and phone alarms and reminders.	Extra screen time from when I complete my routine until I need to leave for school							
Cleaning Bedroom	Organize my desk and nightstand (use checklist) on Sunday Clean out my backpack on Sunday	Can purchase lunch at school one day of the week							
Laundry	Complete my own load of laundry from start to finish on the weekend. Must be put away by Sunday at 5pm.	Clean clothing for the week							
Cooking	Make macaroni and cheese for the family for lunch on the weekend.	Eat the food							
Money	Create a money diary for the past month and then work with Dad to create a monthly budget based on my income and expenses.	Use the car to drive and buy food for myself on the weekend							

____________________ Teen

____________________ Parent / Caregiver

Daily Living Skills Contract

Date ____________

Goal	Expectations	Reward	MONDAY	TUESDAY	WEDNESDAY	THURSDAY	FRIDAY	SATURDAY	SUNDAY
Morning Routine	Wake up on with an alarm clock, wash face, and comb hair with no reminders for 5/5 weekdays. Do all other steps of morning routine.	$2 No reward							
Cleaning Bedroom	Use checklist to complete all steps including vacuuming and dusting. Must be done by Sunday at 9pm.	Choice of snack at the grocery store							
Laundry	Sort laundry into 4 piles (whites, lights, reds, darks), use washer and dryer correctly, & fold clothes and put away by Sat at 6pm. Use Task Analysis.	Book of choice at the bookstore							
Cooking	Cook meal on stovetop (stir fry) with some coaching from Mom. Bake muffins without any help. Help Mom clean the kitchen up.	If ALL cooking goals completed, I get to choose restaurant to eat at. OR $1 per goal met							
Money	Purchase an item using my debit card and then log on to my account to make sure the amount was correct.	No reward							

____________ Teen

____________ Parent / Caregiver

Daily Living Skills Contract

Date ____________________

Goal	Expectations	Reward	MONDAY	TUESDAY	WEDNESDAY	THURSDAY	FRIDAY	SATURDAY	SUNDAY
Morning Routine	Complete 12 out of 13 steps of my morning routine using a checklist that my Mom double checks when I say I am done.	Choice of dessert to pack in his lunch							
Cleaning Bedroom	Strip my bed and wash my sheets. Remake my bed after sheets are washed. Must be done by Sunday at 6pm.	Choice of candy at the grocery store							
Laundry	Wash, dry, and pack my soccer uniform on Tues-Fri before bed at 9pm. Do 1 load of my laundry from start to finish (1 prompt allowed)	Choice of Gatorade for soccer $2 towards Trampoline Park							
Cooking	Make biscuits and gravy for my family on my own. Clean up kitchen using the kitchen checklist with parents' help.	Eat the dinner $1 towards Trampoline Park							
Money	Count up all of the money in the safe in my room and in my wallet. Have parents double check my math.	Open up a checking account at the bank							

____________________ Teen

____________________ Parent / Caregiver

Daily Living Skills Contract

Date ____________________

Goal	Expectations	Reward	MONDAY	TUESDAY	WEDNESDAY	THURSDAY	FRIDAY	SATURDAY	SUNDAY
Morning Routine	Complete 9 out of 9 steps every day with 1 reminder or prompt each day. Must also be out of bed by 6:25am.	$1 per day							
Laundry	Complete 2 loads of laundry (sort, wash, dry, put away) without help. Laundry must be put away on the same day it was started.	$5							
Cooking	Make dinner for the family on Saturday night. Can have some help from parents.	Choice of meal to make and then eat							
Grocery Shopping	Make a grocery list and then pick out items for the family dinner I am cooking.	Choice of dessert for family dinner							
Money	Work with Mom to set a budget for the family dinner by looking up items in the grocery store app.	Purchase the items at the store using Mom's debit card on my own							

____________________ Teen

____________________ Parent / Caregiver

Task Analysis

Skill: Morning Routine

Steps:

Wake up at 6am

Wash face and put lotion on

Brush teeth

Brush hair

Put deodorant on

Clean glasses

Get dressed

Eat breakfast

Take medicine and vitamins

Pack backpack (laptop, lunch, water bottle, phone, wallet, homework folder)

Eat breakfast

In the car by 7:20am

Task Analysis

Skill: Morning Routine

Steps:

Wake up and get out of bed by 645am

Eat breakfast

Take medicine

Use the bathroom

Wash face

Brush teeth

Put on deodorant

Get dressed

Put dirty clothes in hamper

Pack my backpack and lunch

Check weather and put on appropriate coat and shoes

Check that I have everything for school using my checklist and walk out the door by 745 am

Task Analysis

Skill: Nighttime Routine

Steps:

Begin routine at 9pm

Put pajamas on

Put dirty clothes in hamper

Wash face and do acne medicine

Brush teeth

Put retainer in

Lay out clothes for the next day

Charge phone and laptop

Put homework folder in backpack

Lights out at 9:30pm

Task Analysis

Skill: Nighttime Routine

Steps:

Start at 8:30pm

Take a shower

Put dirty clothes and towel in hamper

Put lotion on face and body

Brush hair

Brush teeth

Take contacts out and put them in the case with clean solution

Set alarm to wake up for the next day

Pack backpack and put by my bedroom door

Charge phone

Get in bed and I can read until 10pm

Task Analysis

Skill: Cleaning Bedroom

Steps:

Bring any cups or dishes to the kitchen and put them in the dishwasher

Put all trash (wrappers, papers, empty water bottles) in the trash can

Put all dirty laundry in the hamper

Put all clean laundry away

Pick up items off of the floor and put them where they go

Organize items on my desk (pencils, papers, art supplies)

Put books on bookshelf

Wipe off desk with spray and a rag

Empty trash can and put a new bag in the trash can

Sweep and then vacuum the floor

Have Mom check that I did all of the steps

Task Analysis

Skill: Cleaning Bedroom

Steps:

Put dirty laundry in hamper

Strip sheets and blankets off of my bed and bring to the laundry room

Start a load of laundry with my sheets and blankets

Set a reminder to check the laundry in 60 minutes

Pick up everything off of the floor and put items where they go

Clean off my nightstand and put items where they go

Clean off my desk and put items where they go

Wipe/dust my desk and nightstand

Gather trash and then empty my trash can

Vacuum the carpet (including under my desk)

Switch laundry from the washer to dryer. Set a reminder to take sheets out of dryer and then make my bed.

Have Grandma check that I completed all of the steps

Task Analysis

Skill: Laundry

Steps:

Bring my laundry hamper to the laundry room

Check pockets to make sure they are empty

Put all clothes in washer (make sure you do not overload it!)

Put detergent pod in

Wash clothes on Permanent Press (cold water)

Set alarm on my phone for 75 minutes

Switch clothes to the dryer

Put a dryer sheet in

Dry clothes on Regular cycle

Set alarm on my phone for 45 minutes

Put dry clothes into laundry basket and bring up to my room

Fold clothes and put them away

Task Analysis

Skill: Laundry

Steps:

Bring clothes in the hamper to the laundry room

Sort laundry into light (whites, light grays) and darks (jeans, colors, dark grays)

Put the light laundry load into the washing machine

Measure out detergent for a regular load and pour it into the correct slot

Measure out fabric softener and pour it into the correct slot

Wash clothes on Whites cycle

Set a reminder to check the washer in 60 minutes

Switch clothes to dryer

Put dryer sheet in and dry clothes on Regular cycle

Put the dark laundry load into the washing machine and repeat the same steps as above.

Wash darks on the Permanent Press cycle.

Set a reminder to check the loads of laundry in 60 minutes

Fold clothes from the dryer in a laundry basket.

Switch dark laundry load to the dryer and add in a dryer sheet. Dry them on the Regular Cycle.

Set a reminder to check the dryer in 60 minutes

Fold clothes from the dryer in a laundry basket

Put all clothing away in my bedroom

Have Dad check that I have completed laundry

Strategies Commonly Used to Target Goals on the DLS Contract

- **Morning Routine**
  - Create a morning routine checklist from the steps on the Task Analysis.
    - Electronic (e.g., phone, tablet, smart speaker)
    - Hard copy (e.g., paper, whiteboard)
  - Post the checklist in multiple places (e.g., room, bathroom, kitchen, front door).
  - Post the checklist near the door that the teen will walk out of before going to school so that the caregiver can do a final check.
  - Require the teen to check in with their parent/caregiver at a certain time to double check that all steps have been completed.
  - Create regular alarms and reminders to help the teen with certain steps.
    - Weekday alarm on their phone and alarm clock to wake up in the morning.
    - Multiple alarms to encourage waking up independently (e.g., phone, alarm clock on their dresser, bedroom light turns on at a certain time).
    - Create a daily reminder on a smart speaker (e.g., Amazon Echo) to let teen know how much time they have left ("You have 15 minutes until the bus comes").
    - Create a calendar reminder on the teen's phone that reminds them to pack all of their items in their backpack 10 minutes before they need to leave for school
  - Cluster tasks that are completed in the same area together (e.g., teen does all tasks in their bedroom such as getting dressed and making bed before transitioning to doing all tasks in the bathroom such as brushing teeth and face).
  - Put all hygiene items used during the morning routine in the same spot (e.g., face wash, lotion, toothpaste, toothbrush, and comb are kept in a basket on the bathroom counter).
  - Put all medications/vitamins in a pillbox.
  - Post a menu of possible breakfast foods to make this decision quick and easy.
  - Create a checklist of what items need to be packed in the teen's lunch (e.g., main thing, chips/crackers, granola bar, fruit, and water bottle).
  - Create a checklist for what items need to be packed in the teen's backpack (e.g., phone, laptop, binder, planner, lunch box, and water bottle).
  - Identify steps that the teen needs support in (e.g., packing their lunch) and provide instruction, modeling, and constructive feedback as needed (e.g., help them identify items that they like to pack in their lunch, instruct and model how to make a sandwich or cut up an apple). These supports should be faded after the teen demonstrates that they can complete these steps.
  - Provide a natural reward if the teen has extra time after completing their morning routine (e.g., read a book, screen time, practice driving on the way to school).
  - Do some prep the night before if it is difficult for the teen to complete some steps in the morning (e.g., lay out clothes the night before if the teen struggles to pick out clothes in the morning, pack their backpack at night).

- **Cleaning Bedroom**
  - Create a cleaning bedroom checklist from the steps on the Task Analysis:
    - Electronic (e.g., phone, notes or to do list app, tablet, smart speaker)
    - Hard copy (e.g., paper, whiteboard)
  - Post the checklist in the teen's room.
  - Create a supply list that the teen will need for cleaning their room (e.g., vacuum, all-purpose cleaning spray, rag, garbage bag).
  - Identify a specific day/time that the teen is usually available to clean their room.
  - Create an alarm or reminder to help the teen get started on a specific day/time to clean their room.
    - Calendar reminder on the day/time they are to clean their room
    - Reminder on smart speaker to clean their room
    - Identify some ways that cleaning the room can be fun (e.g., listen to music or a podcast, listen to an audiobook)
  - Identify the steps that the teen needs support in and provide instruction, modeling, and constructive feedback as needed. Caregivers may need to instruct and model/assist teen with cleaning their room until they understand how to complete each step. Some steps the teen may need help with include:
  - Organizing the teen's belongings (e.g., putting all books where they go, putting clothing in the hamper or in the dresser/closet, putting all school materials in their backpack).
    - Using the vacuum to clean the floor or carpet.
    - Dusting and/or cleaning their dresser, nightstand, or desk.
  - Discuss the natural reward for cleaning one's room (e.g., sleeping and living in a clean and organized space, can find things that they need).
  - Require the teen to check in with their parent/caregiver after they have completed the checklist to double check that all steps have been completed.

- **Laundry**
  - Create a laundry checklist from the steps on the Task Analysis.
    - Electronic (e.g., phone, notes or to-do list app, tablet, smart speaker)
    - Hard copy (e.g., paper, whiteboard)
  - Post the checklist in the laundry area near the washer and dryer.
  - Post information on what washing machine and dryer settings the teen will be using regularly so that they can easily refer to this.
  - Put all laundry supplies in one area so that the teen can find them easily.
  - Identify a specific day/time that the teen is available to do one to two loads of laundry.
  - Create an alarm/reminder for starting the teen's laundry on a specific day/time.
    - Calendar reminder on the day/time they are to do their laundry
    - Reminder on smart speaker to start laundry
  - Identify alarms or reminders that the teen can use to remember to complete the steps of laundry.

   - Alarm on their phone to switch laundry from the washer to the dryer
   - Reminder on a smart speaker to take laundry out of the dryer
   - Calendar reminder to have all laundry put away by a certain time
- It can be helpful to require that all steps of laundry be done in one day to encourage the teen to get in the habit of using the washing machine and dryer, and then putting their laundry away in a timely manner.
- Identify some ways that doing laundry can be fun (e.g., do an enjoyable activity while waiting for laundry to finish washing, listen to music or an audiobook while putting laundry away).
- Identify steps that the teen needs support in and provide instruction, modeling, and constructive feedback as needed. Caregivers may need to instruct and model/assist teen with doing laundry until the teen understands the steps and how to complete each step. Common steps teens needs assistance with include:
   - Sorting – removing items from pockets and identifying lights and darks.
   - Washing machine – loading the machine with an appropriate amount of clothing and measuring out the correct amount of detergent.
   - Dryer – ensuring that all clothing is dry before putting it away.
   - Putting clothing away – folding or hanging up clothing items, organizing clothing in a dresser (e.g., all shirts in one drawer, all shorts in another drawer).
- Some teens may benefit from using a folding board or watching videos on how to quickly fold items. This is a way to potentially make this step fun and enjoyable!
- Caregivers may want to identify naturalistic opportunities to continue to build their teen's laundry skills as various situations arise:
   - How to get stains out of clothing before washing them.
   - How to wash delicate items.
   - How to iron or steam clothing.
- Require the teen to check in with their parent/caregiver after they have completed the checklist to double check that all steps have been completed.

♦ **Cooking**
- Identify days/times that the teen can help with cooking.
   - Create a calendar reminder to cook dinner on Thursday nights.
   - Create a calendar reminder to bake cookies on Saturday afternoon.
- Identify recipes that the teen is interested in learning how to cook.
   - Thinking through the meals and snacks that the family regularly cooks.
   - Thinking about recipes the teen wants to learn how to cook.
   - Looking through a cookbook.
   - Researching a cooking blog or website.
- Utilize cooking websites or blogs that also include video demonstrations of how to cook a specific recipe.
- Print recipes out so that the teen can easily refer to them and check off ingredients or cross out steps as they go along.
- Have the teen set alarms or reminders as they are cooking (e.g., set a timer to go off when the cookies should be done cooking).
- It may be easiest to build a teen's motivation and interest in cooking by having them learn how to cook items that they enjoy eating. The natural reward for this will be eating the food after they have cooked it!

- Caregivers may want to have teens cook the same item several times so that they can become confident in their ability to cook it independently without any assistance. For example, a teen may make spaghetti and meatballs each week for their family for 1–2 months before learning a new recipe to cook for dinner.
- Identify the steps that the teen needs support in and provide instruction, modeling, and constructive feedback as needed. Caregivers may need to instruct and model/assist teen with cooking until the teen understands the steps and how to complete each step. Some common challenges for teens include:
  - Using a colander to drain water from a pot.
  - Removing hot items from the oven (e.g., a cookie sheet).
  - Remembering to use a potholder when removing hot items from the oven and microwave.
  - Measuring ingredients accurately.
  - Thoroughly mixing items (e.g., pancake batter).
  - Pouring batter from a bowl into a cake pan or muffin pan.
  - Understanding the settings on a stovetop (e.g., medium vs. high heat).
  - Staying focused when cooking (e.g., not leaving the kitchen, checking items as they are cooking so that they do not burn).
- Caregivers may want to identify naturalistic opportunities to continue to build their teen's cooking skills as various situations arise:
  - When the teen identifies a recipe that they want to cook, have them determine what ingredients are needed and add any ingredients that they do not have to the grocery list.
  - Have the teen help with cooking a meal several times per week (even just for a few minutes!) so that they are exposed to a range of skills such as boiling water, getting items out of the oven, chopping vegetables, understanding how to tell when a meal is done, taking the temperature of meat or fish, and finding various cooking equipment and ingredients in the kitchen.
- For cleaning the kitchen, the caregiver and teen should develop a checklist of steps that need to be completed after cooking.
  - Post the checklist in the kitchen (e.g., on the refrigerator).
  - Put all kitchen cleaning supplies that the teen will be using in one area so that they are able find them easily.
    - Require the teen to check in with their parent/caregiver after they have finished cooking to double check that all steps, including cleaning up have been completed. This is also an opportunity for the caregiver to provide feedback to the teen.

♦ **Grocery Shopping**

- Identify an easy way for the teen to add items to the grocery list that they need (e.g., for their lunch at school, for an after-school snack) or want (e.g., favorite dessert or drink).
- Ideas for keeping a grocery list that your teen can easily access and use include:
  - A piece of paper or whiteboard on the refrigerator.
  - Creating a shared grocery list document or spreadsheet that can be accessed by everyone in the family via phone, tablet, or computer.

- A grocery list app.
- A specific grocery store app.
- Creating a grocery list on a smart speaker that can be added to.

- Specify the expectations for the grocery list (e.g., the teen is responsible for adding items from the grocery list that they need or want by a specific day/time).
- It may be beneficial to also encourage the teen to add any personal hygiene items that they need (e.g., face wash, deodorant) to the grocery list.
- Prior to going grocery shopping, sit down with the teen and review the grocery list items to ensure that all items have been added that are needed for the upcoming week.
- Encourage the teen to think through items that they may need by having them think of what they typically eat for breakfast, lunch, dinner, and snacks.
- Take the teen grocery shopping to allow for an easy and naturalistic opportunity to practice skills such as:
    - Finding items in the grocery store (e.g., using aisle signs, using a specific grocery store's app).
    - Using a list to find and then check off items that they added to the grocery list.
    - Comparing the prices of two items to build understanding of concepts such as quality and quantity.
    - Identifying items that are on sale and evaluating whether it is a good deal.
- Involve the teen in online grocery shopping to build an understanding of skills such as how to find specific items, how to add items to the cart, and how to clip any coupons for items being purchased.
- Online grocery shopping provides an easy way to determine if a budget for grocery shopping is going to be met. For example, if the teen goes over budget, they can look at the items in the cart and remove them to see if they are getting closer to a balanced budget.
- It may be easiest to build the teen's motivation and interest in grocery shopping by allowing them to shop for items that they want/need or are going to be cooking in the next week.
- Provide instruction and feedback during aspects of the check-out process until the teen is ready to be independent including:
    - Taking groceries out of the cart and placing them on the conveyor belt (e.g., being gentle with produce items and bread).
    - Using coupons.
    - Using a debit/credit card or cash to purchase groceries.
    - Checking the receipt to ensure accuracy of items purchased and understand any savings (e.g., coupons, sales).
    - Bagging items (e.g., putting frozen food items in one bag, not overloading bags with heavy items).
    - Using a self-checkout lane (e.g., ensuring an item is placed in a bag before ringing up another item).
    - Loading items into the car.
- Encourage the teen to assist with loading and unloading items into the car so that they understand how to do this (e.g., being gentle when loading/unloading

certain items, arranging bags in the car, carrying items from the car to the house, etc.).

- Provide instruction and feedback on where and how to put grocery items away. Some specific things to address include:
  - Rotating perishable items (e.g., milk, eggs, yogurt) in the fridge so that older items are in front of newer items.
  - The location (e.g., fridge, freezer, pantry) that items that should go in, especially if they could be put away in multiple places (e.g., bread may be stored in the fridge, freezer, or pantry).
  - Checking the expiration date of certain items (e.g., milk, eggs, cheese) and discussing concepts such as "best by" and "use by."
  - Organizing items in the fridge, freezer, and pantry so that items can be easily located.
- It can be beneficial for teens to regularly help with the same steps of grocery shopping (e.g., finding the same items, using a list to check items off) until they have clearly mastered the steps.
- Once teens have demonstrated that they can find items in the grocery store and check out with their caregiver's support, they can be challenged to independently go into the store, find the needed items, and then check out without their caregiver.

♦ **Money Management**

- Increase the teen's awareness of the cost of common items that they use by involving them when shopping (both online and at the store). For example, if purchasing items such as shampoo, conditioner, and toothpaste, discuss the cost with the teen and compare the cost with other similar items.
- When purchasing items at the store or online, involve the teen and talk through your process for choosing the item, researching the cost, and making the choice about when to purchase the item.
- Encourage teens to contribute to their own expenses (e.g., cell phone bill, car insurance, clothing, etc.) – especially if they have regular income from a part-time job or from allowance.
- Use a money diary for a specified period of time (e.g., week, month) to build the teen's understanding of what items they purchase (or their family purchases) on a regular basis.
- Prior to purchasing an item, have the teen research it to make sure that they are getting the best price. For example, if they want to buy a new video game at a store, have them also check the price at other stores or online stores to make sure they are getting the best possible deal.
- Use a savings contract to help the teen set specific savings goals – especially if they have a part-time job that provides them with regular income. Set specific guidelines about saving (e.g., 20% in savings account, 20% towards saving up for a down payment on a car) and re-evaluate as needed.
- Encourage the teen to regularly check the balance on their checking and/or savings accounts so that they get into a routine of doing this regularly. This is particularly important if they are regularly depositing money into their account and/or purchasing items using their debit card.

- Increase the teen's awareness of household costs by showing and reviewing bills such as electric, water, internet/cable, mortgage or rent, and cell phone.
  - It can be particularly helpful for teens to have an understanding of their specific expenses (e.g., cell phone, internet, clothing, food, music lessons, cost of extracurricular activities).
- Use naturalistic opportunities to build budgeting skills including:
  - Saving up for a purchase (e.g., laptop, gaming system, etc.).
  - Upcoming family vacation.
  - Attending a concert or sporting event.
  - Planning for a graduation party, birthday party, and so on.
  - Saving up for a car (e.g., down payment, monthly payment, insurance payment).
  - Attending college (e.g., tuition, books/supplies, room and board).
  - Family's monthly budget (e.g., bills, groceries, etc.)
- Continue to challenge the teen to build increasingly complex money skills as they master skills. It can be helpful to think through the skills that they will need for when they go to college, work a full-time or part-time job, or live on their own.

Motivating Rewards Identified by Teens in the STRW Intervention

- Food
  - Favorite snacks or desserts
  - Choosing an item from the grocery store
  - Cooking a favorite food
  - Eating out at a restaurant
  - Getting a snack at a restaurant or store (e.g., donut, cookie, chips)
  - Ordering a smoothie, coffee, tea, or ice cream at a store
- Money
  - Specific amount of money based on the complexity of the goal
  - Earning money that can be used to save up for an item (e.g., shoes, video game)
  - Earning a weekly allowance (may include money from multiple goals) that can be used as spending money or for saving up for items
- Spending time with family
  - Playing board games
  - Playing outdoor games (e.g., basketball)
  - Going for a hike
  - Making a craft together
  - Family movie night
- Spending time with friends
  - Inviting friends over
  - Going somewhere with friends (e.g., movies, store, restaurant)
- Screen time
  - Extra time to play video games, use phone/computer/tablet, or watch TV
  - Choice of a movie to rent or purchase
- Shopping
  - Purchasing items at a store (e.g., clothing, videogames, crafts, etc.)
  - Purchasing parts to make a computer
  - Purchasing specific apps or subscriptions (e.g., Netflix, Spotify)
  - Purchasing music or books
- Outings (may require saving up)
  - Bowling
  - Movie tickets
  - Concert tickets
  - Museum
  - Amusement park ticket or season pass
  - Arcade
- Privileges
  - Free time
  - Sleeping in or staying up late
  - Earning extra driving time towards driver's license
  - Driving somewhere independently and/or with a parent, sibling, or friend

Recipe Ideas for the STRW Cooking Sessions

- **No-Cook Recipes** (*could also use appliances such as the toaster or blender*)
  - Wrap (e.g., hummus and cheese, turkey and cheese)
  - Sandwich (e.g., peanut butter and jelly, ham and cheese)
  - Bagel with cream cheese
  - Salad (e.g., lettuce, tomatoes, cheese, sunflower seeds, and dressing)
  - Tortilla chips and guacamole
  - Waffles with butter
  - Apple with peanut butter
  - Overnight oats
  - Fruit smoothie

- **Microwave Recipes**
  - Soup
  - Oatmeal
  - Quesadilla (e.g., flour tortilla and cheese)
  - Macaroni and cheese
  - English muffin pizza (e.g., English muffin, sauce, and mozzarella cheese)
  - Hot pocket
  - Pasta or rice pouch
  - Mug recipes (e.g., brownie in a mug, omelet in a mug)

- **Oven Recipes**
  - Brownies, cookies, muffins, or cakes
  - Chex mix
  - Homemade pizza (e.g., crust, sauce, cheese, and pepperoni)
  - Baked potatoes or homemade French fries
  - Pasta bake (e.g., pasta, sauce, and cheese)
  - Frozen foods or meals (e.g., frozen pizza, lasagna, pizza rolls, mac and cheese)
  - Casseroles (e.g., breakfast casserole with eggs, frozen potatoes, peppers, onions)

- **Stovetop Recipes**
  - Spaghetti and sauce
  - Grilled cheese
  - Scrambled eggs
  - Pancakes
  - Chili
  - Fajitas (e.g., chicken, peppers, and onions)
  - Burgers

Other possible kitchen appliances to consider using if the teen has well-developed skills using the microwave, stove, and/or oven include the air fryer, instant pot, crock pot, waffle maker, or grill.

Tips for STRW Therapists: How to Facilitate Achievement of DLS Goals

- *Establish an open and collaborative relationship with the teen and caregiver.* STRW therapists have expertise in how to target the development of age-appropriate daily living skills in adolescents using evidence-based strategies and supports. However, caregivers and teens are truly experts in themselves (e.g., strengths, challenges, what strategies work for them, what motivates them), which is equally critical when creating, targeting, and modifying DLS goals. Some things to keep in mind:
  - Teens should be encouraged to think about what strategies will work best for them when developing or modifying goals and expectations!
  - Caregivers should be given an opportunity to provide their feedback and thoughts about what is working or not working. It can be helpful to discuss this in the caregiver group session so that the caregiver can openly share and then make a plan for how to discuss it with the teen. For example, the therapist may provide ideas on how the caregiver can balance providing honest feedback with praise when discussing the DLS contract.

- *Consider the characteristics of the teen, caregiver(s), and the family to facilitate achievement of DLS goals.* This is particularly important when creating the first several goals on the DLS contract so that there is some initial success and growth. If the teen sees that their strengths, challenges, and thoughts/ideas are considered as they set goals and make progress towards meeting their goals, they will be more likely to continue to be motivated and positive about building their DLS and overall independence. Similarly, it is equally important to ensure that the caregiver and the family environment are considered so that they can provide the instruction, guidance, and motivation that is necessary to support the teen.
- *Explore future goals to build and maintain motivation.* In both the Preparing for STRW Session and Session 1, the caregiver and teen dyad are encouraged to identify future goals (e.g., going to college, getting a job, living in an apartment) and the specific DLS that are needed to reach these goals. The link between acquiring age-appropriate DLS and achieving future goals may increase motivation in both the caregiver and teen. It can also be helpful to revisit these goals over the course of the STRW intervention to remind the dyad of what they are working towards.
- *Review past successes to build confidence.* It can be effective for therapists to take time to remind caregivers and/or teens of their past successes in building DLS or other skills as a way to instill confidence and increase motivation. This can be particularly beneficial when the teen/caregiver are feeling frustrated or impatient about their progress towards DLS goals (e.g., slow progress, plateau in gaining of skills, taking more time to learn and master a new skill than was originally anticipated).
- *Label the teen's progress to instill a sense of pride.* Therapists should identify and describe the teen's progress with a goal to stimulate internal feelings of pride, accomplishment, and independence. Many teens may prefer this to the therapist or caregiver praising them ("Great work!"), labeling emotions ("It must be exciting to make this much progress!"), or stating their own emotions ("I am so proud of you.").

- *Be a guide.* While the therapist may have to be more directive at times by providing instructions and feedback, particularly at the beginning of the STRW intervention, they should be mindful of fading back their support so that the caregiver and teen feel confident to continue to build their DLS and overall independence after completing the STRW intervention.
- *Provide instruction and guidance in a focused and manageable way.* Therapists should let caregivers and teens know when they plan on providing instruction, giving feedback, and/or engaging in problem solving, especially as they work towards increasing independence. It will also be critical for the therapist to ensure that any guidance they provide fits with what the caregiver/teen needs. At times, therapists may find it beneficial to discuss what has worked (or not worked) for other teens as they targeted a DLS goal.
- *Be curious.* As another way to strengthen the collaborative relationship with the caregiver and teen, the therapist should ask questions that will increase their insight and understanding as they target DLS goals. Questions to ask might include "What strategy do you think might work for targeting this goal?", "What do you see as potential obstacles?", or "What ideas do you have?"
- *Be a good listener.* The therapist should take the time to listen to the caregiver and teen as they discuss their progress with the goals on the DLS contract. It can sometimes be easy to rush through parts of the session (e.g., asking the questions in the Real World Practice Check-In), but by really listening and reflecting on the dyad's responses, the therapist will be able to effectively address any obstacles or challenges.
- *Be a good observer.* The therapist has the unique opportunity to "be" in the teen's home while they receive instruction and practice new DLS with the support of their caregiver. It can often be beneficial to observe whether there are any environmental modifications that can easily be made (e.g., how to organize the teen's closet to make putting clothing away easier, where to post visual reminders, how to streamline morning routine steps).
- *Acknowledge differences between teens.* The therapist should be mindful of the different goals, expectations, and rewards of the teens in the group. It may be helpful to directly acknowledge that each teen comes in with different experiences, strengths, and challenges, but the end goal of achieving independence by building age-appropriate DLS is the same for everyone.
- *Create goals that are doable on the DLS contract.* It can be helpful to use the SMART goal framework as a guide to ensure that the goal is written in a way that can be met:
  - **Specific** – be more detailed rather than less detailed when defining the goal and the expectations (e.g., prompts, involvement from caregivers, steps that need to be completed, strategies and supports to be implemented).
  - **Measurable** – it should be clear when the goal has been met or accomplished.
  - **Achievable** – the teen should be challenged, but the goal should also be something that they can realistically meet with the incorporation of specific supports and strategies.
  - **Relevant** – while the goal targets age-appropriate DLS, it may be beneficial to discuss the larger purpose or benefits to both the teen (e.g., meet long-term

goals, build independence) and their caregiver (e.g., build autonomy, decrease involvement, decrease stress).
- **Time-bound** – the goal should include information related to how often (e.g., weekdays only) and when it will start and finish (e.g., starts Monday and ends Friday)
- **Example SMART goal:** I will complete one load of my laundry by Wednesday evening at 8 pm without any help from my parents. I will use the laundry task analysis checklist and alarms on my phone.

- *Affirm the teen's progress towards DLS goals.* During the Real World Practice Check-In, the therapist should actively recognize and acknowledge any positive change or progress made by the teen with the support of their caregiver. Affirming not only communicates that the therapist understands the caregiver and the teen, but also may facilitate continued growth.
- *Emphasize that any progress is good progress.* As the caregiver and teen work towards the goals on their DLS contract, the therapist should emphasize that any progress towards a DLS goal (e.g., becoming more independent, practicing a new skill, effectively implementing a strategy) is a step in the right direction.
- *Identify the individual strategies that work best for a teen.* For many teens, there are likely four to five strategies that they can use over and over again to successfully meet their DLS goals. It is critical for therapists to assist with identifying successful strategies that can be used for current and future DLS goals. The therapist should regularly discuss what strategies work and do not work with the dyad.
- *Assist with building an effective system for reaching goals.* In *Atomic Habits* (2018) by James Clear, he stated the following: "Goals are good for setting a direction, but systems are best for making progress. You fall to the level of your systems." The therapist will need to remind caregivers and teens that the key to achieving DLS goals that last is to build an effective system. Throughout STRW, the therapist will emphasize building an effective system that considers the teen, the caregiver and the family environment, use of evidence-based strategies, and the Four Laws of Behavior Change.
- *Encourage trying out a strategy before choosing another one.* Teens and parents may be resistant to trying out a strategy for a variety of reasons (e.g., it was not effective in the past, it seems too simple, it seems too hard). The therapist should encourage the teen and caregiver to try out a strategy before working to identify a new one. For example, a checklist can be a very effective tool for learning the steps of a task, starting a task, remembering the steps of a task, and completing a task – but the dyad may need to be strongly encouraged to incorporate it!
- *Flexibility is critical when developing goals and expectations.* The therapist, teen, and caregiver will need to be flexible when identifying goals and defining expectations.
- Teens may make progress very quickly such that their expectations may also increase quickly. Conversely, it may take some teens a lot of time to practice a skill such that expectations are changed more slowly. For example, some teens may have an expectation to complete most of their morning routine (e.g., eight out of ten steps), and other teens may only be working on one step at a time (e.g., waking up on their own).

- *Assess motivation continuously.* What is rewarding or motivating to a teen may change quickly, so it is important to regularly evaluate whether a reward for working towards a DLS goal is truly motivating them. The therapist should ask about the effectiveness of rewards at each session and brainstorm additional rewards as needed.
- *Normalize that all teens are different and will make progress at different rates.* Every teen, caregiver, and family environment is unique, and the therapist should consider the individual strengths and challenges when developing DLS goals to target. Additionally, teens will make progress at different rates depending on a range of factors (e.g., motivation, previous experience, commitment, etc.). It can be helpful for therapists to regularly normalize that progress takes time and looks different for everyone.
- *Take a nonjudgmental approach.* Therapists should be aware of how caregivers and teens may be feeling about their progress towards goals and should seek to be open and neutral when engaging in problem solving or providing feedback. Caregivers and teens are more likely to engage in developing and modifying their system for achieving their DLS goals if the therapist is accepting of barriers and challenges.
- *Support caregivers if they need to modify expectations for earning rewards or privileges.* Caregivers may need to adjust or change their own behaviors, expectations, and boundaries in the home to effectively support their teen in building DLS. For example, if teens are able to access all of the things that are rewarding to them (e.g., video games, screen time, privileges) without doing "work" (e.g., laundry, cleaning their room, chores around the home), caregivers may need to edit these expectations so that they are now required to "earn" these rewards. The therapist can provide support and guidance by engaging in problem solving. It can often be helpful to discuss this during the caregiver group session to get ideas and support from other caregivers on how to do this.
- *Be strategic about supporting the caregiver and teen in modifying the DLS contract.* At the beginning of the dyad session, the therapist should intentionally utilize the Real World Practice Check-In to identify how to possibly adapt the DLS contract by incorporating the characteristics of the caregiver and teen, successful evidence-based strategies, and the Four Laws of Behavior Change. These modifications can be discussed further and incorporated when developing the DLS contract at the end of the session in partnership with the caregiver and the teen. The therapist should also utilize the relevant discussion questions (e.g., "What steps of the goal do you need help with?") when developing the new DLS contract to facilitate the likelihood of the teen achieving their goals.
- *Fade support over time.* The therapist needs to be mindful of fading back their support during sessions and when creating and modifying the DLS contract. For example, during the last two or three sessions, the therapist should purposely facilitate the caregiver and teen's independence at creating DLS goals and modifying the DLS contract by letting them take the lead. In Session 14, the therapist will discuss how the caregiver can fade their support when identifying and targeting new DLS goals in the future.
- *Encourage the caregiver to find an accountability partner after the STRW intervention ends.* Many caregivers have reported that meeting with the STRW therapist in both

the caregiver group session and the dyad session provides a level of accountability that motivates them to "do the work" in supporting their teen to build their DLS. It can be beneficial to help the caregiver identify someone (e.g., spouse, partner, family member, friend, another STRW caregiver from the group session) that will check in with them (e.g., via text, email, or in person) as they move forward with targeting their teen's goals on the DLS contract.

Possible Solutions to Common Challenges That Arise for STRW Therapists

- Inattention and/or Distraction
    - Set rules and guidelines when possible to decrease distraction (e.g., limit use of other electronic devices, hold session in a quiet environment, turn off television, wear headphones to increase privacy). It can be helpful to revisit these rules regularly in the caregiver and/or dyad sessions.
    - Problem-solve with the caregiver and teen if they are struggling to maintain focus during the dyad sessions and come up with individualized solutions (e.g., how to manage siblings during dyad sessions, where to hold the session)

- Decreased Participation and/or Engagement
    - Call on the caregiver/teen directly to answer questions, discuss their thoughts, and/or read information from the handout or slide.
    - Allow the teen to write information on the screen (e.g., modify the DLS contract) and/or take notes on their handouts. Many teens may benefit from having a specific task to do during the session, especially during sessions that have significant didactic components (e.g., money management sessions)
    - Encourage caregiver or teen to stand up and move around if they seem tired or have low energy.
    - Move the *Guess the Price* activity to earlier in the session to refocus the dyad or increase engagement.
    - Refer back to the dyad session schedule to provide information about what activities are left in the session to engage the caregiver and/or teen.
    - Emphasize that by actively and consistently participating in the session, the teen will not only get more out of it, but will also finish the session earlier.

- Lack of Commitment
    - Directly address commitment issues such as not completing the weekly Real World Practice assignments or working on goals on the DLS contract by engaging in active problem solving to identify challenges and then brainstorm solutions. For many caregiver/teen dyads, they may need to scale back to make goals more doable so that they can easily be targeted during the week.
    - During the caregiver group session, initiate a group discussion about how the caregivers are finding ways to commit to targeting DLS goals throughout the week to provide additional ideas and support for caregivers.

- Too Much Support and/or Prompting by Caregivers
    - Some caregivers may struggle to decrease the amount of prompting or support that they provide for a variety of reasons (e.g., takes too long for their teen to do a specific skill, become frustrated when instructing the teen, teen is not doing a skill the way that they would like them to do it, caregiver is used to providing multiple prompts for a specific skill and it takes effort to consciously stop this behavior).

- Some possible solutions include:
  - The STRW therapist could bring this issue to the caregiver group session to get general thoughts and feedback on how to decrease involvement. It is often extremely powerful for caregivers to hear from other caregivers about how to fade back support or adjust their expectations of their teen's abilities.
  - The therapist could also address this in the dyad session when modifying the DLS contract (e.g., identifying a day/time to work on a skill when the caregiver has more time or energy). This can be helpful for the teen and caregiver to work together on finding a solution (e.g., set up reminders on a smart speaker rather than the caregiver verbally reminding teen as they get ready for school in the morning). Further, once a set of solutions or strategies is identified, it can likely be used in the future to target other skills (e.g., smart speaker reminder for cleaning the room and getting started on doing laundry).

♦ Family Factors
- Time – many caregivers have competing demands and priorities, and it can be difficult to identify how to find the time to devote to instructing and practicing their teen's DLS. It is essential for the STRW therapist to acknowledge this in a nonjudgmental manner and to work with the caregiver in the group session and/or dyad session to put together a plan that will allow them to be successful in targeting the teen's DLS. Common solutions include:
  - Setting up a system that allows the teen to be as independent as possible once they have learned a new DLS (e.g., phone reminder to start cleaning room, checklist with steps that need to be completed, cleaning products all in one place so that the teen can easily find them).
  - Identifying ways to target DLS that align with tasks that the caregiver is already doing on a daily/weekly basis (e.g., having teen help caregiver with the steps of grocery shopping, having teen help caregiver cook dinner several days per week).
  - Identifying naturalistic opportunities to target skills (e.g., reviewing the teen's cell phone bill before paying it, having the teen pay for groceries at the store using the caregiver's debit card).
- Use of rewards – it is critical to identify rewards that the teen can earn as they are learning a new skill because this increases their motivation and buy-in as they practice and master the DLS. The topic of rewards is particularly important to regularly discuss in the caregiver group sessions and to revisit in each dyad session.

  Some issues that commonly arise include:
  - A teen struggles to identify any rewards. While some teens may state that there is nothing that they would like to earn, this usually just requires some creative brainstorming. Caregivers and teens should discuss the different categories of rewards (e.g., privileges, food, time with friends, entertainment) and may also want to think about if there are large purchases that the teen would like to save up for (e.g., amusement park pass, laptop, guitar class).

- A teen already has the opportunity to engage in the activities (e.g., several hours of video games or screen time per day) and privileges (e.g., caregiver gives them money to go see a movie) that motivate them. If the caregiver/teen dyad is unable to identify other types of rewards, it may be beneficial to alter the current system at home such that the teen now has to earn access to activities or privileges. Teens may be very resistant to this, so the therapist can provide support as needed (e.g., instead of having 3–4 hours of screen time per day, the teen gets 1 hour each day and must earn any additional screen time).
- A caregiver is not willing to provide specific rewards that the teen would like to earn. This issue often arises when a caregiver does not think that the teen should earn rewards for doing the skills that they should be doing anyways. It will be important for the therapist to discuss the link between learning new DLS and earning rewards but also to assist the caregiver in brainstorming rewards that they are willing to allow the teen to earn. Oftentimes, caregivers may provide activities and privileges to their teen (e.g., spending money when going out with friends, purchasing a movie rental on the weekend), and they can now require their teen to "earn" these privileges and activities by working towards their DLS goals.
- It can be beneficial to discuss the concept of "first work, then play" with DLS. For example, many caregivers likely have to "work" in the evening (e.g., make dinner, do the laundry, take the trash out) before they are able to "play" (e.g., watch a television show, eat a dessert). Similarly, it can be helpful to point out that if teens get their DLS "work" done (e.g., get ready for school in the morning), they can then have time to "play" (e.g., read a book, play a game on their phone). This concept may help teens to identify natural self-rewards that can be earned after they "work" on their DLS goals.

- Caregiver/teen relationship – the STRW therapist may need to provide support around actions that will strengthen the caregiver/teen relationship in dyad sessions.
  - Providing praise for the teen's effort towards DLS goals – the therapist should model and encourage the caregiver to praise the teen as they make progress towards building various DLS.
  - Coaching the teen on learning new skills – the therapist should provide constructive feedback on how to instruct and give support and guidance in a patient and neutral manner as the teen is learning new DLS.
  - Showing respect for their caregiver's input – the therapist should give feedback to the teen if they are disregarding and/or being disrespectful to their caregiver during the session. For example, the therapist may need to be explicit about the caregiver's role in the DLS Teaching Method such that the caregiver will first demonstrate a new skill and then the teen will have ample opportunities to practice and do it independently.
  - Showing respect for the teen's input – similarly, the therapist may need to discuss that the teen's input is essential when building DLS and that their thoughts, ideas, and concerns need to be heard. The therapist may often need to mediate if issues or disagreements arise, and then demonstrate how to problem-solve and compromise (e.g., agreeing that the teen should be allowed to choose a recipe to cook for the family dinner, but that the caregiver has input on the day/time that they will be cooking).

Index